11ᵀᴴ EDITION

FIRST AID

MANUAL

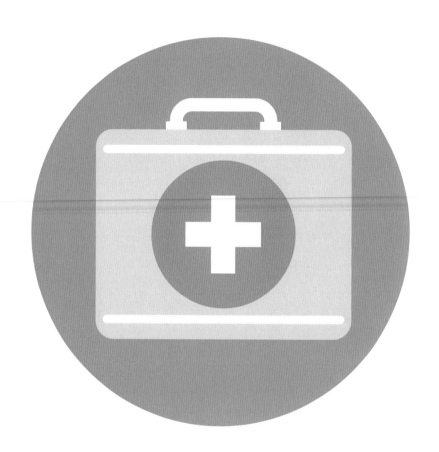

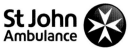

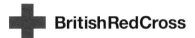

St Andrew's First Aid

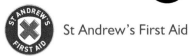

BritishRedCross

11TH EDITION

FIRST AID MANUAL

The Authorised Manual of St John Ambulance, St Andrew's First Aid and the British Red Cross

St John Ambulance
Dr Margaret Austin DStJ LRCPI LRCSI LM
Chief Medical Adviser

St Andrew's First Aid
Mr Rudy Crawford MBE BSc (Hons) MB ChB FRCS (Glasg) FRCEM
Chairman of the Board

British Red Cross
Dr Barry Klaassen BSc (Hons) MB ChB FRCS (Edin) FRCEM
Chief Medical Adviser

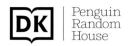

DORLING KINDERSLEY

Consultant editor
Jemima Dunne

Production editor
Kavita Varma

Managing editor
Angeles Gavira Guerrero

Associate Publishing Director
Liz Wheeler

Publishing director
Jonathan Metcalf

Senior art editor
Sharon Spencer

Senior jacket designer
Surabhi Wadhwa

Jacket design development manager
Sophia M.T.T

Senior production controller
Meskerem Berhane

Photography
Gerard Brown, Vanessa Davies,
Ruth Jenkinson, Nigel Wright

Managing art editor
Michael Duffy

Art director
Karen Self

Text revised in line with the latest guidelines from the
Resuscitation Council (UK)

11th edition first published in Great Britain in 2021 by
Dorling Kindersley Limited, DK, One Embassy Gardens,
8 Viaduct Gardens, London SW11 7BW

The authorised representative in the EEA is
Dorling Kindersley Verlag GmbH. Arnulfstr. 124,
80636 Munich, Germany

A Penguin Random House Company
10 9 8 7 6 5 4 3 2 1
001–319130–July/2021

Text copyright © 2021 St John Ambulance;
St Andrew's First Aid; The British Red Cross Society
Illustration copyright © 2021 Dorling Kindersley Limited,
except as listed in acknowledgments on p.296

A CIP catalogue record for this book is
available from the British Library
ISBN: 978-0-2414-4630-0

Printed and bound in Slovakia

For the curious
www.dk.com

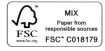

This book was made with Forest Stewardship
Council™ certified paper – one small step
in DK's commitment to a sustainable future.
For more information go to
www.dk.com/our-green-pledge

THE FIRST AID SOCIETIES

Drawing on 100s of years of combined experience, the First Aid Societies are the acknowledged experts in training and practising first aid. Each society offers distinct charitable, voluntary and training services, but all work together to raise standards in first aid. Our medical advisers have based the advice in this book on the most up-to-date research, and our training experts have presented it in a way that is both easy to learn and easy to recall.

ST JOHN AMBULANCE

St John Ambulance responds to health emergencies, supports communities, and saves lives. Compassionate care is not just part of our heritage, it is in our hearts.

Our clinical expertise and the skills of St John people make us unique; a volunteer-led health and first aid charity, with national presence, reach and scale.

From our vibrant youth programmes to our world-class training, we empower people of all ages with lifesaving skills and the confidence to use them, every day. St John volunteers treat and transport thousands of patients each year, and in times of crisis we are England's national health reserve. As a charity with a long history of serving humanity, we are proud of our past and excited about creating a healthier, safer, more resilient future.

St John Ambulance has relieved people from illness, injury, distress and suffering for over 140 years and, with the public's support, will do so for decades to come.
● We are your St John Ambulance
www.sja.org.uk

ST ANDREW'S FIRST AID

St Andrew's First Aid (St. Andrew's Ambulance Association) is Scotland's dedicated first aid charity and provider of first aid training, services and supplies. Our volunteers provide essential first aid services including cover for events large and small, and our trainers teach life-saving skills to communities, schools and industry.

We also supply a full range of first aid products and training materials to first aid professionals, industry and the general public.
● Visit *www.firstaid.org.uk*
● Email *info@firstaid.org.uk*
● Call 0800 4 666 999

BRITISH RED CROSS

As part of the world's largest humanitarian organisation and provider of first aid training and education, we are a recognised leader and standard setter globally. The British Red Cross trains tens of thousands of people in the UK every year, building resilience within communities and preparing them to cope with all types of emergencies. Our courses provide training for every need, including treatment for adult, baby and child and first aid at work. For the last 150 years, the British Red Cross has been helping millions of people in the UK and around the world get the support they need when crisis strikes, putting kindness into action.
● The British Red Cross – the power of kindness
● For more information and to learn about first aid, visit: *redcross.org.uk/firstaid* or call us on 0344 871 8000

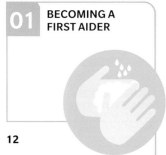

01 BECOMING A FIRST AIDER

12

02 MANAGING AN INCIDENT

26

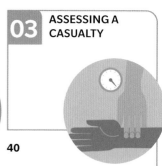

03 ASSESSING A CASUALTY

40

CONTENTS

04 THE UNRESPONSIVE CASUALTY

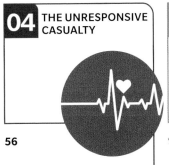

56

05 RESPIRATORY PROBLEMS

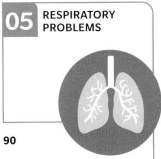

90

06 WOUNDS AND BLEEDING

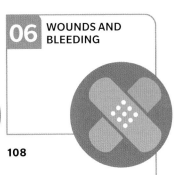

108

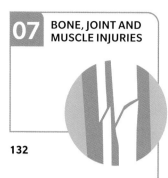

07 BONE, JOINT AND MUSCLE INJURIES

132

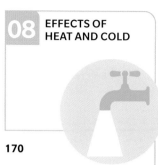

08 EFFECTS OF HEAT AND COLD

170

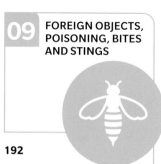

09 FOREIGN OBJECTS, POISONING, BITES AND STINGS

192

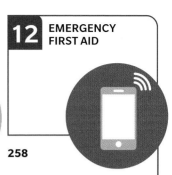

INTRODUCTION

This publication, now in its 11th edition, is the authorised manual of the First Aid Societies – St John Ambulance, St Andrew's First Aid and the British Red Cross. Together, they have endeavoured to ensure that this manual reflects the relevant guidance from informed authoritative sources, current at the time of publication. While the material contained here provides guidance on initial care and treatment, it must not be regarded as a substitute for medical advice.

The First Aid Societies do not accept responsibility for any claims arising from the use of this manual when the guidelines have not been followed. First aiders are advised to keep up-to-date with developments, to recognise the limits of their competence and to obtain first-aid training from a qualified trainer.

The first three chapters provide background information to help you examine your role as a first aider, manage a situation safely and learn how to assess a sick or injured person effectively. Treatment for injuries and conditions is given in specific chapters that follow. Life-saving treatment for an unresponsive casualty has an entire chapter. In other chapters, injuries and conditions are grouped either by body system, for example *Respiratory Problems* or by the type of injury, such as *Wounds and Bleeding* and *Effects of Heat and Cold*.

HOW TO USE THIS BOOK

ANATOMY

The chapters are grouped by body system or cause of injury. Within the chapters there are easy-to-understand anatomical feature pages that explain the risks involved with particular injuries or conditions and how and why first aid can help.

Colour-coded chapters help you find relevant sections easily

Introduction gives an overview of the anatomy for the section

Simple, clear artworks of body systems illustrate essential anatomy

Additional artworks provide extra information

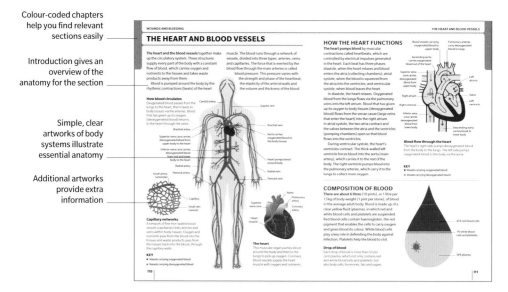

CONDITIONS AND INJURIES

The main part of the book features seven colour-coded chapters that outline first aid for more than 112 conditions or injuries. For each entry there is an introduction that describes the risks and the likely cause, then first aid treatment is shown in clear step-by-step instructions.

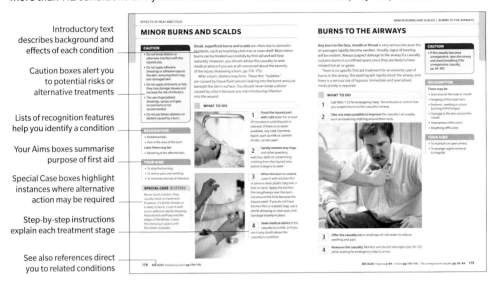

Introductory text describes background and effects of each condition

Caution boxes alert you to potential risks or alternative treatments

Lists of recognition features help you identify a condition

Your Aims boxes summarise purpose of first aid

Special Case boxes highlight instances where alternative action may be required

Step-by-step instructions explain each treatment stage

See also references direct you to related conditions

EMERGENCY ADVICE

At the back of the manual is a quick-reference emergency section. This provides additional at-a-glance action plans summarising treatment for potentially life-threatening injuries and conditions ranging from unresponsiveness and bleeding to asthma and heart attack.

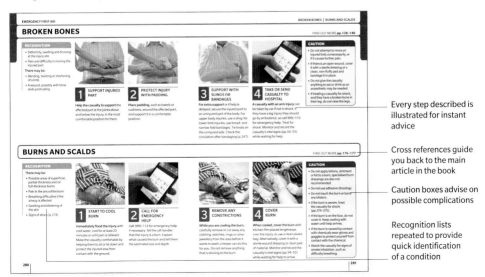

Every step described is illustrated for instant advice

Cross references guide you back to the main article in the book

Caution boxes advise on possible complications

Recognition lists repeated to provide quick identification of a condition

01 BECOMING A FIRST AIDER

First aid is the initial assistance or treatment given to a person who is injured or taken ill. The person who provides this help is a first aider. This chapter prepares you for being a first aider, psychologically and emotionally, as well as giving practical advice on what you should and should not do in an emergency.

The information given throughout this book will help you deliver effective first aid to any casualty in any situation. However, to become a fully competent first aider, you should complete a recognised first aid learning programme. Completing this will strengthen your skills and increase your confidence. St John Ambulance, St Andrew's First Aid and the British Red Cross are all able to provide first aid education tailored to your needs.

AIMS AND OBJECTIVES

- To understand your own abilities and limitations
- To stay safe and calm at all times
- To assess a situation quickly and calmly and summon help if necessary
- To assist the casualty and provide the necessary treatment, with the help of others if possible
- To pass on relevant information to the emergency services, or the person who takes responsibility for the casualty
- To be aware of your own needs

WHAT IS A FIRST AIDER?

"First aid" in this book refers to the actions that a person takes to assist someone who is injured or taken ill (the casualty). A first aider is a person who takes this action while taking care to keep everyone involved safe (p.28) and to cause no further harm to anyone while doing so. By using the guidelines set out here, you – the first aider – can take actions that most benefit the casualty, but always take into account your own skills, knowledge and experience.

The aim of this chapter is to prepare you for the role of first aider. It explains how best to respond to a situation where first aid is needed and how to assess the priorities for one or more casualties. There is also advice on the psychological aspect of giving first aid and information showing how to protect yourself and a casualty. Chapter 2, Managing an Incident (pp.26–39), provides guidelines on dealing with traffic incidents, water incidents or fires, and what you should do in the event of a major incident involving large numbers of casualties. Chapter 3, Assessing a Casualty (pp.40–55), looks at the practical steps to take when assessing a sick or injured person.

The first rule is to ensure that an area is safe for you before you approach a casualty (p.28). Do not attempt heroic rescues in hazardous circumstances. If you put yourself at risk, you are unlikely to be able to help others and you could become a casualty. If it is not safe to approach a casualty **call 999/112 for emergency help.**

FIRST AID PRIORITIES
- **Assess a situation** quickly and calmly.
- **Protect yourself** and any casualties from danger – never put yourself at risk (p.28).
- **Prevent cross infection** between yourself and the casualty as far as possible (pp.16–18).
- **Comfort and reassure** casualties at all times.
- **Assess the casualty:** identify, as far as you can, the injury or nature of illness affecting a casualty (pp.38–53).
- **Give early treatment,** and treat the casualties with the most serious (life-threatening) conditions first (pp.40-41).
- **Arrange for appropriate help. Call 999/112 for emergency help** immediately if you suspect serious injury or illness. For advice for a less serious condition, or you are unsure, you or the casualty should consult 111.nhs.uk online, or if this is not possible, call 111. You can take or send the casualty to hospital, advise them to seek medical advice, or take them home. Always stay with the casualty until the right care is available.

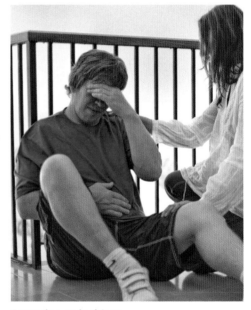

Assessing an incident
When you come across an incident stay calm and support the casualty. Ask them what has happened. Try not to move the casualty; if possible, treat them in the position you find them.

HOW TO PREPARE YOURSELF

When you respond to an emergency it is important to recognise both the emotional and physical needs of all involved, especially your own. You should look after your own psychological health and be able to identify stress if it develops (pp.24–25).

A calm, considerate response from you that builds trust and respect from those around you is fundamental to you being able to give or receive information from a casualty or witnesses effectively. You should be aware of, and be able to manage, your reactions, so that you can focus on the casualty and make an assessment. By talking to a casualty in a kind, considerate, gentle but firm manner, you will inspire their confidence in your actions, which will generate trust between you and the casualty (and bystanders). Without this confidence they may not want to tell you about an important event, injury or symptom, and the casualty may remain in a highly distressed state.

The steps and plans described in this chapter aim to help you build this trust, minimise distress and provide support to promote the casualty's ability to cope and recover. The key steps to being an effective first aider are:

- **Be calm** in your approach.
- **Be aware of risks** (to yourself and others).
- **Build and maintain trust** (from the casualty and the bystanders).
- **Give early treatment,** always dealing with the most serious (life-threatening) conditions first.
- **Call appropriate help.**
- **Remember your own needs.**

BE CALM

It is important to be calm when you approach any casualty. To convey confidence to others and encourage them to trust you, you need to be able to control your own emotions and reactions. Consider what situations might challenge you, and how you would deal with them.

People often fear the unknown. If you familiarise yourself with first aid priorities and the key techniques in this book you can help yourself feel more comfortable and confident. By identifying your fears in advance, you can also take steps to overcome them. Find out as much as you can, for example, by completing a first aid training programme with one of the Societies. For additional reassurance, talk to other people about how they dealt with similar situations or talk through your fears with a person you trust.

STAY IN CONTROL

In an emergency situation, the body responds by releasing hormones that may cause a "fight-flight-or-freeze" response. When this happens, your heart beats faster, your breathing speeds up and you may sweat more. You may also feel more alert, but you may want to run away or feel as if you are "frozen" to the spot.

If you feel overwhelmed and/or slightly panicky, you may feel pressured to do something before you are clear about what is really required. Pause. Take a few slow breaths. Consider who or what might help you feel calmer, and remind yourself of the first aid priorities (opposite). If you are still overwhelmed, take another breath and quietly say to yourself "be calmer" as a cue. When you are calm, you will be better able to think more clearly and plan your response.

The thoughts you have are linked to the way you behave and how you feel. If you think that you cannot cope, you may find it more difficult to work out what to do and will feel more anxious – more ready to "fight, flee or freeze". If you know how to calm yourself, you will be better able to deal with your anxiety and so help the casualty.

PROTECTION FROM INFECTION

When you give first aid, it is important to protect yourself (and the casualty) from infection as well as injury. Take steps to avoid cross-infection (transmitting bacterial or viral infections to a casualty or contracting infection from a casualty).

Blood-borne viruses may be transmitted by contact with blood, so cross-infection is a risk when you are treating any wound, even a minor one. In practice the risk is low and it should not deter you from carrying out first aid. The risk does increase if an infected person's blood makes contact with yours, for example through a cut or graze. Usually, taking measures such as hand washing and wearing disposable gloves will provide sufficient protection for you and the casualty. There is no known evidence of blood-borne viruses being transmitted during rescue breathing, and you can use a face shield or pocket mask if available (p.71 and p.81). Take care not to prick yourself with a needle found on or near a casualty, or cut yourself on glass. If you accidentally prick or cut your skin, or splash your eye, wash the area thoroughly and seek medical help immediately. If you are providing first aid on a regular basis, it is advisable to seek guidance on additional protection, such as immunisation.

Some viral infections, such as flu and diseases like Covid-19, can be transmitted through the air. In a pandemic (when disease is prevalent over a whole country, or the world), delivering first aid can be challenging as distancing yourself from

CAUTION
To help protect yourself from infection you can carry protective equipment: • Latex-free disposable gloves, a face mask and a disposable apron.   • Hand sanitiser to clean your hands.   • Pocket mask or face shield for rescue breathing.

a casualty is impossible. You can reduce the chances of cross-infection by taking precautions such as frequent hand washing, or using hand sanitiser, and wearing a face mask, disposable gloves and a plastic apron.

MINIMISING THE RISK OF CROSS INFECTION

- **Do not** breathe, cough or sneeze over wounds.
- **Do not** touch a wound or any part of a dressing that will come into contact with a wound with your bare hands.
- **Do** wash your hands and wear latex-free disposable gloves. If gloves are not available, enclose your hands in clean plastic bags or ask the casualty to dress their own wound.
- **Do** cover cuts and grazes on your hands with waterproof dressings.
- **Do** wear a plastic apron if dealing with large quantities of body fluids and wear plastic glasses to protect your eyes.
- **Do** dispose of all waste safely (p.18).

SPECIAL CASE PROTECTING YOURSELF IN A PANDEMIC

Always follow guidance from your local and/or international health authorities.

- Maintain physical distancing: stay 1–2 m (3–6 ft) away from those outside your home. Avoid crowded or narrow places where this is difficult.
- Wear a face covering such as a mask when in public spaces and on public transport.
- Avoid touching your eyes, nose and mouth (or mask if worn) with your hands.

- Follow good respiratory hygiene: cough or sneeze into a tissue, or if none is available into your elbow. Dispose of the tissue immediately and re-wash hands.
- Self-isolate at home if you have symptoms such as a fever or cough, and/or loss of taste or smell, or when advised to do so. Follow local guidelines for recommended quarantine period, permitted activities and guidance on being tested.

HAND WASHING

If you can, wash your hands thoroughly with soap and water before and after contact with a casualty. Wash your hands for at least 20 seconds every time, paying attention to all parts of your hands – palms, wrists, fingers, thumbs and fingernails. If no soap and water is available, rub your hands with hand sanitiser, then wash them with soap and water as soon as possible.

HOW TO WASH YOUR HANDS

1 **Wet your hands** under running water. Put some soap into the palm of a cupped hand. Rub the palms of your hands together.

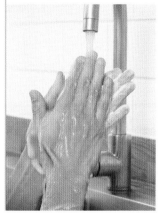

2 **Rub the palm** of your left hand against the back of your right hand, then rub the right palm on the back of your left hand.

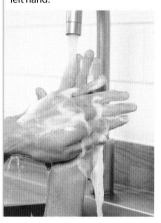

3 **Interlock the fingers** of both hands and work the soap between them.

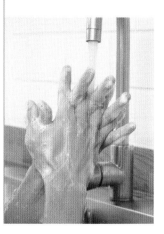

4 **Rub the back** of the fingers of your right hand against the palm of your left hand, then repeat with your left hand in your right palm.

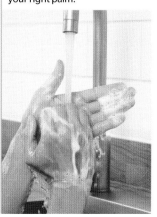

5 **Rub your right thumb** in the palm of your left hand, then your left thumb in the right palm.

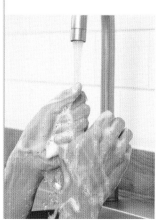

6 **Rub the fingertips** of your left hand in the palm of your right hand and vice versa. Rinse thoroughly, then pat dry with a disposable paper towel.

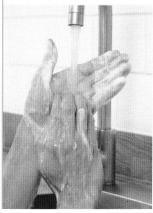

continued ⟫

◀◀ PROTECTION FROM INFECTION

USING PROTECTIVE GLOVES

In addition to hand washing, disposable gloves give added protection against infection in a first aid situation. If possible, you should carry protective, disposable, latex-free gloves with you at all times. Wear them whenever there is a likelihood of contact with blood or other body fluids. If in doubt, put them on anyway.

Gloves should only be used to treat one casualty. Wash or sanitise your hands, then put

> ### CAUTION
> - Always use latex-free gloves. Some people have a serious allergy to latex, and this may cause anaphylactic shock (p.227). Nitrile gloves (often blue or purple) are recommended.

the gloves on just before you approach the person. Remove them as soon as the treatment is completed without touching the outside. Dispose of the gloves and any other personal protective equipment as described below.

PUTTING ON AND REMOVING DISPOSABLE GLOVES

1 Ideally, wash or sanitise your hands before putting on the gloves. Hold one glove by the top edge and pull it on. Do not touch the main part of the glove with your fingers.

3 To remove the gloves, first grasp the outside cuff of one glove with a gloved hand and peel it off. Without touching the outer side put this glove in your other (gloved) hand.

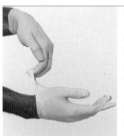

2 Pick up the second glove with your gloved hand. Put your fingers under the top edge, and pull the glove on to your other hand. Your gloved fingers should not touch your skin.

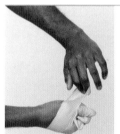

4 Insert two fingers beneath the top edge of the second glove and peel it off over the first one so that the first glove is inside the second one. Without touching the outer surfaces, place both gloves in a waste bag.

DEALING WITH WASTE

Once you have treated a casualty, all soiled material, including personal protective equipment (PPE), must be disposed of safely to prevent the spread of infection.

Place items such as dressings in a waste bag, ideally a yellow clinical waste bag. If possible ask the attending emergency service how to deal with this type of waste. Seal the bag and label it "clinical waste".

Put sharp objects, such as needles, in a special yellow plastic container called a sharps box. If you do not have one, put used needles in a jar with a screw top and dispose of it safely.

Carefully remove PPE without touching the outward-facing surfaces and put it in a waste bag.
- Take off the gloves as described above, then wash or sanitise your hands.
- Snap or unfasten your apron ties at the neck and let the top fall forward, then repeat at the waist; fold it inwards so you do not touch the outer surface and dispose of it.
- Remove any eye protection by the side arms, then wash or sanitise your hands again.
- Remove your mask using the earpieces; do not touch the main part of the mask.
- Wash or sanitise your hands thoroughly.

DEALING WITH A CASUALTY

Casualties are often frightened because of what is happening to them, and what may happen next. Your role is to stay calm and take charge of the situation – be ready to stand back if there is someone better qualified. If there is more than one casualty, use the primary survey (pp.46–47) to identify the most seriously injured casualties and treat in the order of priority.

BUILDING TRUST

Establish trust with your casualty by first introducing yourself. Find out what they like to be called, and use their name when you talk to them. Crouch or kneel down so you are at the same level and can make eye contact with the person. Treat them with dignity and respect at all times. Explain what is happening and why – you will inspire trust if you tell them what you are doing before you do it. If possible, give them choices, for example, ask whether they would prefer to sit or lie down and/or who they would like with them. Also, if possible, gain their consent before you begin treatment by asking if they agree with whatever you are going to do.

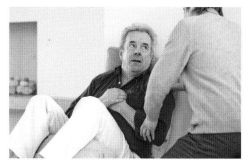

Reassure the casualty
When treating a casualty, stay calm and do not do anything without explaining your actions first. Always answer their questions honestly and clearly.

DIVERSITY AND COMMUNICATION

It is important to consider the age and appearance of a casualty when you talk to them, as different people need different responses. Always respect a person's wishes and accept the fact that they might want to be treated in a particular way. Communication can be difficult if a person speaks a different language or cannot hear you. Use simple language or signs or you can write questions down and show them. Also ask if anyone nearby speaks the same language, knows the person and/or saw the incident and can describe what happened.

SPECIAL CASE TREATING CHILDREN

You will need to use simpler, shorter words when talking to children. If possible, their parents or carers should be with them. Keep them involved at all times. It is important to establish the carer's trust as well as the child's. Talk first to the parent/carer and get their permission to continue. Once the parent/carer trusts you, the child will also feel more confident.

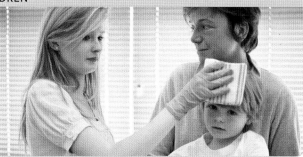

continued ≫

DEALING WITH A CASUALTY

LOOK AND LISTEN CAREFULLY

Use your eyes and ears when attending a casualty so you are aware of how they respond. Use both verbal and non-verbal skills.

- **Make eye contact,** but look away now and then so it does not look like you are staring.
- **Use a calm, confident voice.** Speak loudly enough to be heard but do not shout.
- **Do not speak too quickly.**
- **Keep your instructions simple.** Use short sentences and simple words.
- **Use affirming nods** and "mmms" to show you are listening when the casualty speaks.
- **Check that the casualty understands** what you mean – ask them to tell you what they think you said so you can make sure.
- **Use simple hand gestures** and movements.
- **Do not interrupt the casualty,** and always acknowledge what they tell you. For example, summarise what a casualty has told you so they know that you understand.

WHEN A CASUALTY RESISTS HELP

If someone is ill or injured they may be upset, confused, tearful, angry and/or keen to get away. Be sensitive to their feelings and let them know that their reactions are understandable. Also accept that you may not be able to help, or even that the casualty might see you as a threat. Stay at a safe distance until you have gained the person's consent to move closer, so that they do not feel crowded. Do not argue or disagree, or be judgemental. A casualty may refuse help for example if they have a head injury or hypothermia. If you think a person needs something other than what they ask for, explain why. For example, you could say, "I think someone should look at where you're hurt before you move, in case moving makes it worse". If someone refuses first aid, but you think they need urgent medical attention, **call 999/112 for emergency help.** A casualty has the right to refuse help, even if it causes further harm. Tell the emergency services that you have offered help and been refused. If you are worried that a person's condition is deteriorating, observe them from a distance until help arrives.

TREATING THE CASUALTY

When you are treating a casualty, always remain calm and act thoughtfully to gain and maintain their trust. Think about how they might be feeling. Check that you have understood what the casualty has said and consider the impact of your actions, for example, are they becoming more (or less) upset, angry and tense? A change in emotional state can also indicate that a casualty's condition is worsening.

Be prepared to change your manner, depending on what the person feels comfortable with – for example, ask fewer questions or talk about something else. Keep a casualty updated and give them options rather than telling them what to do. Ask them if anyone else, such as their next-of-kin or friends can assist, and help them to make contact with them if necessary. Ask if you can help to make arrangements so that any other responsibilities the casualty may have can be taken care of.

Always stay with the casualty until appropriate help arrives. Do not leave someone who may be dying, or who is seriously ill or injured on their own, unless it is unavoidable because you have to call for emergency help. Talk to the casualty and, if they feel comfortable with it, touch their shoulder or arm, or hold their hand. Never let a casualty feel alone.

ENLISTING HELP FROM OTHERS

In an emergency situation you may be faced with several tasks at once – for example, to maintain safety, call for help and start giving first aid. People at the scene may be able to help. Bystanders can be asked to do the following:

- **Make the area safe**, for example, control traffic and keep onlookers away.
- **Call 999/112 for emergency help** (p.23).
- **Fetch first aid equipment**, for example an AED (automated external defibrillator).
- **Control bleeding** with direct pressure (p.116), or support an injured limb (pp.138–141).
- **Help maintain the casualty's privacy** by holding a blanket around the scene and/or encouraging onlookers to move away.
- **Transport the casualty** to a safe place if their life is in immediate danger. Only ever do this if it is safer to move someone than to leave them where they are, and you have the necessary help and equipment (p.238).

The reactions of bystanders may cause you concern or anger. Be aware that they may have had no first aid training and feel helpless or frightened themselves – your response can reassure them. If they have seen or been involved in the incident, they too may be injured and/or distressed. Always bear this in mind if you need to ask bystanders to help you. Talk to them gently but firmly. If you remain calm, you will gain their trust and help them stay calm.

CARE OF A CASUALTY'S BELONGINGS

Make sure their belongings remain with them at all times. If you have to search their belongings for identification or clues to their condition (medication, for example), do so in front of a reliable witness. If possible, ask the casualty's consent before you do this. Once the emergency services arrive, ensure that all of the clothing, personal belongings and medication accompany the casualty to hospital in the ambulance or are handed over to the police.

KEEPING NOTES

Make a note of any information you obtain about a casualty and/or the incident, so that you can refer to it later. A record of the timing of events is particularly valuable to medical personnel. You can note, for example, the length of time a casualty is unresponsive, the duration of a seizure, the time of any changes in the casualty's condition (improvement or deterioration), and the time of any intervention or treatment given. Hand the information to the emergency services or give them to the casualty. Useful facts to provide are:

- **Casualty's details,** including their name, date of birth and contact details.
- **History** of the incident or illness – from the casualty and/or bystanders.
- **Brief description** of any injuries observed.
- **Unusual behaviour**, or a change in behaviour.
- **Treatment** – what, when and where given.
- **Casualty's vital signs** – breathing, pulse and level of response (pp.54–55).
- **Medical history** from casualty or bystanders.
- **Medication** taken by the casualty. Give details of how much and when they took it (p.24).
- **Next-of-kin/friends** contact details.
- **Your contact details** – include the date, time and place of your involvement.

Remember that any information you obtain is confidential. Never share it with anyone not involved in the casualty's care without their agreement. Let the casualty know why you are recording information and who you will give it to. When you are asking the casualty for this information, be sensitive to who is around them and of their privacy and dignity. Always delete or destroy your notes after the event.

REQUESTING HELP

Further help is available from a range of sources. First you must decide both on the type of help and how to access it. Carry out a primary survey (pp.46–47) to ascertain the severity of the casualty's condition. If it is not serious, explain the options and allow them to choose where to go, see below. If a casualty's condition is serious, call 999/112 for emergency help. Throughout the book the treatment steps provide guidance for choosing an appropriate level of help:

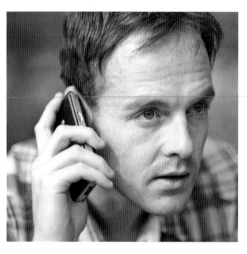

- Call 999/112 for emergency help if the casualty needs urgent medical attention; for example, when you suspect a heart attack or stroke.
- **Take or send the casualty to hospital.** Choose this option when a casualty needs hospital treatment, but their condition is unlikely to worsen on the journey – for example, with a finger injury. You can take them yourself if you can arrange transport in your car or in a taxi.
- **Seek medical advice.** Depending on what is available locally, advise the casualty to call their doctor's surgery or nearest NHS walk-in centre. Or the casualty (or you) can consult the NHS online service 111.nhs.uk or call 111, for example, if there are symptoms such as earache or diarrhoea; if a serious condition is indicated you will be diverted.

Calling for help
Use your phone to call for help. Stay calm, be clear and concise, and give as much detail as possible. Put the device on speaker phone if you need to give first aid at the same time. Stay with the casualty once the call has been made.

TELEPHONING FOR HELP
You can telephone for help from any of the following sources.
- **Emergency services,** including police, fire and ambulance services; mine, mountain, cave and fell rescue; and HM Coastguard by calling 999 or 112. Calls to the emergency services are free from any phone.
- **Utilities,** including gas, electricity or water. The phone number will be online or in the local telephone directory.
- **Health services,** including the casualty's doctor, dentist, nurse or midwife, or consult the NHS online advice service, 111.nhs.uk, or call the helpline on 111.

On motorways, there are also emergency phones every 1.6 km (1 mile) – arrows on marker posts indicate the direction of (and distance to) the nearest one. To summon help using these telephones, simply pick up the receiver and your call will be answered.

Keep time away from the casualty to a minimum. Ideally, tell someone else to make the call while you stay with the casualty. Ask the person to come back to confirm that the call has been made. If you have to leave a casualty to make a call, carry out a primary survey first (pp.46–47) and take any necessary vital action before making the call.

MAKING AN EMERGENCY CALL

When you dial 999 **or** 112, you will be asked which service you require. If there are casualties, ask for the ambulance service. Stay on the line until the emergency services clear it; you will be asked a number of questions and be given information about what to do for the casualty while you wait. If someone else makes the call, ensure they are aware of the importance of the call and that they report back to you. The call should be made by someone who is at the scene and from a phone that can remain with the casualty until help arrives. Ask whoever makes the call to put the device on speaker phone so that you can hear first aid instructions given by the call handler. Identify a point of contact to receive information from the emergency services and to direct the ambulance personnel to where they are needed when they arrive.

TALKING TO THE EMERGENCY SERVICES

State your name clearly and say that you are helping at the scene of an incident. It is essential to provide the following information:

- **Your telephone number** and/or the number you are calling from.
- **The exact location** of the incident; give the road name or number and postcode, if possible – some street signs include the postcode. Your call can be traced if you are unsure of your exact location. It can be helpful to mention any junctions or other landmarks in the area. If you are on a motorway, say which direction the vehicles are travelling in.
- **The type and gravity** of the emergency. For example, "Traffic incident, two cars, road blocked, three people trapped".
- **Number, gender and age** of casualties. For example, "One man, early sixties, breathing difficulties, suspected heart attack".
- **Details of any hazards,** such as gas, toxic substances, power-line damage, or adverse weather conditions, such as fog or ice.
- **Follow instructions** such as first aid guidance given by the emergency services.

WHEN THE EMERGENCY SERVICES ARRIVE

The emergency services will take over the care of the casualty as soon as they arrive. Tell them what has happened and what treatment has been given. Hand over any notes you made, or information you gained, while attending the casualty (p.21). You may be asked to continue helping, for example, by assisting relatives or friends of the casualty while the paramedics provide emergency care.

You may be asked to contact a relative on the casualty's behalf. Explain as simply and honestly as you can what has happened and where the casualty has been taken, but do not cause unnecessary alarm. It is better to admit ignorance than to give someone misleading information. However, the information you give may cause distress; if so, remain calm and be clear about what they need to do next.

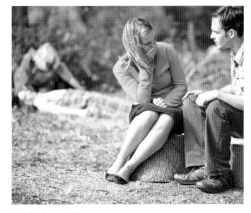

Assisting at the scene
Once the emergency services arrive, tell the team everything that you know. While they assess and treat the casualty, you may be asked to look after or reassure friends.

23

THE USE OF MEDICATION

In first aid, the administration of medication is largely confined to relieving general aches and pains. It usually only involves helping a casualty to take their own painkillers.

A variety of medications can be bought without a doctor's prescription. However, you must never buy or borrow medication to administer to a casualty yourself.

If you advise the casualty to take any medication other than that stipulated in this manual, they may be put at risk, and you could face legal action as a consequence. Whenever a casualty takes their own medication, it is essential to make sure that:

- **It is for the condition.**
- **It is not out of date.**
- **It is taken as advised.**
- **Any precautions** are strictly followed.
- **The recommended dose** is not exceeded.
- **You keep a record** of the name and dose of the medication as well as the time and method of administration.

> **CAUTION**
>
> - Aspirin should never be given to anyone under the age of 16 years.

REMEMBER YOUR OWN NEEDS

Most people who learn first aid gain significantly from doing so. By completing a course you will not only acquire new skills and meet new people, but also in learning first aid you can make a difference to other people's lives.

Being able to help people who are ill or injured often results in a range of positive feelings. However, you may also feel stressed when you are called upon to administer first aid, and feel emotional once you have finished treating a casualty, whatever the outcome. Occasionally, that stress accumulates and can interfere with your physical and mental well-being. Everyone responds to stress in different ways, and some people are more susceptible to it than others. It is important to learn how to deal with any stress in order to maintain your own health and effectiveness as a first aider. Gaining an understanding of your needs can help you be better prepared for future situations, too.

IMMEDIATELY AFTER AN INCIDENT

An emergency is an emotional experience. Many first aiders experience satisfaction, or even elation, and cope well. However, after you have treated a casualty, depending on the type of incident and the outcome, you might experience a mix of emotions such as:

- **Satisfaction.**
- **Confusion, worry, doubt.**
- **Anger, sadness, fear.**

You may go through what happened again and again in your mind, so it can be helpful to talk to someone you trust about what you did at the scene and how you feel about it. Consider talking to someone else who was there, or a friend or colleague who you know has had a similar experience. Never reproach yourself for any negative feelings or hide your feelings – talk to someone. This is especially important if the outcome was not as you had hoped. Even with the correct treatment, and however hard you try, there are occasions when a casualty may not recover from the injury or illness.

LATER REACTIONS

Delivering first aid can lead to positive feelings as you discover new things about yourself, such as, for example, your ability to deal with a crisis. Occasionally, your response and feelings will depend not only on your experience, but also the nature of the incident.

The majority of the incidents you will deal with will be of a minor nature and probably involve people you know. However, if you have witnessed an incident that involved a threat to life or you have experienced a feeling of helplessness at the time, you may find yourself suffering from feelings of stress after the incident. While stress is a normal part of living, it can become harmful when excessive, or sustained. In most situations, your feelings should disappear over time, but it is important to seek help if they persist.

WHEN TO SEEK HELP

If you experience persistent or distressing symptoms, such as nightmares and flashbacks, associated with an incident, it is important to seek further help from someone you trust and feel you can confide in.

If you feel overwhelmed by your symptoms, seek professional help. Make an appointment with your doctor and/or ask to be referred to a counsellor. They can talk through your feelings with you and together you can decide what is best for you. Seeking help is nothing to be embarrassed about, and is not a sign of weakness – quite the opposite. It is important to be able to manage these feelings. Doing this will not only help you deal with your current reactions, but it will also help you learn how to respond to situations in the future.

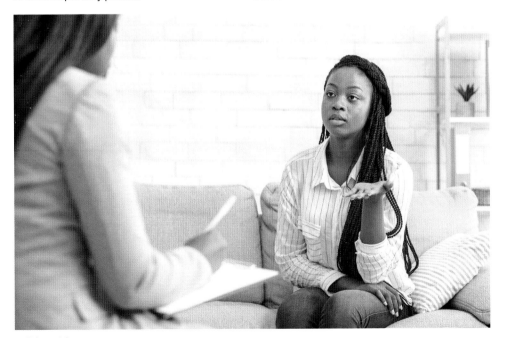

Talking things over
Confiding in a friend or relative is often useful. Ideally, talk to someone who also attended the incident so you can share experiences – they may have the same feelings about it as you. If you are unable to deal with the effects of an event, seek professional help from your doctor or a counsellor.

02 MANAGING AN INCIDENT

The scene of any incident can present many potential dangers, whether someone has become ill or has been injured, whether in the home or outside. Before first aid can be provided you must make sure that approaching the scene does not present unacceptable danger to you, the casualty or anyone else who may be helping.

This chapter provides advice for first aiders on how to ensure safety in an emergency situation. There are specific guidelines for emergencies that pose a particular risk. These include fire, traffic and electrical incidents and water rescue.

The procedures used by the emergency services for major incidents, where particular precautions are necessary and where first aiders may be called on to help, are also described here.

AIMS AND OBJECTIVES

- To protect yourself from danger and make the area safe
- To assess the situation quickly and calmly and summon help if necessary
- To assist any casualties and provide necessary treatment with the help of bystanders
- To call 999 / 112 for emergency help if you suspect serious injury or illness
- To be aware of your own needs

ACTION AT AN EMERGENCY

In any emergency it is important that you follow a clear plan of action. This will not only enable you to prioritise the demands that may be made upon you, but also help you to decide on your best response to the incident.

The principal steps are: to assess the situation, to make the area safe (if possible) and to give first aid. Use the primary survey (pp.46–47) to identify the most seriously injured and treat casualties in the order of priority.

ASSESSING THE SITUATION

Evaluating the scene accurately is one of the most important factors in the management of an incident. You should stay calm. State that you have first aid training and, if there are no medical personnel in attendance, calmly take charge of the situation.

Identify any safety risks and assess the resources available to you. Action for key dangers you may face, such as fire, are dealt with later in this chapter, but be aware, too, of trip hazards, sharp objects, chemical spills and falling masonry.

All incidents should be managed in a similar manner. Consider the following:
- **Safety** What are the dangers and do they still exist? Are you wearing protective equipment? Where are you and is it safe to approach?
- **Scene** What factors are involved at the incident? What are the mechanisms of the injuries (pp.44–45)? How many casualties are there? What are the potential injuries?
- **Situation** What happened? How many people are involved? Are any of them children or elderly?

MAKING AN AREA SAFE

The conditions that give rise to an incident may still present a danger and must be eliminated if possible. It may be that a simple measure, such as turning off the ignition of a car to reduce the risk of fire, is sufficient. As a last resort, move the casualty to safety. Usually specialist help and equipment is required for this (p.238).

When approaching a casualty make sure you protect yourself: wear high-visibility clothing, gloves, face covering and head protection if you have them. Remember, too, that a casualty faces the risk of injury from the same hazards that you face. If extrication from the scene is delayed, try to protect the casualty from additional hazards – without endangering yourself.

If you cannot make an area safe, then **call 999 / 112 for emergency help.** Stand clear of the incident, observing from a distance, until the emergency services have secured the scene, then follow their instructions.

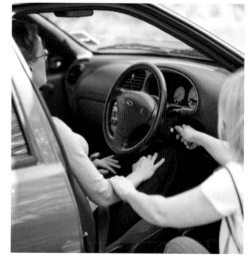

Making a vehicle safe
Wear a high-visibility jacket if you have one to alert others of your presence. Switch off the ignition (even if the engine is no longer running); this reduces the risk of a spark causing a fire.

GIVING EMERGENCY HELP

Once an area has been made safe, use the primary survey (pp.46–47) to quickly carry out an initial assessment of the casualty to establish treatment priorities. If there is more than one casualty, attend to those with life-threatening conditions first. If possible, treat casualties in the position in which you find them. Move them only if they are in immediate danger or if it is necessary for you to be able to provide life-saving treatment, and even then only if it is safe for you to do so.

Enlist help from others if possible. Ask bystanders to call for the emergency services (p.23). They can also help to protect a casualty's privacy, put out warning triangles in the event of a vehicle incident (p.30), or fetch equipment such as an AED (automated external defibrillator, pp.86–87), while you begin life-saving first aid.

ASSISTING THE EMERGENCY SERVICES

Hand over any notes you have made to the emergency services when they arrive (p.21). Answer any questions they may have and follow any instructions. As a first aider you may be asked to assist, for example, with moving a casualty using specialist equipment. If so, you should always follow their instructions. Occasionally, helicopter rescue is required. If a casualty is being rescued in this way, there are a number of safety rules to follow, see below.

SPECIAL CASE HELICOPTER RESCUE

The emergency services may already be in attendance, in which case you should keep clear unless they give you specific instructions. If the emergency services have not arrived take the following steps.

- Clear all loose items from the landing area.
- Stay clear of the landing area. Move yourself and bystanders to the edge of the field or landing area; make sure everyone is at least 50 m (55 yd) away from the landing site and in a position where the pilot can see them.
- If the helicopter is landing on a slope, ensure you remain on the downward slope, below the level of the aircraft.
- Make sure no-one is smoking.
- A helicopter creates a strong "down wash" as it lands so kneel or crouch down with your back to the helicopter as it approaches.
- Once a helicopter has landed do not approach unless requested to by the emergency services, and then only after the blades have stopped turning and the pilot has left the aircraft.
- If a helicopter is leaving the scene, remain well clear of the landing site (where the pilot can see you) until the helicopter is in forward flight, just in case the pilot needs to abort the take off.

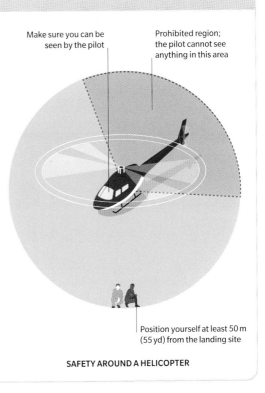

Make sure you can be seen by the pilot

Prohibited region; the pilot cannot see anything in this area

Position yourself at least 50 m (55 yd) from the landing site

SAFETY AROUND A HELICOPTER

TRAFFIC INCIDENTS

The severity of traffic incidents can range from a fall from a bicycle to a major vehicle crash involving many casualties. Often, the incident site will present serious risks to safety, largely because of passing traffic.

It is essential to make the incident area safe before you attend any casualties (p.30); this not only protects you, but also the casualties and any other road users. Once the area is safe, quickly assess the casualty or casualties and prioritise treatment (pp.46–47). Give first aid to those with life-threatening injuries before treating anyone else. **Call 999/112 for emergency help,** giving as much detail as you can about the incident, indicating the number and age of the casualties, and types of injury.

MAKING THE INCIDENT AREA SAFE

Do not put yourself or others in further danger. Take the following precautions.

- **Park safely,** well clear of the incident site, set your hazard lights flashing and put on a high-visibility jacket/vest if you have one.
- **Set up warning triangles** (or another vehicle with hazard lights) at least 45 m (49 yd) from the incident in each direction; bystanders can do this while you attend to the casualty. Send helpers who are wearing high-visibility jackets to warn other drivers to slow down.
- **Make vehicles safe.** For example, switch off the ignition of any damaged vehicle and, if you can, disconnect the battery. Pull the supply cut-off on large diesel vehicles; this is normally found on the outside of the vehicle and will be marked.
- **Stabilise vehicles.** If a vehicle is upright, apply the handbrake, put it in gear and/or place blocks in front of the wheels. If it is on its side, do not attempt to right it, but try to prevent it from rolling over further.
- **Watch out for physical dangers,** such as traffic. Make sure that no-one smokes anywhere near the incident.
- **Alert the emergency services** to damaged power lines, spilt fuel or any vehicles with Hazchem signs (opposite).

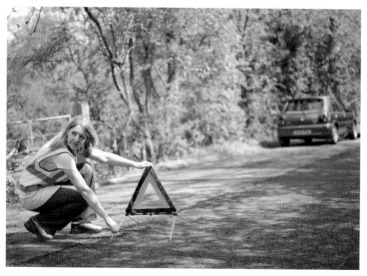

Warn other road users
Ask a bystander to set up warning triangles at least 45 m (49 yd) away from the vehicles in both directions. Advise the person to wear a hi-visibility jacket and watch out for other vehicles while they do this.

SPECIAL CASE HAZARDOUS SUBSTANCES

Traffic incidents may be complicated by spillages of toxic substances or vapours. Keep bystanders away from the scene and stand upwind of the vehicle. Hazchem signs on the back of the vehicle indicate that it may be carrying a potentially dangerous substance. Give the details to the emergency services so they can assess the risks involved. If in doubt about your safety or the meaning of a symbol, keep your distance. If the top left panel of a sign contains the letter "E", the substance is a public safety hazard.

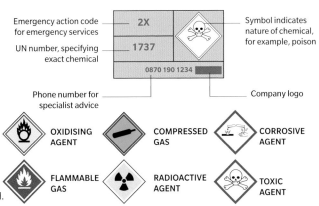

Emergency action code for emergency services

UN number, specifying exact chemical

2X

1737

0870 190 1234

Symbol indicates nature of chemical, for example, poison

Phone number for specialist advice

Company logo

OXIDISING AGENT

COMPRESSED GAS

CORROSIVE AGENT

FLAMMABLE GAS

RADIOACTIVE AGENT

TOXIC AGENT

ASSESSING THE CASUALTIES

Quickly assess any casualties by carrying out a primary survey (pp.46–47). Deal first with those who have life-threatening injuries. If a casualty can move freely and can get out of a vehicle allow them to do so. Otherwise treat them in the position in which you find them. A casualty who has been involved in a road-traffic incident may have a neck or spinal injury (pp.159–161) so support the head and neck and wait for the emergency

services. Search the area around the incident thoroughly to make sure you do not overlook anyone who may have been thrown clear, or who has wandered away from the site. Bystanders can help. If a person is trapped inside or under a vehicle, they will need to be released by the fire service. Monitor and record the casualty's vital signs (pp.54–55) while you are waiting for the emergency services to arrive.

CAUTION

- Only cross a motorway to attend to an incident or casualty if you are officially informed that it is safe to do so.
- At night, wear or carry something light or reflective, such as a high-visibility jacket, and use a torch.
- Do not move the casualty unless it is absolutely necessary. If you do have to move them, the method will depend on their condition and available help.
- Be aware that road surfaces may be slippery because of fuel, oil or even ice.
- Be aware that undeployed air bags and unactivated seat-belt tensioners may be a hazard.
- Find out as much as you can about the incident and relay this information to the emergency services when they arrive.

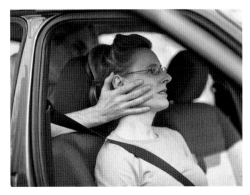

Casualty in a vehicle

If you suspect a neck injury and a casualty is unable to get out of a vehicle, support their head and neck while you await help and reassure them. Make sure that their ears are uncovered so they can hear you.

FIRES

Fire spreads very quickly, so your first priority is to warn any people at risk. If you are in a building, activate the nearest fire alarm, **call 999/112 for emergency help**, then leave the building. However, if doing this delays your escape, make the call when you are out of the building. As a first aider, try to keep everyone calm. Encourage and assist people to evacuate the area as quickly and calmly as possible.

When arriving at an incident involving fire, stop, observe, think: do not enter the area. A minor fire can escalate in minutes to a serious blaze. **Call 999/112 for emergency help** and wait for it to arrive.

THE ELEMENTS OF FIRE

A fire needs three components to start and maintain it: ignition (a spark or flame); a source of fuel (petrol, wood or fabric); and oxygen (air). Removing one of these elements can break this "triangle of fire".

- **Remove combustible materials,** such as paper or cardboard, from the path of a fire, as they can fuel the flames.
- **Cut off a fire's oxygen** supply by shutting a door on a fire or smothering the flames with a fire blanket. This will cause the fire to suffocate and go out.
- **Switch off a car's ignition,** or pull the fuel cut-off on a large diesel vehicle (this is normally marked on the outside of the vehicle), or turn off the gas supply.

LEAVING A BURNING BUILDING

If you see or suspect a fire in a building, activate the first fire alarm you see. Try to help people out of the building without putting yourself at risk. Close doors behind you as you leave to help prevent the fire from spreading. If you are in a public building, use the fire exits and look for assembly points outside.

You should already know the evacuation procedure at your workplace. If, however, you are visiting other premises you are not familiar with, follow the signs for escape routes and obey any instructions you are given by the fire marshals in that building.

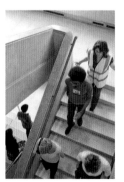

Evacuating other people
Encourage people to leave the building calmly but quickly by the nearest exit. If they have to use the stairs, make sure they do not rush and risk falling down.

> **CAUTION**
>
> **When escaping from a fire:**
> - Do not re-enter a burning building to collect personal possessions.
> - Do not use lifts.
> - Do not go back to a building until cleared to do so by a fire officer.
>
> **Fire precautions:**
> - Do not move anything that is on fire.
> - Do not smother flames with flammable materials.
> - Do not fight a fire if it puts your own safety at risk.
> - If your clothes catch fire and help is not available, wrap yourself up tightly in suitable material and roll along the ground to extinguish the flames.
> - Do not put water on an electrical fire: pull the plug out or switch the power off at the mains.
> - Smother a pan fire with a fire blanket; never water.

CLOTHING ON FIRE

If a person's clothing is on fire always follow this procedure: Stop, Drop and Roll.

- **Stop** the casualty panicking, running around or going outside – any movement or breeze will fan the flames.
- **Drop** the casualty to the ground. If possible, wrap them tightly in a fire blanket, or heavy fabric such as a coat, curtain, blanket (not an open-weave type or one made from synthetic materials) or rug.
- **Roll** the casualty along the ground until the flames have been smothered. Treat any burns (pp.176–183): help the casualty to lie down, burned side uppermost, and start cooling the burn as soon as possible.

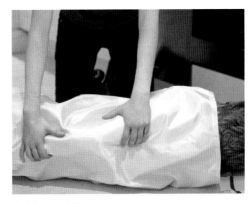

Putting out flames
Help the casualty on to the ground to stop flames rising towards their face. Wrap them in a fire blanket to starve flames of oxygen, and roll them on the ground until the flames are extinguished.

SMOKE AND FUMES

Any fire in a confined space creates a highly dangerous atmosphere that is low in oxygen and may also be polluted by carbon monoxide and other toxic fumes. Never enter a smoke- or fume-filled building or open a door that leads to a fire. Let the emergency services do this.

- **If you are trapped** in a burning building, if possible go into a room at the front of the building with a window and shut the door behind you. Block gaps under the door by placing a rug or similar heavy fabric across the bottom of the door to minimise smoke coming in to the room. Open the window and shout for help.
- **Stay low** if you have to cross a smoke-filled room as the air is clearest at floor level.
- **If escaping through a high window,** climb out backwards feet first – lower yourself to the full length of your arms before you drop down.

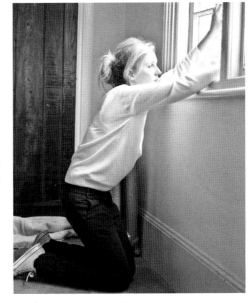

Avoiding smoke and fumes
Shut the door of the room you are in and put a rug or blanket against the door to keep smoke out. Open the window and shout for help. Keep as low as possible to avoid fumes in the room.

ELECTRICAL INCIDENTS

When a person is electrocuted, the passage of electrical current through the body may stun them, causing their breathing and heartbeat to stop (cardiac arrest, p.59). The electrical current can also cause burns both where it enters and where it exits the body to go to "earth". An electrical burn may appear very small or may not even be visible on the skin, however, the damage the burn causes can extend deep into the body tissues (p.178).

The factors that affect the severity of the injury are: the voltage; the type of current; and the path of the current. A low voltage of 240 volts is found in a home or workplace, a high voltage of 440–1,000 volts is found in industry, and voltage of more than 1,000 volts passes along power lines. The type of current will either be alternating (AC) or direct (DC), and the path of the current can be hand-to-hand, hand-to-foot or foot-to-foot.

Most low-voltage and high-tension currents are AC, which causes muscular spasms (known as tetany) and the "locked-on" phenomenon –

the casualty's grasp is "locked" on to the object, which prevents them from letting go, so they may remain electrically charged ("live"). In contrast, DC tends to produce a single large muscular contraction that often throws the person away from the source of electricty. Be aware that the jolt may cause the casualty to be thrown or to fall, which can result in injuries such as spinal injuries and fractures.

CAUTION

- Do not touch the casualty if they are in contact with the electrical current.
- Do not use anything metallic to break the electrical contact.
- Do not approach high-voltage wires until the power is turned off.
- Do not move a person with an electrical injury unless they are in immediate danger and they are no longer in contact with the electricity.
- If the casualty is unresponsive, and it is safe to touch them, open the airway and check breathing (The unresponsive casualty, pp.56–89).

HIGH-VOLTAGE CURRENT

Contact with a high-voltage current found in power lines and overhead cables is usually immediately fatal. Anyone who survives will have severe burns, since the temperature of the electricity may reach up to 5,000°C (9,032°F). Furthermore, the shock produces a muscular spasm that propels the casualty some distance, causing additional injuries.

High-voltage electricity may jump ("arc") up to 18 m (20 yd) from its source. The power must be cut off and isolated before anyone can approach the casualty. A casualty who has suffered this type of shock is likely to be unresponsive. Once you have been officially informed that it is safe to approach, assess the casualty, open the airway and check breathing (The unresponsive casualty, pp.56–89).

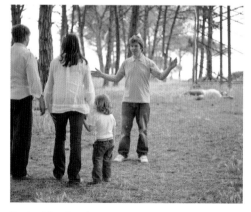

Protect bystanders
Keep everyone away from the incident. Bystanders should stay at least 18 m (20 yd) from the damaged cable and/or casualty.

LOW-VOLTAGE CURRENT

Domestic current, as used in homes and workplaces, can cause serious injury or even death. Incidents are usually due to faulty or loose switches, frayed flexes or defective appliances. Young children are at risk since they are naturally curious, and may put fingers or other objects into electrical wall sockets.

Water is also a very efficient conductor of electricity, so presents additional risks to both you and the casualty. If you handle an otherwise safe electrical appliance with wet hands, or when you are standing on a wet floor, you greatly increase the risk of an electric shock.

BREAKING CONTACT WITH ELECTRICITY

1 **Before beginning any treatment,** look at the area first – do not touch the casualty. If they are still in contact with the electrical source, they will be "live" and you risk electrocution.

2 **Turn off the source of electricity,** if possible, to break the contact between the casualty and the electrical supply. Switch off the current at the mains or meter point if possible. Otherwise remove the plug or wrench the cable free.

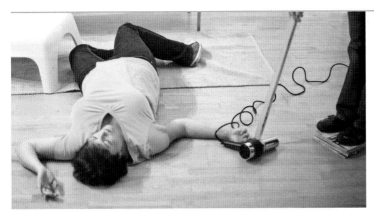

3 **Alternatively, move the source** away from both you and the casualty. Stand on some dry insulating material, such as a wooden box, plastic mat or pile of magazines or books. Using a wooden pole or broom, push the casualty's limb away from the electrical source or push the source away from the casualty.

4 **If it is not possible to break the contact** using a wooden object, loop a length of rope around the casualty's ankles or under the arms, taking great care not to touch them, and pull them away from the source of the electrical current.

5 **Once you are sure that the contact** between the casualty and the electricity has been broken, perform a primary survey (pp.46–47) and treat injuries in order of priority. **Call 999/112 for emergency help.**

LIGHTNING

A natural burst of electricity discharged from the atmosphere, lightning forms an intense trail of light and heat. Lightning seeks contact with the ground through the nearest tall feature in the landscape and, sometimes, through anyone standing nearby. However, because the duration of a lightning strike is short it usually precludes serious thermal injury. It may, however, set

clothing on fire, knock the casualty down or cause the heart and breathing to stop (cardiac arrest, p.59). Cardiopulmonary resuscitation/ CPR (adult, pp.68–73; child, pp.78–81; infant, pp.84–85) must be started promptly.

Always clear everyone from the site of a lightning strike since, contrary to popular belief, it can strike again in the same place.

WATER INCIDENTS

Incidents around water can involve people of any age. However, drowning is one of the most common causes of accidental death among young people under the age of 16. Young children can drown in fish ponds, paddling pools, baths and even in the toilet if they fall in head first, as well as in swimming pools, in the sea and in open water. Many cases of drowning have also involved people who have been swimming in strong currents or very cold water, or who have been swimming or boating after drinking alcohol.

There are particular dangers connected with incidents involving swimmers in cold water. Open water around Great Britain and Ireland is cold, even in summer. Sea temperatures range from 5°C (41°F) to 15°C (59°F); inland waters, such as lakes or reservoirs may be even colder. The sudden immersion in cold water can result in an overstimulation of nerves, causing the heart to stop (cardiac arrest, p.59). Submersion in cold water may cause hypothermia (pp.188–189) and exacerbate shock (pp.114–115). Spasm in the throat and inhalation of water can block the airway leading to hypoxia (p.94) and drowning (p.102). Inhaled or swallowed water may be absorbed into the circulatory system, causing water overload to the brain, heart or lungs. The exertion of swimming can also strain the heart.

CAUTION

- If the casualty is unresponsive, lift them clear of the water. Try to keep the casualty horizontal, supporting the head and neck and maintaining an open airway. When you reach land, lay them down on the ground and open the airway and check breathing. Begin CPR if necessary (The unresponsive casualty, pp.56–89).

Drowning chain of survival

This describes the five linked steps that, when enacted by professional or lay responders, can significantly improve the chances of preventing incidents in water as well as survival and recovery from drowning.

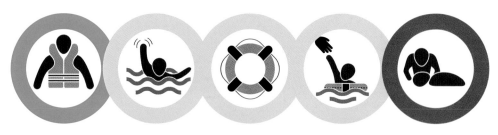

Prevent drowning
Always be safe in and around water.

Recognise distress
Ask someone to call for help.

Provide flotation
This can prevent submersion.

Remove from water
Do this only if it is safe to do so.

Provide care as needed
Seek medical attention and treat as necessary.

RESCUING A PERSON FROM WATER

1 **Your first priority** is to get the casualty on to dry land with the minimum of danger to yourself. Stay on dry land, hold out a stick, a branch or a rope for them to grab, then pull them from the water. Alternatively, throw them a float.

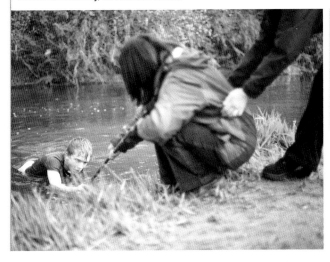

2 **If you are a trained life-saver** and the casualty is unresponsive, wade or swim to the casualty and tow them ashore – try to keep them horizontal. If you cannot do this safely, or you are not a trained lifesaver, call 999/112 for emergency help.

3 **Once the casualty is out of the water,** shield them from the wind, if possible. Treat them for drowning (p.102) and the effects of severe cold (hypothermia, pp.188–190). If possible, replace any wet clothing with dry clothing.

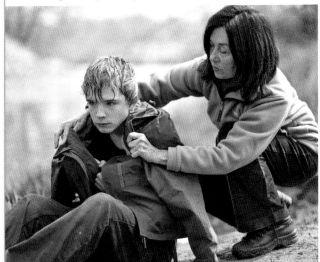

4 **Monitor and record** the casualty's vital signs (pp.54–55). Seek medical help if necessary.

MAJOR INCIDENTS

A major incident is one that presents a serious threat to the safety of a community or where the number of casualties, location, nature or severity requires special arrangements to manage the situation. Incidents of this kind can overwhelm the normal resources of the emergency services, but they continuously plan and train personnel for these events. It is the emergency services' responsibility to declare a situation to be a major incident, which then activates their combined services major incident plan in the locality. In recent years such events have included incidents considered to be acts of terrorism. Although acts of terrorism are rare compared to the other incidents described this chapter, if you are caught up in such an event the prompt actions of a first aider can save lives.

If you are the first person on the scene of what may be considered a major incident do not approach it. **Call 999/112 for emergency help** immediately (pp.22–23). The control officer will need to know the type of incident, for example, a fire, traffic incident or explosion; the location and access route if known; any particular hazards; and an estimate of the approximate number of casualties.

EMERGENCY SERVICE SCENE ORGANISATION

When a major incident is declared the emergency services will establish cordons around the area to ensure safety of all involved. The first, or inner, cordon is placed directly around the incident site, and a second, outer, cordon is placed around this to establish a minimum safe area for all emergency personnel (police, fire and ambulance). Only those with correct identification and adequate personal protective equipment (PPE) will be granted access to these areas. Other important areas to be established will be: a casualty clearing station, where emergency treatment takes place; a survivor reception centre, where the uninjured assemble; and ambulance parking and loading areas.

TRIAGE
This is a dynamic process used to prioritise the casualties needing emergency treatment. It is repeated many times during the care of each casualty in a major incident. Triage principles are applied when the number of casualties exceeds the skilled help available to treat them. In most situations this is the responsibility of the emergency services attending, primarily the ambulance service aided by available medical support – the aim is to do the greatest good for the greatest number of individuals. Triage can also be used to identify treatment priorities in other situations such as road traffic incidents, for example, where there may be several casualties but only one or two people available to give first aid before emergency services arrive.

At a major incident the emergency services activate a "triage sieve". Casualties who cannot walk undergo a primary survey assessment (pp.46–47) – based on airway, breathing and circulation (or ABCs) – at the scene to establish treatment priorities. When they arrive at the casualty clearing station a more detailed assessment is made to ensure each person receives the treatment they need. This is repeated at regular intervals until they reach the medical team in hospital.

- **Casualties who cannot walk** will undergo further assessment at the clearing station and, depending on the findings, will be assigned to the priority one (immediate) or priority two (urgent) areas, and be given life and/or limb-saving treatment prior to transfer to hospital by ambulance as soon as possible.

- **Walking casualties** will be assigned to priority three (delayed treatment) and will be taken to hospital if necessary when transport is available.
- **Uninjured people** will be directed to the survivor reception area, where they are comforted and observed for signs of delayed injury.

WHAT A FIRST AIDER CAN DO

As a first aider you can only enter the cordoned area if you have the correct identification and adequate PPE. Once there, you may be asked to assist the emergency services by, for example, helping casualties with minor injuries, making note of casualties' names and addresses and/or helping to contact relatives.

FIRST AID AT A TERRORIST INCIDENT

Despite high-profile examples, and apart from areas of the world considered active war zones, acts of terrorism remain very rare and so it is extremely unlikely that you will ever be faced with one. However, if you are involved in one be aware that the scene may be more chaotic than with other major incidents. It may take the emergency services longer to reach any casualties because of concerns around safety and security in the vicinity. Your overriding priority is to ensure your own safety by removing yourself from the source of danger.

You should:

- **Run** to a safe place away from the incident and call **999/112 for emergency help.**

If you cannot get away:

- **Hide** in a safe place if possible.
- **Tell** the emergency services about the incident; call **999/112 for emergency help.**

If you are alone with casualties prior to the arrival of the emergency services and you are able to deliver first aid without further endangering yourself, perform an initial triage assessment using the primary survey (pp.46–47) to determine who to treat first. Always remember that the quiet, still casualty might be the one most in need of urgent help. Extreme events such as these may require an exceptional level of improvised first aid. Life-threatening conditions such as severe bleeding can be dealt with using whatever material is available, for example, clothing for applying pressure to a wound (p.116), or in the case of life-threatening uncontrolled bleeding from a limb, the application of an improvised tourniquet (p.117).

> **CAUTION**
> - Always consider your safety before helping others.

WHAT TO DO

1 Stay calm and take control (p.15). Call 999/112 for emergency help immediately. The emergency services will advise you on how you can assist them as their response develops. When they arrive, hand over any relevant information such as emergency treatment given.

2 If you are on your own and faced with multiple casualties – and it is safe to do so – perform an initial triage to determine who you treat first. Be prepared to use life-saving first aid techniques such as opening and clearing the airway (p.47) and control of major bleeding by direct pressure (p.116) or, if that fails, the application of a tourniquet (p.117).

03 ASSESSING A CASUALTY

When a person is suddenly taken ill or has been injured, it is important to find out what is wrong as quickly as possible. As a first aider your immediate priority is to make sure that you are not endangering yourself in any way by approaching the scene.

Once you are sure that an incident area is safe, you need to begin your assessment of the casualty (or casualties). This chapter explains how to approach each casualty and plan your assessment using a methodical two-stage system, first to identify and treat life-threatening conditions according to their priority (primary survey), then to carry out a detailed assessment looking for injuries that are not immediately apparent (secondary survey).

There is advice on deciding treatment priorities, managing more than one casualty and arranging their aftercare. A casualty's condition may also improve or deteriorate while they are in your care, so there is guidance on how to monitor and record changes in their condition.

AIMS AND OBJECTIVES

- To assess a situation quickly and calmly, while first protecting yourself and the casualty from any danger
- To assess each casualty and treat life-threatening injuries first
- To carry out a more detailed assessment of each casualty
- To seek appropriate help. Call 999/112 for emergency help if you suspect serious injury or illness
- To be aware of your own needs

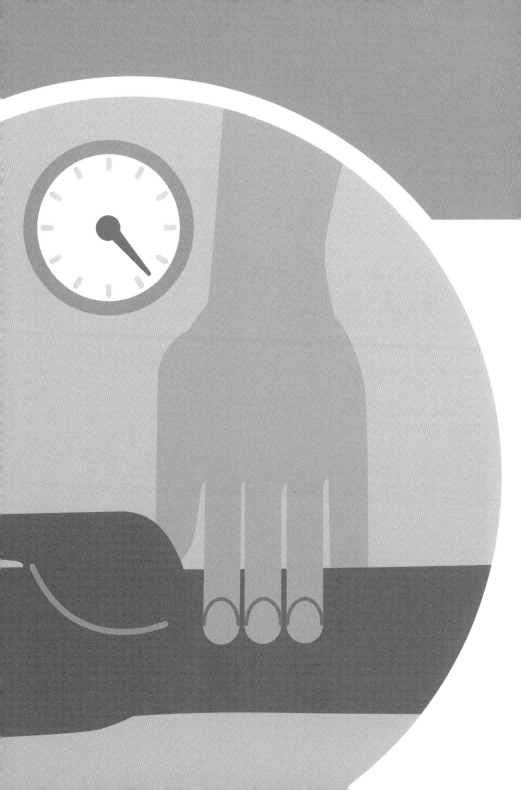

ASSESSING THE SICK OR INJURED

From reading the previous chapters you will now know that to ensure the best possible outcome for anyone who is injured or suddenly becomes ill you need to take responsibility for making assessments. Tell those at the scene that you are a trained first aider and calmly take control. However, as indicated in Chapter 2 (pp.26–39), resist the temptation to begin dealing with any casualty until you have assessed the overall situation, ensured that everyone involved is safe and, if appropriate, have taken steps to organise the necessary help.

As you read through this chapter, look back at Chapter 1 (pp.12–25) as well and remember the following:

- **Be calm**
- **Be aware of risks**
- **Build and maintain the casualty's trust**
- **Call for appropriate help**
- **Remember your own needs**

MANAGING THE SICK OR INJURED

There are three aspects to managing a sick or injured person. It is important to work quickly and systematically to avoid unnecessary delay.

- **First,** find out what is wrong with the casualty.
- **Second,** treat conditions found in order of severity – life-threatening ones first.
- **Third,** arrange for the next step of a casualty's care. You will need to decide what type of care a casualty needs. You may need to call for emergency help, suggest the casualty seeks medical advice or allow them to go home, accompanied if necessary.

Other people at the incident can help you. For example, ask one of them to **call 999/112 for emergency help** while you attend a casualty. Alternatively, they may be able to help support injured limbs, look after less seriously injured casualties, or fetch first aid equipment (pp.21, 22–23 and 29).

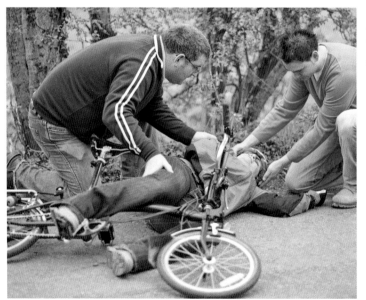

First actions
Support the casualty; a bystander may be able to help. Ask the casualty what happened, and try to identify their most serious injury.

METHODS OF ASSESSMENT

When you assess a casualty you first need to identify and deal with any life-threatening conditions or injuries as quickly as possible with a primary survey. Deal with each life-threatening condition as you find it, working in the following order – airway, breathing, then circulation – before you progress to the next stage.

Depending on your findings you may or may not move on to the next stage of the assessment. If the life-threatening injuries are successfully managed, or there are none, continue the assessment by performing a secondary survey.

THE PRIMARY SURVEY

This is an initial rapid assessment of a casualty to establish and treat conditions that are an immediate threat to life (pp.46–47).

If a casualty is suffering from minor injuries and responding to you, for example, talking, then this survey will be completed very quickly. If, however, a casualty is more seriously injured and/or not responding to you (unresponsive), the assessment may take longer.

Follow the ABC principle: Airway, Breathing and Circulation.

- **Airway** Is the airway open and clear? The airway is not open and clear if the casualty is unable to speak. An obstructed airway will prevent breathing, causing hypoxia (p.94) and ultimately death. The airway is open and clear if the casualty is talking to you.
- **Breathing** Is the casualty breathing normally? If the casualty is not breathing normally, **call 999 / 112 for emergency help,** then start chest compressions with rescue breaths (cardiopulmonary resuscitation/CPR). If this

happens, you are unlikely to move on to the next stage.

If the casualty is breathing, check for and treat any breathing difficulty such as asthma, then move on to the next stage: circulation.

- **Circulation** Is the casualty bleeding severely? If they are bleeding this must be treated immediately since it can lead to the life-threatening condition, shock (pp.114–115). **Call 999 / 112 for emergency help.** If there is no bleeding, continue to the secondary survey.

THE SECONDARY SURVEY

This is a detailed examination of a casualty to look for other injuries or conditions that may not be immediately apparent (pp.48–53). To do this, carry out a head-to-toe examination (pp.51–53). Your aim is to find out:

- **History** What actually happened and any relevant medical history.
- **Symptoms** Injuries or abnormalities that the casualty tells you about.
- **Signs** Injuries or abnormalities that you can see.

By checking the recognition features of the different injuries and conditions explained in the later chapters of this book you can identify what may be wrong. Record your findings and pass on any relevant information to the medical team.

LEVEL OF RESPONSE

You will initially have noted whether or not a casualty is responding to you. They may have spoken to you or made eye contact or some other gesture (p.46). Or perhaps there has been no response to your questions such as "Are you all right?" or "What happened?". Next, establish the casualty's level of response (p.54). This is important since some illnesses and injuries cause a deterioration in a person's level of response. Note the response level when you first attend them, then monitor them for changes.

SPECIAL CASE SEVERAL CASUALTIES

If there is more than one casualty, you need to prioritise those that must be treated first according to the severity of their injuries. Use the primary survey ABC principles (above and overleaf) to do this; unresponsive casualties are at greatest risk.

MECHANISMS OF INJURY

The injury that a person sustains is directly related to how it is caused. In addition, whether a casualty sustains a single or multiple injury is also determined by the mechanisms that caused it. This is the reason why a history of the incident itself, and therefore the injury mechanism, is important. In many situations, this vital information can only be obtained by those people who deal with the casualty at the scene – often first aiders. Look, too, at the circumstances in which an injury was sustained and the forces involved.

The information is useful because it also helps the emergency services and medical team predict the type and severity of injury, as well as the treatment a casualty requires. This in turn helps the diagnosis, treatment and likely outcome for the casualty.

CIRCUMSTANCES OF INJURY

The extent and type of injuries sustained due to impact – for example, a fall from a height or the impact of a car crash – can be predicted if you know exactly how the incident happened. For example, a car occupant is more likely to sustain serious injuries in a side-impact collision than in a frontal collision at the same speed. This is because the side of the car provides less protection and cannot absorb as much energy as the front of the vehicle. Unrestrained occupants of a vehicle are at even greater risk of injury. For a driver wearing a seatbelt whose vehicle is struck either head-on or from behind, a specific pattern of injuries can be suspected. The driver's body will be suddenly propelled one way, but the driver's head will lag behind briefly before moving. This results in a "whip-like" movement of the neck (below). The casualty may also have injuries caused by the seatbelt restraint; for example, fracture of the breastbone and collarbone and possibly bruising of the heart or lungs. There may also be injuries to the face due to contact with the steering wheel or an inflated airbag.

Whiplash injury

The head may be "whipped" backwards and then rapidly forwards, or vice versa, due to sudden forces on the body, such as in a car crash. This produces a whiplash injury, with strained muscles and stretched ligaments in the neck.

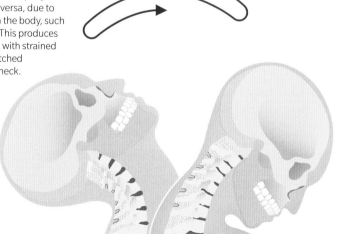

FORCES EXERTED ON THE BODY

The energy forces exerted during an impact are another important indicator of the type or severity of any injury. For example, if a person falls from a height of 1 m (3 ft 3 in) or less on to hard ground, they will probably suffer bruising but no serious injury. A fall from a height of more than 2 m (6 ft 6 in), however, is likely to produce more serious injuries, such as a pelvic fracture and internal bleeding. But an apparently less serious fall can mask a more severe injury. If a person falls down the stairs, for example, they may tell you that they injured their ankle. If they have fallen awkwardly on to a hard surface, however, they may have sustained a spine and/or head injury. A fall down more than five stairs is associated with a greater risk of injury than a fall down fewer than five stairs. Be aware too that the elderly or those suffering from bone disorders such as osteoporosis are at greater risk of serious injury from minor knocks or falls.

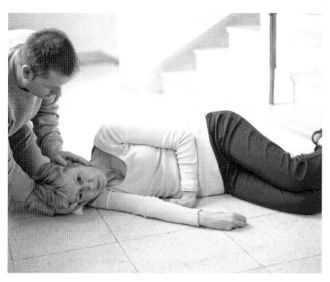

Most serious injury may be hidden
Advise the casualty not to move. If they cannot remain still, support their head and ask someone to **call 999/112 for emergency help.**

QUESTIONS TO ASK AT THE SCENE

When you are attending a casualty, ask the casualty, or any witnesses, questions to try to find out the mechanism of the injury. Witnesses are especially important if the casualty is unable to talk to you. Possible questions include:

- **Was the casualty ejected from a vehicle?**
- **Was the casualty wearing a seatbelt?**
- **Did the vehicle roll over?**
- **Was the casualty wearing a helmet?**
- **How far did the casualty fall?**
- **What type of surface did they land on?**
- **Is there evidence of body contact** with a solid object, such as the floor or a vehicle's windscreen or dashboard?
- **How did they fall?** (For example, twisting falls can stretch or tear the ligaments or tissues around a joint such as the knee or ankle.)

Pass on all the information that you have gathered to the emergency services (pp.21 and 23).

PRIMARY SURVEY

The primary survey is a quick, systematic assessment of a casualty to establish if any conditions or injuries sustained are life threatening. By following a methodical sequence using established techniques, each life-threatening condition can be identified in a priority order and dealt with on a "find and treat" basis. The sequence should be applied quickly and systematically to every casualty you attend. You should not allow yourself to be distracted from it by other events. If there is a high risk of infection or contamination, put on your PPE before you begin this assessment (pp.16–19).

Use the chart opposite to guide you through the assessment sequence. Depending on your findings you may or may not move on to the next stage of the assessment. Only when any life-threatening conditions are successfully managed, or you have established that there are none, should you perform a secondary survey (pp.48–53).

RESPONSE

At this point you need to make a quick assessment to find out whether a casualty is responding to you or is unresponsive (not responding). Observe the casualty as you approach. Introduce yourself even if they do not appear to be responding to you. Ask the casualty some questions, such as, "What happened?" or "Are you all right?" or give a command, such as "Open your eyes!". If there is no initial response, gently shake the casualty's shoulders. If the casualty is a child, tap their shoulder; if they are an infant, tap their foot. If there is still no response, they are described as unresponsive. If the casualty makes eye contact or some other gesture, they are responsive.

Unresponsive casualties take priority and require urgent treatment (pp.56–89).

AIRWAY

The first step is to check that a casualty's airway is open and clear. If a casualty is alert and talking to you, it follows that the airway is open and clear. If, however, a casualty is unresponsive, the airway may be obstructed (p.61). You need to open and clear the airway (adult, p.65; child, p.75; infant, p.82) – do not move on to the next stage until the airway is open and clear.

BREATHING

Is the casualty breathing normally? Look, listen and feel for breaths. If they are alert and/or talking to you, they will be breathing. However, it is important to note the rate, depth and ease with which they are breathing. For example, conditions such as asthma (p.104) that cause breathing difficulty require urgent treatment.

If an unresponsive casualty is not breathing, the heart will stop. Chest compressions and rescue breaths (cardiopulmonary resuscitation/CPR) must be started immediately (adult, pp.68–73; child, pp.78–81; infant, 84–85).

CIRCULATION

Conditions that affect the circulation of blood can also be life threatening. Injuries that result in severe bleeding (pp.116–117) can cause blood loss from the circulatory system, so must be treated immediately. In some instances this may need to take priority over checking airway and circulation. Successful control of bleeding can be life-saving and minimise the risk of a life-threatening condition known as shock (pp.114–115) developing.

Only when life-threatening conditions have been stabilised, or there are none present, should you begin to carry out a detailed secondary survey of the casualty (pp.48–53).

THE ABC CHECK

Work through these checks quickly and systematically to establish treatment priorities.

AIRWAY
Is the casualty's airway open and clear (adult, pp.64–65; child, pp.74–75; infant, p.82)?

NO

YES

RESPONSIVE

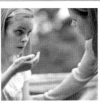

- If a casualty is responsive, treat conditions such as choking or suffocation that cause the airway to be blocked.
  Go to the next stage, **BREATHING**, when the airway is open and clear.

UNRESPONSIVE

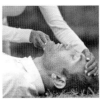

- If a casualty is unresponsive, tilt the head and lift the chin to open the airway (adult, p.65; child, p.75; infant, p.82).
  Go to the next stage, **BREATHING**, when the airway is open and clear.

BREATHING
Is the casualty breathing normally?
Look, listen and feel for breaths.

NO

YES

RESPONSIVE

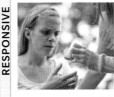

- If a casualty is responsive, treat any difficulty found; for example, asthma.
  Go to the next stage, **CIRCULATION**.

UNRESPONSIVE

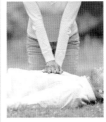

- If a casualty is unresponsive and not breathing, **call 999/112 for emergency help.** Begin chest compressions and rescue breaths (adult, pp.68–73; child, pp.78–81; infant, pp.84–85). If this happens, you are unlikely to move on to the next stage.

CIRCULATION
Are there any signs of severe bleeding?

YES

NO

- Control the bleeding (pp.116–117); this may take priority over checking airway and breathing. **Call 999/112 for emergency help.** Treat the casualty to minimise the risk of shock developing (pp.114–115).

If life-threatening conditions are managed, or there are none, move on to the **secondary survey** (pp.48–53) to check for other injury or illness.

SECONDARY SURVEY

Once you have completed the primary survey and dealt with any life-threatening conditions, start the methodical process of checking for other injuries or illnesses by performing a head-to-toe examination. This is called the secondary survey. Question the casualty as well as the people around them. Make a note of your findings if you can, and make sure you pass all the details to the emergency services or hospital, or whoever takes responsibility for the casualty (pp.23 and 29).

Ideally, the casualty should remain in the position found, at least until you are satisfied that it is safe to move them into a more comfortable position appropriate for their injury or illness.

This survey includes two further checks beyond the ABC (pp.43 and 46–47).

● **Disability** This is the casualty's level of response (p.54).
● **Examine the casualty** You may need to remove or cut away clothing to examine and/or treat the injuries.

By conducting this survey you are aiming to discover the following:

● **History** What happened in the moments leading up to the injury or sudden illness and any relevant medical history.
● **Symptoms** Information that the casualty gives you about their condition.
● **Signs** These are what you find on examination of the casualty.

HISTORY

There are two important aspects to the history: what happened and any medical history.

EVENT HISTORY

The first consideration is to find out what happened. Your initial questions should help you to discover the immediate events leading up to the incident. The casualty can usually tell you this, but sometimes you have to rely on information from people nearby so it is important to verify that they are telling you facts and not just their opinions. There may also be clues, such as the impact on a vehicle, which can indicate the likely nature of the casualty's injury. These are often referred to as the mechanisms of injury (pp.44–45).

PREVIOUS MEDICAL HISTORY

The second aspect to consider is a person's medical history. While this may have nothing to do with their present condition, it could be a clue to the cause. Clues to the existence of such a condition may include a medical bracelet or medication in the casualty's possessions (p.50).

TAKING A HISTORY

● **Ask what happened;** for example, establish whether the condition is due to illness or an injury.
● **Ask about medication** the casualty is taking currently.
● **Ask about medical history.** Find out if there are ongoing and previous conditions.
● **Find out if a person has any known allergies.**
● **Check when the person last** had something to eat or drink.
● **Note the presence of a medical warning bracelet** – this may indicate an ongoing medical condition, such as epilepsy, diabetes or risk of anaphylactic shock.

SYMPTOMS

These are the sensations that the casualty feels and describes to you. When you talk to the casualty, ask them to give you as much detail as possible. For example, if they complain of pain, ask where it is. Ask them to describe the pain (for example, is it constant or intermittent, sharp or dull, as well as severity). Ask them what makes the pain better or worse, for example whether it is affected by movement or breathing and, if it did not result from an injury, where and how it began. The casualty may describe other symptoms, too, such as nausea, giddiness, heat, cold or thirst. Listen very carefully to the casualty's answers (p.20) and do not interrupt them while they are speaking.

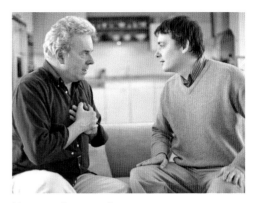

Listen to the casualty
Make eye contact with the casualty as you talk to them. Keep your questions simple, and listen carefully to the symptoms they describe.

SIGNS

These are features such as swelling, bleeding, discolouration, deformity and smells that you can detect by observing and feeling the casualty. Use all of your senses – look, listen, feel and smell. Conduct a head-to-toe survey (pp.51–53). Always compare the injured and uninjured sides of the body. You may also notice that the person is unable to perform normal functions, such as moving their limbs or standing. Make a note of any obvious superficial injuries, but do not treat them until you have completed the examination, as there may be other conditions or injuries that need attention first.

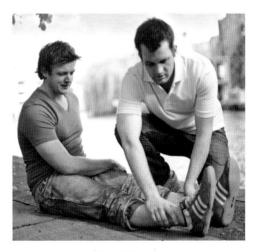

Compare both sides of the body
Always compare the injured part of the body with the uninjured side. Check for swelling, deformity and/or discolouration.

« SECONDARY SURVEY

LOOK FOR EXTERNAL CLUES

As part of your assessment, look for external clues to a casualty's condition. If you need to search a casualty's belongings, always try to ask the casualty first and then carry out the search in front of a reliable witness (p.21). If you suspect drug abuse, take care as they may be carrying needles and syringes. You may find an appointment card for a hospital or clinic, or a card indicating a history of allergy, diabetes or epilepsy. Horse-riders or cyclists may carry such a card inside their riding hat or helmet. Food or medication may also give valuable clues about the casualty's condition; for example, people with diabetes may carry sugar lumps or glucose gel as well as insulin. A person with a known disorder may also have medical warning information on a special locket, bracelet, medallion or key ring (such as a "MedicAlert" or "SOS Talisman"). Make sure these stay with the casualty or give it to the emergency services.

MEDICAL CLUES	
	MEDICATION A casualty may be carrying medication such as pain relief for back pain or tablets or a spray for angina.
	MEDICAL WARNING BRACELET This may be inscribed with information about a casualty's medical history (for example, epilepsy, diabetes or risk of anaphylaxis), or there may be a number to call.
	INHALER The presence of an inhaler usually indicates that the casualty has asthma or a chronic lung disease; reliever inhalers are generally blue; preventive inhalers are usually brown or white.
	INSULIN PEN The presence of an insulin pen or injector usually indicates that a person has diabetes. The casualty is also likely to carry a glucose testing kit.
	AUTO-INJECTOR This contains adrenaline for use by people at risk of anaphylactic shock. The pens are colour-coded for adult and child doses.

HEAD-TO-TOE EXAMINATION

Once you have taken the casualty's history (p.46) and asked about any symptoms they have (p.47), you should carry out a detailed examination, or head-to-toe survey. Use all of your senses when you examine a casualty: look, listen, feel and smell. Always start at the casualty's head and work down; this "head-to-toe" routine is both easily remembered and thorough. You may have to sensitively loosen, open, cut away or remove clothing where necessary to examine the casualty (p.236). Always be sensitive to a casualty's privacy and dignity, and ask their permission before you begin the survey.

Protect yourself and the casualty by putting on your disposable gloves, and if necessary a face mask/covering and apron if you have them. Make sure that you do not move the casualty more than is absolutely necessary. If possible, examine a casualty in the position in which you find them, or one that best suits their condition, unless their life is in immediate danger. If an unresponsive breathing casualty has been placed in the recovery position, leave them in this position while you carry out the head-to-toe examination.

Check the casualty's breathing and pulse rates (pp.54–55), then work from the head downwards (see overleaf). Initially, note any minor injuries found, but continue your examination to make sure that you do not miss any concealed potentially serious conditions that need attention; only return to the minor injuries when you have completed your examination.

POSSIBLE FINDINGS ON CARRYING OUT AN EXAMINATION

METHOD OF IDENTIFICATION	SYMPTOMS OR SIGNS
The casualty may tell you of these symptoms	● Pain ● Anxiety ● Heat ● Cold ● Loss of sensation ● Abnormal sensation ● Thirst ● Nausea ● Tingling ● Pain on touch or pressure ● Faintness ● Stiffness ● Weakness ● Memory loss ● Dizziness ● Sensation of broken bone ● Sense of impending doom
You may see these signs	● Temporary unresponsiveness ● Anxiety and painful expression ● Unusual chest movement ● Burns ● Sweating ● Wounds ● Bleeding from orifices ● Response to touch ● Response to speech ● Bruising ● Abnormal skin colour ● Muscle spasm ● Swelling ● Deformity ● Foreign bodies ● Needle marks ● Vomit ● Incontinence ● Loss of normal movement ● Containers and other circumstantial evidence
You may feel these signs	● Dampness ● Abnormal body temperature ● Swelling ● Deformity ● Irregularity ● Grating bone ends
You may hear these signs	● Noisy or distressed breathing ● Groaning ● Sucking sounds from a penetrating chest injury ● Response to touch ● Response to speech ● Grating bone (crepitus)
You may smell these signs	● Acetone ● Alcohol ● Burning ● Gas or fumes ● Solvents or glue ● Urine ● Faeces ■ Cannabis

continued ⟫ | **51**

« SECONDARY SURVEY

WHAT TO DO: COMPLETING A HEAD-TO-TOE EXAMINATION

1 **Start the physical examination** at the casualty's head. Run your hands carefully over the scalp to feel for bleeding, swelling, tenderness or depression of the bone, which may indicate a fracture. Do not move the casualty if you suspect that they may have injured their neck.

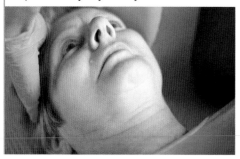

2 **Speak clearly to the casualty** in both ears to find out if they respond or if they can hear. Look for bleeding, clear fluid or watery blood coming from either ear; discharges may be signs of a serious head injury (pp.146).

3 **Examine both eyes.** Note whether they are open. Check the size of the pupils (the black area). If the pupils are not the same size it may indicate head injury (p.146). Look for any foreign object, blood or bruising in the whites of the eyes.

4 **Check the nose for discharges** as you did for the ears. Look for bleeding, clear fluid or watery blood coming from either nostril. Any of these discharges may also indicate serious head injury (p.146).

5 **Look in the mouth** for anything that might obstruct the airway. If the casualty has dentures that are intact and fit firmly, leave them. Look for mouth wounds or burns and check for irregularity in the line of the teeth.

6 **Assess breathing** (p.54). Check the rate (fast or slow), depth (shallow or deep) and nature (is it easy or difficult, noisy or quiet).

7 **Look at the skin.** Note the colour and temperature: is it pale, flushed or grey-blue (cyanosis); is it hot or cold, dry or damp? Pale, cold, sweaty (clammy) skin suggests shock (pp.114–115); a flushed, hot face suggests fever (p.221) or heatstroke (p.187). A blue tinge indicates lack of oxygen; look for this in the lips, ears and face.

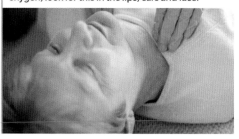

8 **Loosen clothing around the neck,** and look for signs such as a medical warning medallion (p.50) or a hole (stoma) in the windpipe. Run your fingers gently along the spine from the base of the skull down as far as possible without moving the casualty; check for irregularity, swelling, tenderness or deformity.

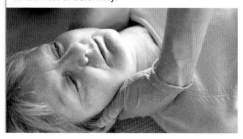

9 **Check the pulse** (p.55). Assess the rate (fast or slow), rhythm (regular or irregular) and strength (strong or weak).

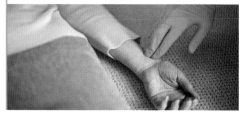

10 **Look at the chest.** Ask the casualty to breathe deeply, and note whether the chest expands evenly, easily and equally on both sides. Feel the ribcage to check for deformity, irregularity or tenderness. Ask the casualty if they are aware of grating sensations when breathing, and listen for unusual sounds. Note whether breathing causes any pain. Look for any external injuries, such as bleeding or stab wounds.

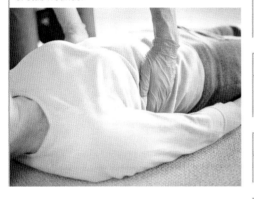

11 **Feel along the collar bones,** shoulders, upper arms, elbows, hands and fingers for any swelling, tenderness or deformity. Check the movements of the elbows, wrists and fingers by asking the casualty to bend and straighten each joint.

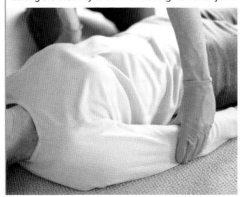

12 **Check that the casualty** has no abnormal sensations in the arms or fingers. If the fingertips are pale or grey-blue there may be a problem with blood circulation. Look out for needle marks on the arms or hands, or a medical warning bracelet (p.50).

13 **If there is any impairment** in movement or loss of sensation in the limbs, do not move the casualty to examine the spine, since these signs suggest spinal injury. Otherwise, gently pass your hand under the hollow of the back and check for swelling and tenderness.

14 **Gently feel the casualty's abdomen** to detect any evidence of bleeding, and to identify any rigidity or tenderness of the abdomen's muscular wall, which could be a sign of internal bleeding. Compare one side of the abdomen with the other.

15 **Feel both sides of the hips,** and examine the pelvis for signs of fracture. Check clothing for any evidence of incontinence, which suggests spinal or bladder injury, or bleeding from orifices (p.118), which suggests pelvic fracture (p.157).

16 **Check the legs.** Look and feel for bleeding, swelling, deformity or tenderness. Ask the casualty to raise each leg in turn, and to move their ankles and knees.

17 **Check the movement** and feeling in the casualty's toes. Check that they have no abnormal sensations in their feet or toes. Compare both feet. Look at the skin colour: grey-blue skin may indicate a circulatory disorder or there may be an injury due to cold.

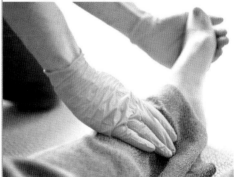

MONITORING VITAL SIGNS

When treating a casualty, you may need to assess and monitor their breathing, pulse and level of response. This information can help you to identify problems and indicate changes in a casualty's condition. Monitoring should be repeated regularly, and your findings recorded and handed over to whoever is responsible for taking over (p.21).

In addition, if a casualty has a condition that affects their body temperature, such as fever, heat stroke or hypothermia, you will also need to check, then monitor, their temperature.

LEVEL OF RESPONSE

You need to assess and monitor a casualty's level of response and make a note of any change in their condition (deterioration or improvement) while they are in your care. Any injury or illness that affects the brain may alter a person's ability to respond, and any deterioration is potentially serious. Assess the casualty's level of response using the list, right, only moving to the next point if needed. Repeat your assessment again at regular intervals.

- **Is the casualty alert?** Are their eyes open and do they respond to questions?
- **Does the casualty respond to your voice?** Can they open their eyes, answer simple questions and obey commands?
- **Does the casualty respond to pain?** Do they open their eyes, move or groan if you pinch the ear lobe?
- **Is the casualty not responding** to any stimulus (unresponsive)?

BREATHING

When assessing a casualty's breathing, check the rate of breathing and listen for any breathing difficulties or unusual noises.

An adult's normal breathing rate is 12–16 breaths per minute; in babies and young children, it is 20–30 breaths per minute. When checking breathing, listen for breaths and watch the casualty's chest movements. For a baby or young child, it might be easier to place your hand on the chest and feel for movement of breathing. Record the following information:

- **Rate** – count the number of breaths per minute.
- **Depth** – are the breaths deep or shallow.
- **Ease** – are the breaths easy, difficult or painful.
- **Noise** – is the breathing quiet or noisy, and if noisy, what are the types of noise.

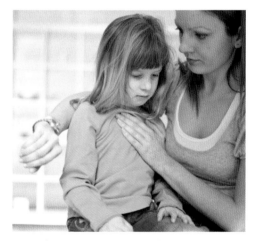

Checking a casualty's breathing rate
Observe the chest movements and count the number of breaths per minute. Use a watch to time breaths. For a baby or young child, place your hand on the chest and feel for movement.

PULSE

Each heartbeat creates a wave of pressure as blood is pumped along the arteries (pp.110–111). Where arteries lie close to the skin surface, such as on the inside of the wrist and at the neck, this pressure wave can be felt as a pulse. The normal pulse rate for an adult is 60–80 beats per minute. The pulse rate is faster in children and may be slower in very fit adults. An abnormally fast or slow pulse rate may be a sign of illness or injury.

The pulse may be felt at the wrist (radial pulse), or if this is not possible, the neck (carotid pulse). In babies, the pulse in the upper arm (brachial pulse) is easier to find.

When checking a pulse, use your fingers (not your thumb) and press lightly against the skin. Record the following points:

- **Rate** (number of beats per minute).
- **Strength** (strong or weak).
- **Rhythm** (regular or irregular).

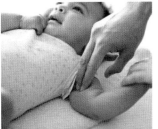

Brachial pulse
Place the pads of two fingers on the inner side of an infant's upper arm.

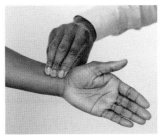

Radial pulse
Place the pads of three fingers just below the wrist creases at the base of the thumb.

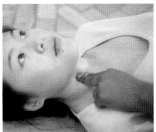

Carotid pulse
Place the pads of two fingers in the hollow between the large neck muscle and the windpipe.

BODY TEMPERATURE

Although not a vital sign, you may sometimes need to assess body temperature. You can feel exposed skin on the forehead for example, but use a thermometer to obtain an accurate reading. Normal body temperature is 37°C (98.6°F). A temperature above this (fever) is usually caused by infection, but can also be the result of heat exhaustion or heatstroke (pp.186–187). A lower body temperature may result from exposure to cold and/or wet conditions – hypothermia (pp.188–190) – or it may be a sign of life-threatening infection or shock (pp.114–115). There are several different types of thermometer, see below.

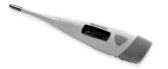

Digital thermometer
Used to measure temperature under the tongue or armpit. Leave it in place until it makes a beeping sound (about 30 seconds), then read the display.

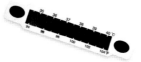

Forehead thermometer
A heat-sensitive strip for use on a young child. Hold it against the child's forehead for about 30 seconds. The colour on the strip indicates temperature.

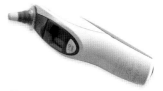

Ear sensor
Place the probe inside the ear. Press the measurement key and wait for a beeping sound, then read the display. This type can be used while a person is asleep.

04 THE UNRESPONSIVE CASUALTY

To stay alive we need an adequate supply of oxygen to enter the lungs and be transferred to all cells in the body by the circulating blood. If a person is deprived of oxygen for any length of time, the brain will begin to fail. As a result, the casualty will eventually become unresponsive, breathing will cease, the heart will stop and death results.

The casualty's airway must be kept open so that breathing can occur, allowing oxygen to enter the lungs and be circulated in the body.

Therefore, the priority of a first aider when treating any collapsed casualty is to establish an open airway and maintain breathing and circulation. An AED (automated external defibrillator) may be used to "shock" a fibrillating heart back into a normal rhythm. This chapter outlines the priorities to remember when dealing with an unresponsive adult, child or infant.

There are important differences in the treatment for unresponsive infants, children and adults; this chapter gives separate step-by-step instructions for dealing with each of these groups.

AIMS AND OBJECTIVES

- To maintain an open airway, to check breathing and resuscitate if required
- To call 999/112 for emergency help

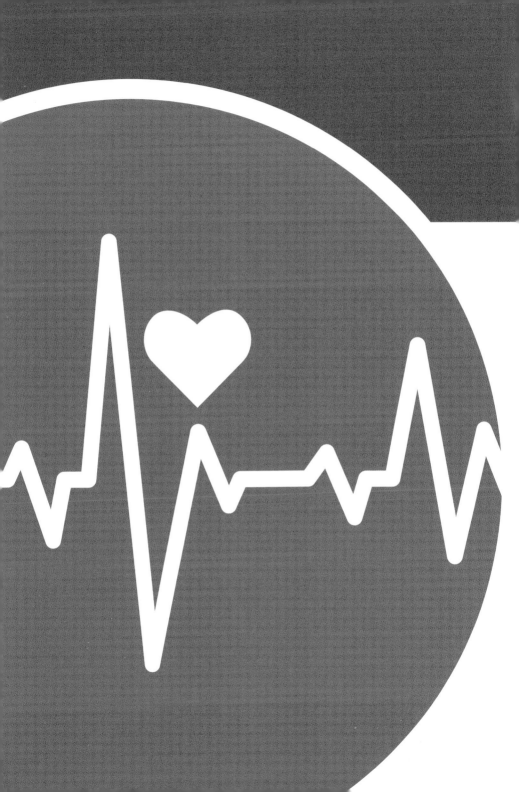

BREATHING AND CIRCULATION

Oxygen is essential to support life. Without it, cells in the body die – those in the brain survive only a few minutes without oxygen. Oxygen is taken in when we breathe in (pp.92–93), and it is then circulated to all the body tissues via the circulatory system (p.110). It is vital to maintain breathing and circulation in order to sustain life.

The process of breathing enables air, which contains oxygen, to be taken into the air sacs (alveoli) in the lungs. Here, the oxygen is transferred across blood vessel walls into the blood, where it combines with blood cells. At the same time, the waste product of breathing,

carbon dioxide, is released and exhaled in the breath. When oxygen has been transferred to the blood cells it is carried from the lungs to the heart through the pulmonary veins. The heart then pumps the oxygenated blood to the rest of the body via blood vessels called arteries.

After oxygen is given up to the body tissues, deoxygenated blood is brought back to the heart by blood vessels called veins (p.110). The heart pumps this blood to the lungs via the pulmonary arteries, where the carbon dioxide is released and the blood is reoxygenated before circulating around the body again.

How the heart and lungs work together

Air containing oxygen is taken into the lungs via the mouth and nose. Blood is pumped from the heart to the lungs, where it absorbs oxygen. Oxygenated blood is returned to the heart before being pumped around the body.

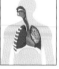

Exchange of gases in the air sacs (alveoli)

Carbon dioxide passes out of blood cells into air sacs (alveoli). Oxygen crosses the walls of alveoli into blood cells.

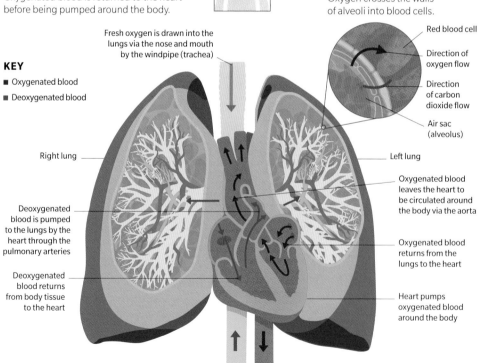

Fresh oxygen is drawn into the lungs via the nose and mouth by the windpipe (trachea)

KEY
- ■ Oxygenated blood
- ■ Deoxygenated blood

Right lung

Deoxygenated blood is pumped to the lungs by the heart through the pulmonary arteries

Deoxygenated blood returns from body tissue to the heart

Red blood cell

Direction of oxygen flow

Direction of carbon dioxide flow

Air sac (alveolus)

Left lung

Oxygenated blood leaves the heart to be circulated around the body via the aorta

Oxygenated blood returns from the lungs to the heart

Heart pumps oxygenated blood around the body

LIFE-SAVING PRIORITIES

The procedures set out in this chapter can maintain a casualty's circulation and breathing.

With an unresponsive casualty your priorities are to maintain an open airway, to maintain blood circulation (to get oxygenated blood to the tissues), and to breathe for the casualty (to get oxygen into the body). In an adult during the first minutes after the heart stops (cardiac arrest), the blood oxygen level remains constant, so chest compressions are more important than rescue breaths in the initial phase of resuscitation. After about two to four minutes, the blood oxygen level falls and rescue breathing becomes more important. The combination of chest compressions and rescue breaths is known as cardiopulmonary resuscitation, or CPR.

In addition to CPR, a machine called an AED (automated external defibrillator) can be used to deliver an electric shock that may restore a normal heartbeat (pp.86–89). In children and infants, a problem with breathing is the most likely reason for the heart to stop. Because of this they should therefore be given FIVE initial rescue breaths before you begin chest compressions.

CHEST-COMPRESSION-ONLY CPR

If you have not had any training in CPR, you are unwilling or unable to give rescue breaths, or current guidelines advise against giving them, you can give chest compressions only. The emergency services call handler will give instructions for chest-compression-only CPR (pp.72–73).

KEY ELEMENTS FOR SURVIVAL

If all of the following elements are complete, the casualty's chances of survival are as good as they can possibly be:

- **Emergency help** is called quickly.
- **CPR** is used to provide circulation and oxygen to the body tissues.
- **AED** is used promptly.
- **Specialised treatment** and advanced care arrive quickly.

CHAIN OF SURVIVAL

EARLY HELP
Call 999/112 for emergency help so that an AED and expert help can be brought to the casualty.

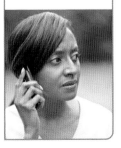

EARLY CPR
Chest compressions and rescue breaths are used to "buy time" until expert help arrives.

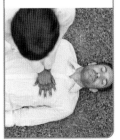

EARLY DEFIBRILLATION
A controlled electric shock from an AED is given. This can "shock" the heart into a normal rhythm.

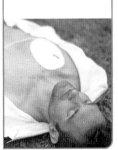

EARLY ADVANCED CARE
Specialist treatment and hospitalisation can stabilise the casualty's condition.

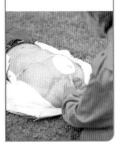

continued »

⟨⟨ LIFE-SAVING PRIORITIES

IMPORTANCE OF MAINTAINING CIRCULATION

If the heart stops beating, blood does not circulate through the body. As a result, vital organs – most importantly the brain – become starved of oxygen. Brain cells are unable to survive for more than 3 to 4 minutes without a supply of oxygen.

Some circulation can be maintained artificially with chest compressions (pp.68–69). These act as a mechanical aid to the heart in order to get blood flowing around the body. Pushing vertically down on the centre of the chest increases the pressure in the chest cavity, expelling blood from the heart and forcing it into the tissues. As pressure on the chest is released, the chest recoils, or comes back up, and more blood is "sucked" into the heart; this blood is then forced out of the heart by the next compression. It is possible to find the hand position for chest compressions without removing clothing.

To ensure that the blood is supplied with enough oxygen, chest compressions should be combined with rescue breathing (opposite).

RESTORING HEART RHYTHM

A machine called an AED (automated external defibrillator) will be used to attempt to restore normal heart rhythm (pp.86–89). The earlier the AED is used, the greater the chance of the casualty surviving. With each minute's delay, the chances of survival fall – however, do not leave a casualty to search for an AED; always ask a bystander to fetch one (pp.62 and 86). AEDs can be used safely and effectively without any prior training in their use.

AEDs are found in many public places, such as railway stations, shopping centres, airports, coach stations and ferry ports. They are generally housed in cabinets, often marked with a recognised symbol (p.87), and placed where they can be easily accessed – on station platforms for example. Many cabinets are not locked. Some are fitted with an alarm that is activated when the door is opened and a code may be required to gain access.

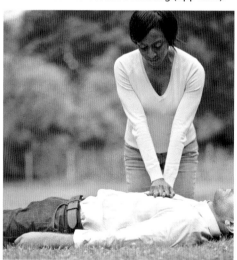

GIVING CHEST COMPRESSIONS

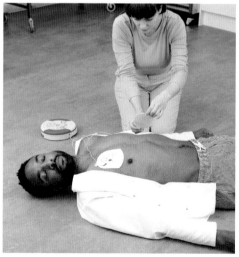

USING AN AED

AN OPEN AIRWAY

An unresponsive casualty's airway can become narrowed or blocked. This can be the result of muscular control being lost, which allows the tongue to fall back and block the airway. When this happens, the casualty's breathing becomes difficult and noisy and may stop altogether. Lifting the casualty's chin and tilting the head back lifts the tongue away from the entrance of the air passage, which allows the casualty to breathe.

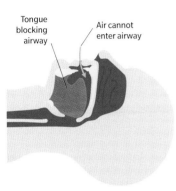

Tongue blocking airway

Air cannot enter airway

Blocked airway

In an unresponsive casualty, the muscle control in the tongue is lost so it falls back, blocking the throat and airway.

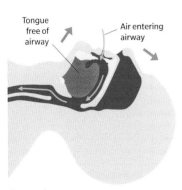

Tongue free of airway

Air entering airway

Open airway

In the head-tilt, chin-lift position, the tongue is lifted from the back of the throat and the trachea is open, so the airway will be clear.

BREATHING FOR A CASUALTY

Exhaled air contains about 16 per cent oxygen (only 5 per cent less than inhaled air) and a small amount of carbon dioxide. Your exhaled breath therefore contains enough oxygen to supply another person with oxygen – and potentially keep them alive – when it is forced into their lungs during rescue breathing.

By giving a casualty rescue breaths (p.69), you force air into their air passages. This reaches the air sacs (alveoli) in the lungs, and oxygen is then transferred to the blood vessels in the lungs.

When you take your mouth away from the casualty's, their chest falls, and air containing waste products is pushed out, or exhaled, from their lungs. This process, performed together with chest compressions (pp.68–69), can supply the tissues with oxygen until help arrives.

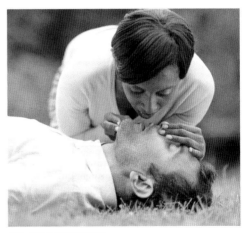

GIVING RESCUE BREATHS

CAUTION

AGONAL BREATHING
This type of breathing usually takes the form of short, irregular gasps for breath. It is common in the first few minutes after a cardiac arrest. It should not be mistaken for normal breathing and, if it is present, chest compressions and rescue breaths (cardiopulmonary resuscitation/CPR) should be started without hesitation.

continued >> | **61**

« LIFE-SAVING PRIORITIES

ADULT RESUSCITATION

This action plan is a summary of the techniques to use when attending a collapsed adult. There are more detailed instructions given on the following pages. Carry out the following steps in rapid succession to minimise interruption to CPR.

CHECK CASUALTY'S RESPONSE

- Try to get a response by asking questions and gently shaking the shoulders (p.64).

Is there a response?

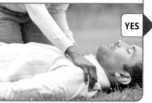

YES Leave the casualty in the position found. Use the primary survey (pp.46–47) to identify the most serious injury and treat in order of priority.

NO

OPEN THE AIRWAY; CHECK FOR BREATHING

- Tilt the head back and lift the chin to open the airway (p.65).
- Check for breathing (p.65).

Are they breathing normally?

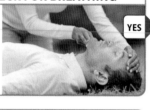

YES If possible, leave the casualty in the position found. Use the primary survey (pp.46–47) to identify the most serious injury and treat in order of priority. If necessary, place the casualty in the recovery position (pp.66–67). **Call 999/112 for emergency help.**

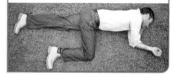

NO

Ask a helper to **call 999/112 for emergency help** and fetch an AED.
- If you are on your own, make the call yourself.

BEGIN CPR

- Give 30 chest compressions (pp.68–69).
- Give TWO rescue breaths (p.69).
- Alternate 30 chest compressions with TWO rescue breaths (30:2) until help arrives; the casualty shows signs of becoming responsive, for example, coughing, opening their eyes, speaking, or moving purposefully, and starts to breathe normally; or you are too exhausted to continue.

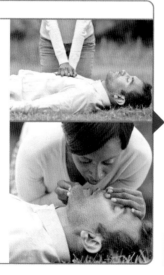

- If you are on your own, start CPR straight away; do not leave the casualty in search of an AED.
- If you have not had training in CPR, you are unwilling or unable to give rescue breaths, or guidelines advise against rescue breaths, you can give chest compressions only (pp.72–73). The emergency services give instructions for chest-compression-only CPR.
- If the casualty starts breathing normally, but remains unresponsive, monitor them closely and await the arrival of emergency services.

CHILD/INFANT RESUSCITATION

This action plan shows the order for the techniques you should use when attending a child over the age of one year or an infant under one year.

CHECK CHILD'S RESPONSE

- Try to get a response by asking questions and gently tapping the child's shoulder or an infant's foot.

Is there a response?

NO

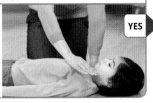

YES ▶ Leave the child in the position found. Use the primary survey (pp.46–47) to identify the most serious injury and treat in order of priority.

OPEN THE AIRWAY; CHECK FOR BREATHING

- Tilt the head back and lift the chin to open the airway (child, p.75; infant, p.82).
- Check for breathing (child, p.75; infant, p.83).

Are they breathing normally?

NO

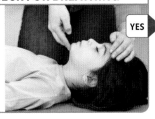

YES ▶ If possible, leave the casualty in the position found. Use the primary survey (pp.46–47) to identify the most serious injury and treat in order of priority. If necessary, place the child in the recovery position (pp.76–77), or hold an infant (p.83). **Call 999/112 for emergency help.**

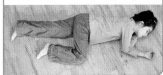

Ask a helper to **call 999/112 for emergency help** and, for a child, fetch an AED, ideally with paediatric pads.
- Do not use an AED on an infant.

GIVE INITIAL RESCUE BREATHS

- Carefully remove any visible obstruction from the mouth.
- Give FIVE initial rescue breaths (child, p.78; infant, p.84).

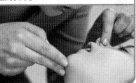

BEGIN CPR

- Give 30 chest compressions (child, p.79; infant, p.85).
- Follow with TWO rescue breaths.
- Alternate 30 chest compressions with TWO rescue breaths (30:2) until emergency help arrives; the child shows signs of becoming responsive, such as coughing, opening their eyes, speaking, or moving purposefully, and starts to breathe normally; or you are too exhausted to continue.

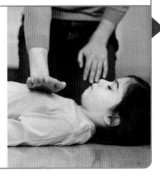

- It is better to give a combination of rescue breaths and chest compressions. However, if you have not had training in CPR, you are unwilling or unable to give rescue breaths, or guidelines advise against rescue breaths, you may give chest compressions only (pp.72–73). The emergency services will give you instructions for chest-compression-only CPR.

- If you are alone, carry out CPR for one minute before calling for emergency help. Take the child with you to the phone if possible – never leave a child unattended to fetch an AED.

- If the child starts breathing normally, but remains unresponsive, monitor them closely and await the arrival of emergency services.

UNRESPONSIVE ADULT

The following pages describe techniques for the management of an unresponsive adult who may require resuscitation.

Always approach and treat the casualty from the same side, kneeling down next to their head or chest. You will then be in the correct position to perform all the stages of resuscitation: opening the airway; checking breathing; and giving chest compressions and rescue breaths (together called cardiopulmonary resuscitation, or CPR). At each stage you will have decisions to make, for example, is the casualty breathing? The steps on these pages tell you what to do; work through them in rapid succession.

Your first priority is to check that the airway is open and clear. If the casualty is not breathing, begin CPR straightaway (pp.68–69). The early use of an AED may increase their chance of survival (pp.86–89). If the casualty is breathing normally, check for conditions affecting circulation (p.46) and, if necessary, place them in the recovery position (pp.66–67).

CAUTION

- Always assume that there is a neck injury and shake the shoulders very gently.

HOW TO CHECK THE RESPONSE

On discovering a collapsed casualty, you should first make sure the scene is safe and then establish whether they are responsive or unresponsive. Do this by gently shaking the casualty's shoulders. Ask "What has happened?" or give a command such as, "Open your eyes". Always speak loudly and clearly to them.

IF THERE IS A RESPONSE

1 If there is no further danger, leave the casualty in the position in which they were found. Use the primary survey (pp.46–47) to identify the most serious injury and treat conditions in order of priority. Summon help if needed.

2 Monitor and record vital signs (pp.54–55) until help arrives or the casualty recovers.

IF THERE IS NO RESPONSE

1 Shout for help. Leave the casualty in the position in which they were found and open the airway.

2 If you are unable to open the airway in the position in which they were found, roll them on to their back and open the airway. Go to How to open the airway (opposite).

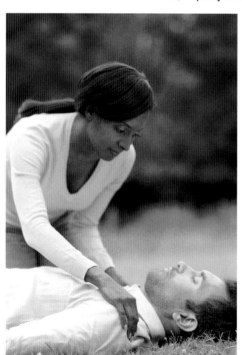

HOW TO OPEN THE AIRWAY

1 **Place one hand on the casualty's forehead.** Gently tilt their head back. As you do this, the mouth will fall open slightly.

2 **Place the fingertips** of your other hand on the point of the casualty's chin and lift the chin. Check the casualty's breathing. Go to *How to check breathing*, below.

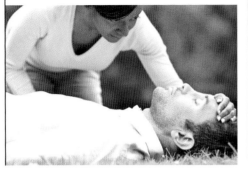

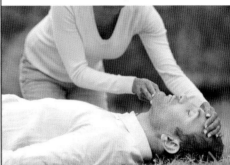

HOW TO CHECK BREATHING

Keeping the airway open, look, listen and feel for normal breathing: look for chest movement; listen for sounds of breathing; and feel for breaths on your cheek. Do this for no more than 10 seconds before deciding whether or not the casualty is breathing normally. Breathing may be agonal (p.61). If there is any doubt, act as if it is not normal.

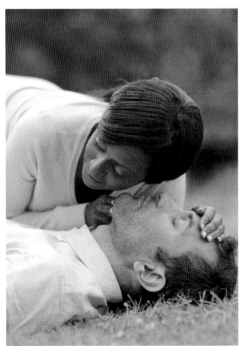

IF THE CASUALTY IS BREATHING

1 **Use the primary survey** (pp.46–47) to identify the most serious injury and treat conditions in order of priority.

2 **Place the casualty in the recovery position,** if necessary, and **call 999/112 for emergency help.** Go to *How to place casualty in recovery position* (pp.66–67).

3 **Monitor and record the casualty's vital signs** (pp.54–55) while waiting for help to arrive.

IF THE CASUALTY IS NOT BREATHING

1 **Ask a helper to call 999/112 for emergency help.** Ask the person to bring an AED if one is available. If you are alone, make the call yourself, ideally use your mobile device set to speaker phone to make the call.

2 **Begin CPR with chest compressions** – do not leave a casualty in search of an AED. Go to *How to give CPR* (pp.68–69).

continued ⟩⟩ | **65**

⟪ UNRESPONSIVE ADULT

HOW TO PLACE CASUALTY IN RECOVERY POSITION

If the casualty is found lying on their side or front, rather than their back, not all the following steps will be necessary to place them in the recovery position. If the mechanism of injury suggests a spinal injury, treat as described opposite and on pp.159–161.

WHAT TO DO

1 Kneel beside the casualty. Remove their spectacles and bulky objects, such as mobile phones or large bunches of keys, from their pockets. Do not search the pockets for small items.

2 Make sure that both of the casualty's legs are straight. Place the arm that is nearest to you away from the casualty's body, with the elbow bent and the palm facing upwards.

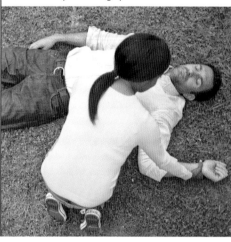

3 Bring the arm that is farthest from you across the casualty's chest, and hold the back of their hand against the cheek nearest to you. With your other hand, grasp the far leg just above the knee and pull it up, keeping the foot flat on the ground.

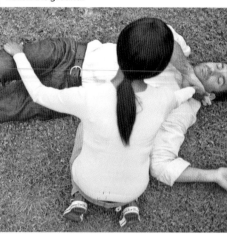

4 Keeping the casualty's hand pressed against their cheek, pull on the far leg and roll the casualty towards you and on to their side.

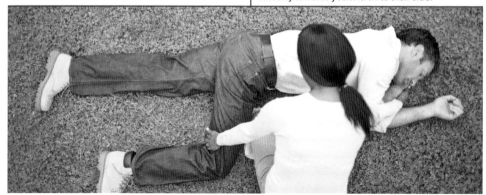

5 Adjust the upper leg so that both the hip and the knee are bent at right angles.

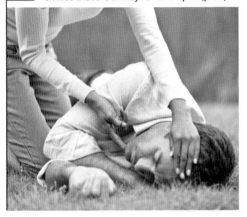

6 Tilt the casualty's head back and tilt their chin so that the airway remains open (p.65).

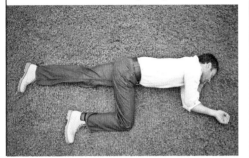

7 If necessary, adjust the hand under the cheek to keep the head tilted and the airway open to allow fluid to drain from the mouth.

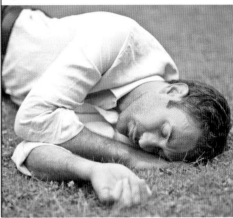

8 If it has not already been done, call 999/112 for emergency help. Monitor and record vital signs (pp.54–55) while waiting for help to arrive.

9 If the casualty is likely to remain in the recovery position for a while, after 30 minutes roll them on to their back, and then roll them on to the opposite side – unless other injuries prevent you from doing this.

SPECIAL CASE RECOVERY POSITION FOR SUSPECTED SPINAL INJURY

If you suspect a spinal injury (pp.159–161) and need to put the casualty in the recovery position because you cannot maintain an open airway, try to keep the spine straight using the following guidelines:

- If you are alone, use the technique shown opposite and above.
- If you have one helper, one of you should steady the head while the other turns the casualty (right).
- With three people, one person should steady the head while another turns the casualty. The third person should keep the back straight during the manoeuvre.
- If there are four or more people in total, use the log-roll technique (p.161).

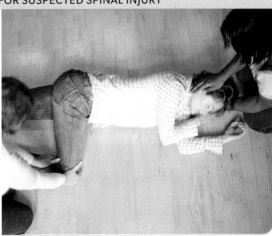

continued ⟩⟩

« UNRESPONSIVE ADULT

HOW TO GIVE CPR

WHAT TO DO

1 **Kneel beside the casualty** level with their chest. Place the heel of one hand on the centre of the casualty's chest. You can identify the correct hand position for chest compressions through a casualty's clothing.

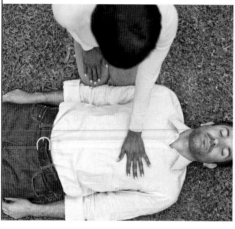

HAND POSITION

Place the heel of your hand on the casualty's breastbone as indicated here. Make sure that you do not press on the casualty's ribs, the lower tip of the breastbone or the upper abdomen.

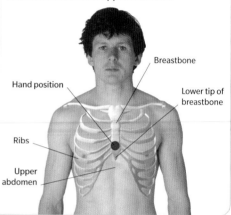

Hand position

Ribs

Upper abdomen

Breastbone

Lower tip of breastbone

2 **Place the heel of your other hand** on top of the first hand, and interlock your fingers, making sure the fingers are kept off the ribs.

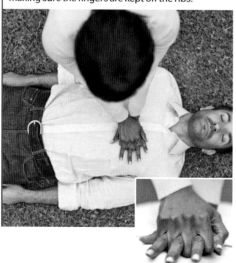

3 **Leaning over the casualty,** with your arms straight, press down vertically on the breastbone and depress the chest by 5–6 cm (2–2½ in). Release the pressure without removing your hands from the casualty's chest. Allow the chest to come back up fully (recoil) before giving the next compression.

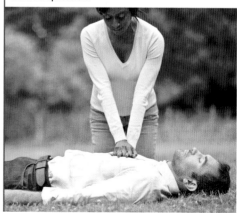

4 **Compress the chest** 30 times at a rate of 100–120 compressions per minute. The time taken for compression and release should be about the same.

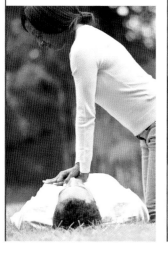

5 **Move to the casualty's head** and make sure that the airway is still open. Put one hand on their forehead and two fingers of the other hand under the tip of their chin. Move the hand that was on the forehead down to pinch the soft part of the nose with the finger and thumb. Allow the casualty's mouth to fall open.

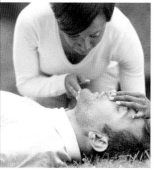

CAUTION

- If there is more than one rescuer, change over every 1–2 minutes, with minimal interruption to chest compressions.
- If the casualty starts to breathe normally, but remains unresponsive leave them on their back. Monitor them closely and await the arrival of the emergency services.

6 **Take a breath** and place your lips around the casualty's mouth, making sure you have a good seal. Blow into the casualty's mouth until the chest rises. A complete rescue breath should take one second. If the chest does not rise, you may need to adjust the head position (How to open the airway, p.65).

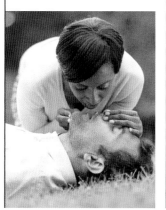

7 **Maintaining head tilt** and chin lift, take your mouth off the casualty's mouth and look to see the chest fall. If the chest rises visibly as you blow and falls fully when you lift your mouth away, you have given a rescue breath – one rescue breath should take one second. Give a second rescue breath.

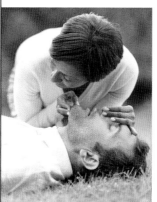

8 **Continue the cycle** of 30 chest compressions followed by TWO rescue breaths (30:2) until: emergency help arrives and takes over; the casualty shows signs of becoming responsive – such as coughing, opening their eyes, speaking, or moving purposefully – and starts to breathe normally; or you are too exhausted to continue.

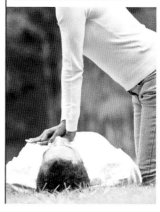

UNRESPONSIVE ADULT

SPECIAL CONSIDERATIONS FOR CPR

There are circumstances when it may be more difficult to deliver CPR:

- If national guidelines advise use of gloves and face coverings (p.16) for protection from cross infection, put them on before you start.
- If you have not been trained in CPR, are unwilling or unable to give rescue breaths, or guidelines advise against giving them, you can give chest compressions only (pp.72–73). The emergency services call handler will give instructions for chest-compression-only CPR.
- If there is more than one rescuer, change over every 1–2 minutes, with minimal interruption to chest compressions.

- If the casualty vomits during CPR, roll them away from you onto their side, ensuring that their head is turned towards the floor to allow vomit to drain away. Clear any residual debris from the mouth, then immediately roll them onto their back again and recommence CPR.
- If a casualty in the late stage of pregnancy requires CPR, raise the right hip off the ground by tilting it upwards before you begin compressions, see below.
- Modified rescue breathing may be necessary if there are chemicals around mouth or if there is a stoma (opposite). You can use a pocket mask or face shield when giving rescue breaths.

CPR IN LATE STAGES OF PREGNANCY

If a heavily pregnant casualty is lying on their back, the pregnant uterus will press against the large blood vessels in the abdomen. This restricts blood from the lower part of the body returning to the heart, which reduces the amount of blood circulation that can be achieved with chest compressions. To prevent this from happening, tilt their right hip upwards.

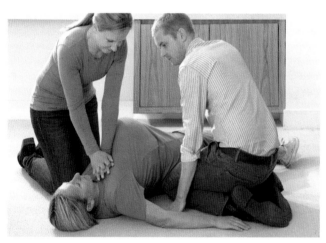

Positioning the person
Keep the person's upper body as flat on the floor as possible in order to give good-quality compressions. Raise their right hip and ask a helper to kneel beside them so that their knees are underneath the raised hip. If you are on your own, place tightly rolled up clothing or towels under the casualty's hip to lift it.

PROBLEMS WITH RESCUE BREATHING

If a casualty's chest does not rise when giving rescue breaths:

- Re-check the head tilt and chin lift.
- Re-check the casualty's mouth and remove any obvious obstructions, but do not do a finger sweep of the mouth.

Make no more than two attempts to achieve rescue breaths before continuing compressions.

VARIATIONS FOR RESCUE BREATHING

There are some situations where mouth-to-mouth rescue breaths are not possible and you need to use a mouth-to-nose or mouth-to-stoma technique.

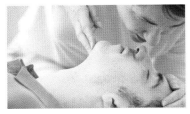

Mouth-to-nose rescue breathing
If a casualty has injuries to the mouth that make it impossible to achieve a good seal, you can use the mouth-to-nose method for giving rescue breaths. With the casualty's mouth closed, form a tight seal with your lips around the nose and blow steadily into the casualty's nose. Then allow the mouth to fall open to let the air escape.

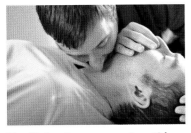

Mouth-to-stoma rescue breathing
A casualty who has had their voice-box surgically removed breathes through an opening in the front of the neck (a stoma), rather than through the mouth and nose. Always check for a stoma before giving rescue breaths. If you find a stoma, close off the mouth and nose with one hand and then breathe into the stoma.

FACE SHIELDS AND POCKET MASKS

Face shields are plastic barriers with a filter that is placed over the casualty's mouth. A pocket mask has a mouthpiece through which breaths are given. If you have one of these barrier devices, avoid unnecessary interruptions to CPR when you use it.

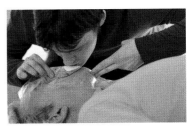

Using a face shield
Tilt the casualty's head back to open the airway. Place the shield over the casualty's face so that the filter is over the mouth and pinch the nostrils shut. Deliver rescue breaths through the filter.

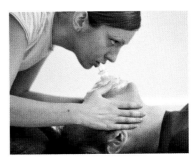

Using a pocket mask
Kneel behind the casualty's head. Open the airway and place the mask, narrow end towards you, over the casualty's mouth and nose. Deliver rescue breaths through the mouthpiece.

WHEN THE AMBULANCE ARRIVES

The ambulance service may initially send a sole responder in a fast-response vehicle or a community first responder ahead of the ambulance. If an AED is not already attached to the casualty, the ambulance personnel will do that. They will also use additional drugs and equipment to provide advanced care (p.59). If you are asked to help you should listen carefully and follow the instructions given (p.23).

The ambulance personnel will make a decision whether to transfer the casualty to hospital immediately or to continue treatment at the scene. Any decision to stop resuscitation can only be made by a healthcare professional.

continued ›› **71**

« UNRESPONSIVE ADULT

CHEST-COMPRESSION-ONLY CPR

Healthcare professionals and trained first aiders will deliver CPR using chest compressions combined with rescue breaths (pp.68–69). However, if you have not had training in CPR, you are unwilling or unable to give rescue breaths, or you have been advised against giving rescue breaths, chest-compression-only CPR has been shown to be of great benefit. The emergency services will give instructions for chest-compression-only resuscitation when advising an untrained person by telephone. Put your device on speaker-phone mode so that you can deliver first aid and talk to the call handler. Start chest compressions as soon as possible and continue them until: emergency help arrives and takes over; the casualty shows signs of becoming responsive – such as coughing, opening their eyes, speaking or moving purposefully – and starts breathing normally; or you are too exhausted to continue.

WHAT TO DO

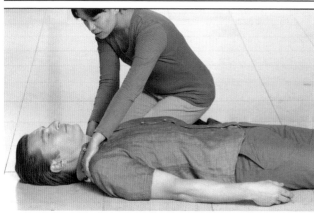

1 Check for a response. Gently shake the casualty's shoulders, and talk to them or give a command (p.64).

IF THERE IS A RESPONSE
Use the primary survey (pp.46–47) to identify the most serious injury and treat conditions in order of priority.

IF THERE IS NO RESPONSE
Shout for help and open the airway, step 2.

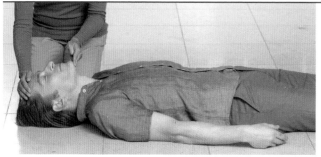

2 Open the casualty's airway. Place one hand on the forehead and gently tilt the head – the mouth should fall open. Place the fingertips of your other hand on the chin and lift it.

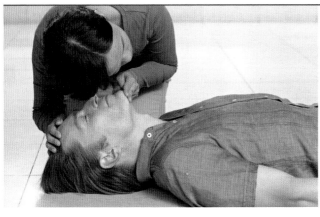

3 **Check breathing:** look, listen and feel for signs of breathing for no more than 10 seconds.

IF THEY ARE BREATHING
Use the primary survey (pp.46–47) to identify the most serious injury and treat conditions in order of priority. Place in the recovery position if necessary (pp.66–67).

IF THEY ARE NOT BREATHING
Call 999/112 for emergency help then begin chest compressions, step 4.

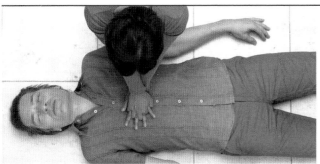

4 **Kneel beside the casualty,** level with their chest. Place the heel of one hand on the centre of the chest (p.68) – you can identify the position through clothing. Put the heel of your other hand on top of the first and interlock your fingers. Make sure your fingers are not in contact with the casualty's ribs.

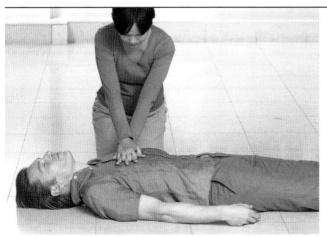

5 **Begin chest compressions.** Lean over the casualty, with your arms straight and press down vertically on the breastbone, depressing the chest by about 5–6 cm (2–2½ in). Release the pressure – but do not take your hands off the chest – and let the chest come back up. The time taken for compression and release should be about the same.

6 **Continue with chest compressions** at a rate of 100–120 per minute until: emergency help arrives; the casualty shows signs of becoming responsive – such as coughing, opening their eyes, speaking or moving purposefully – and starts breathing normally; or you are too exhausted to continue.

UNRESPONSIVE CHILD ONE YEAR AND OVER

The following pages describe the techniques that may be needed for the resuscitation of an unresponsive child over the age of one year; see pp. 82–85 for infants under one year.

When treating a child, always approach and treat them from the same side, kneeling down next to the head or chest. You will then be in the correct position to carry out all the different stages of resuscitation: opening the airway, checking breathing and giving rescue breaths and chest compressions (together known as cardiopulmonary resuscitation, or CPR). At each stage you will have decisions to make depending on what you find, for example,

is the child breathing? The steps on the following pages tell you what to do; work through them in rapid succession.

Your first priority is to check that the airway is open and clear. If the child is not breathing, begin CPR (pp.78–79). If they are breathing normally, check for conditions affecting circulation (p.46) and, if necessary, place them in the recovery position (pp.76–77).

If a child with a known heart condition collapses, **call 999/112 for emergency help** immediately and ask for an AED to be brought (pp.86–89). Early access to advanced care can be life-saving.

HOW TO CHECK RESPONSE

On discovering a collapsed child, you should first establish whether they are responsive or unresponsive. Do this by speaking loudly and clearly to the child. Ask "What has happened?"

or give a command such as, "Open your eyes". Place one hand on their shoulder, and gently tap them to see if there is a response.

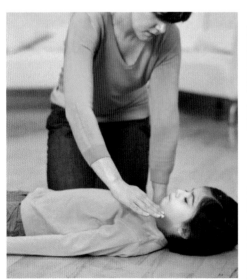

IF THERE IS A RESPONSE

1 **If there is no further danger,** leave the child in the position in which they were found. Use the primary survey (pp.46–47) to identify the most serious injury and treat conditions in order of priority.

2 **Monitor and record vital signs** (pp.54–55) until help arrives or the child recovers.

IF THERE IS NO RESPONSE

1 **Shout for help.** Leave the child in the position in which they were found; open the airway.

2 **If you are unable to open the airway** in the position in which they were found, roll the child on to their back and open the airway. Go to *How to open the airway* (opposite).

HOW TO OPEN THE AIRWAY

1 **Place one hand** on the child's forehead. Gently tilt the head back. As you do this, the mouth will fall open slightly.

2 **Place the fingertips of your other hand** on the point of the chin and lift. Do not push on the soft tissues under the chin since this may block the airway. Now check to see if the child is breathing. Go to *How to check breathing* (below).

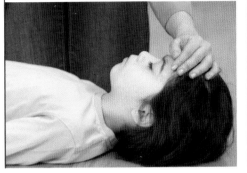

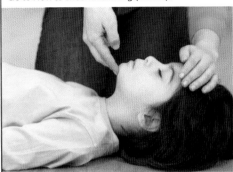

HOW TO CHECK BREATHING

Keep the airway open and look, listen and feel for normal breathing – look for chest movement, listen for sounds of normal breathing and feel for breaths on your cheek. Do this for no more than 10 seconds.

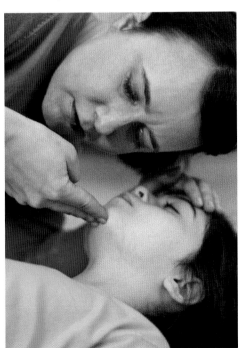

IF THE CHILD IS BREATHING

1 **Use the primary survey** (pp.46–47) to identify the most serious injury and treat conditions in order of priority.

2 **Place the child in the recovery position** if necessary. **Call 999/112 for emergency help.** Go to *How to place a child in the recovery position* (pp.76–77)

3 **Monitor and record vital signs** (pp.54–55) while waiting for help to arrive.

IF THE CHILD IS NOT BREATHING

1 **Ask a helper to** call 999/112 for emergency help. If you are on your own, perform CPR for one minute and then make the emergency call yourself. Use your mobile device set to speaker phone to make the call. If you need to go to a telephone take the child with you if possible.

2 **Begin CPR** with FIVE initial rescue breaths. Go to *How to give CPR* (pp.78–79).

continued >>

« UNRESPONSIVE CHILD ONE YEAR AND OVER

HOW TO PLACE CHILD IN RECOVERY POSITION

If the child is found lying on their side or front, rather than their back, not all of these steps will be necessary to place them in the recovery position. If the mechanisms of injury suggest a spinal injury, treat as described opposite and on pp.159–161.

WHAT TO DO

1 Kneel beside the child. Remove their spectacles and any bulky objects from their pockets, but do not search them for small items.

2 Make sure that both of the child's legs are straight. Place the arm nearest to you away from the child's body, with the elbow bent and the palm facing upwards.

3 Bring the arm that is farthest from you across the child's chest, and hold the back of their hand against the cheek nearest to you. With your other hand, grasp the far leg just above the knee and pull it up, keeping the foot flat on the ground.

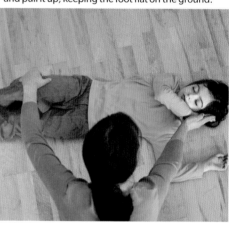

4 Keeping the child's hand pressed against their cheek, pull on the far leg and roll the child towards you and on to their side.

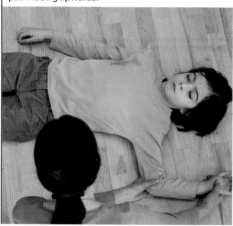

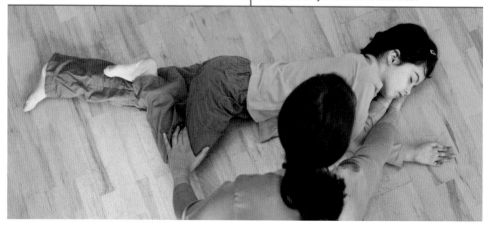

5 Adjust the upper leg so that both the hip and the knee are bent at right angles. Tilt the child's head back and lift the chin so that the airway remains open.

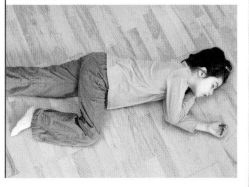

6 If necessary, adjust the hand under the cheek to make sure that the head remains tilted and the airway stays open so that any fluid can drain from the mouth. If it has not already been done, call 999/112 for emergency help. Monitor and record the child's vital signs (pp.54–55) until emergency help arrives.

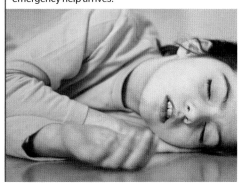

7 If the child is likely to remain in the recovery position for a while, after 30 minutes you should roll them on to their back, then turn them on to the opposite side – unless other injuries prevent you from doing this.

SPECIAL CASE RECOVERY POSITION FOR SUSPECTED SPINAL INJURY

If you suspect a spinal injury (pp.159–161) and need to place the child in the recovery position because you cannot maintain an open airway, try to keep the spine straight using the following guidelines:

- If you are on your own, use the technique shown opposite and left.
- If there are two of you, one person should steady the head while the other turns the child, see below.
- If there are three of you, one person should steady the head while one person turns the child. The third person should keep the child's back straight during the manoeuvre.
- If there are four or more people in total, use the log-roll technique (p.161).

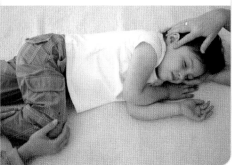

continued ⟩⟩

« **UNRESPONSIVE CHILD** ONE YEAR AND OVER

HOW TO GIVE CPR

WHAT TO DO

1 **Ensure the airway is still open** by keeping one hand on the child's forehead and two fingers of the other hand on the point of their chin.

2 **Pick out any visible obstructions** from the mouth. Do not sweep the mouth with your finger to feel for obstructions.

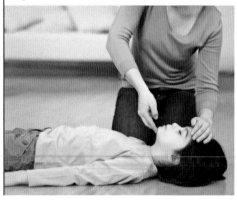

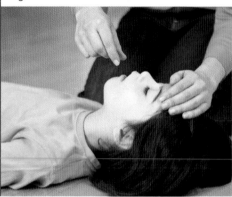

3 **Pinch the soft part** of the child's nose with the finger and thumb of the hand that was on the forehead. Make sure that their nostrils are closed to prevent air from escaping. Allow their mouth to fall open.

4 **Take a breath** before placing your lips around the child's mouth, making sure that you form an airtight seal. Blow steadily into the child's mouth; the chest should rise.

5 **Maintaining head tilt** and chin lift, take your mouth off the child's mouth and look to see the chest fall. If the chest rises visibly as you blow and falls fully when you lift your mouth, you have given a rescue breath. Each complete rescue breath should take one second. If the chest does not rise you may need to adjust the head (p.75). Give a child FIVE initial rescue breaths.

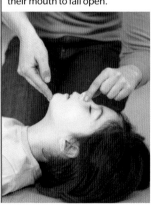

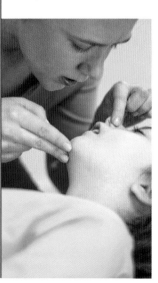

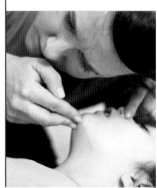

6 **Kneel level with the child's chest.** Place the heel of one hand on the centre of their chest. This is the point at which you will apply pressure.

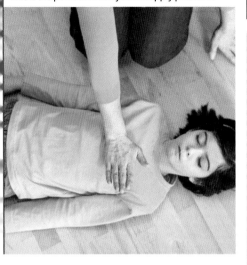

7 **Lean over the child,** with your arm straight, and then press down vertically on the breastbone with the heel of your hand. Depress the child's chest by at least one-third of its depth. Release the pressure without removing your hand from the chest. Allow the chest to come back up completely (recoil) before you give the next compression. Compress the chest 30 times, at a rate of 100–120 compressions per minute. The time taken for compression and release should be about the same.

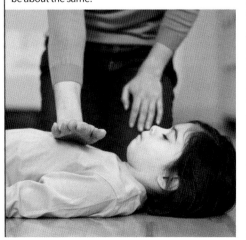

CAUTION

- With more than one rescuer, change every 1–2 minutes with minimal interruption to compressions.

HAND POSITION

Place the heel of one hand on the child's breastbone as indicated here. Make sure that you do not apply pressure over the child's ribs, the lower tip of the breastbone or the upper abdomen.

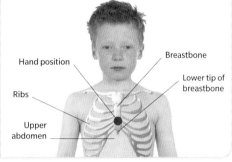

Hand position

Breastbone

Lower tip of breastbone

Ribs

Upper abdomen

8 **Return to the child's head,** open the airway and give TWO further rescue breaths.

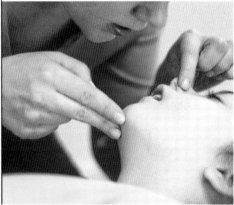

9 **If you are on your own,** alternate 30 chest compressions with TWO rescue breaths (30:2) for one minute, then stop to call 999/112 for emergency help. Continue CPR until: emergency help arrives and takes over; the child shows signs of becoming responsive – such as coughing, opening their eyes, speaking, or moving purposefully – and starts to breathe normally; or you become too exhausted to continue.

continued »

⟨⟨ UNRESPONSIVE CHILD ONE YEAR AND OVER

SPECIAL CONSIDERATIONS FOR CPR

There are circumstances when it may be more difficult to deliver CPR.

- If national guidelines advise use of gloves and face coverings (p.16) for protection from cross infection, put them on before you start.
- While it is better to give a combination of rescue breaths and chest compressions for children, if you have not been formally trained in CPR, you are unwilling or unable to give rescue breaths, or guidelines advise against giving them you can give chest compressions only. The emergency services call handler will give instructions for chest-compression-only resuscitation when you call them.
- If there is more than one rescuer, change over

every 1–2 minutes, with minimal interruption to compressions.

- If the child vomits during CPR, roll them away from you onto their side, ensuring that their head is turned towards the floor to allow vomit to drain away. Clear the mouth, then immediately roll them onto their back again and recommence CPR.
- If the child is large, or the rescuer is small, you can give chest compressions using both hands, as for an adult casualty (pp.68–69). Place the heel of one hand on the chest, cover it with the heel of your other hand and interlock your fingers, keeping them clear of the child's chest.

GIVING CHEST-COMPRESSION-ONLY CPR

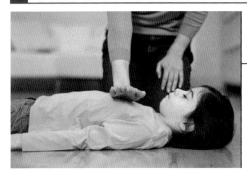

1 Kneel beside the child, level with their chest. Place the heel of one hand on the centre of their chest.

2 Lean over the child with your arm straight and depress the chest by at least one third of the depth, and release the pressure (but do not remove your hand).

3 Repeat compressions at a rate of 100–120 per minute until: emergency help arrives and takes over; the child shows signs of becoming responsive – such as coughing, opening their eyes, speaking, or moving purposefully – and starts to breathe normally; or you become too exhausted to continue.

PROBLEMS WITH RESCUE BREATHING

If a child's chest does not rise when giving rescue breaths:

- Re-check the head tilt and chin lift;
- Re-check the mouth. Remove any obvious obstructions, but do not do a finger sweep of the mouth.

Make no more than FIVE attempts to achieve rescue breaths before commencing the chest compressions.

VARIATIONS FOR RESCUE BREATHING

There are some cases where mouth-to-mouth rescue breaths are not possible and you can use a mouth-to-nose technique.

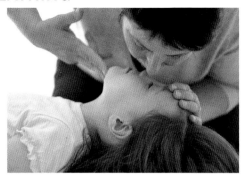

Mouth-to-nose rescue breathing

If a child has been rescued from water (pp.36–37), or injuries to the mouth make it impossible to achieve a good seal, you can use the mouth-to-nose method for giving rescue breaths. With the child's mouth closed, form a tight seal with your lips around the nose and blow steadily into the child's nose. Then allow the mouth to fall open to let the air escape.

FACE SHIELDS AND POCKET MASKS

A face shield is a plastic barrier with a filter that is placed over the child's mouth. A pocket mask is more substantial and has a valve through which breaths are given. If you have one of these barrier devices, avoid unnecessary interruptions when giving CPR to the child.

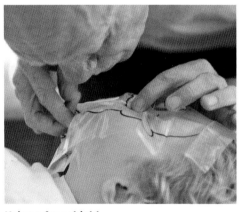

Using a face shield
Tilt the child's head back to open the airway and lift the chin. Place the plastic shield over the child's face so that the filter is over their mouth. Pinch the nose and deliver breaths through the filter.

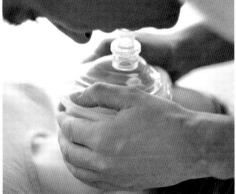

Using a pocket mask
Kneel behind the child's head. Open the airway and place the mask, broad end towards you, over the child's mouth and nose. Deliver breaths through the mouthpiece.

WHEN THE AMBULANCE ARRIVES

The ambulance service may initially send a sole responder in a fast response vehicle or a community first responder ahead of the ambulance. If an AED is not already attached to the child the ambulance personnel will do that. They will also use additional drugs and equipment to provide advanced care (p.59).

If you are asked to help you should listen carefully and follow the instructions given (p.23).

The ambulance personnel will make a decision whether to transfer the child to hospital immediately or to continue treatment at the scene. Any decision to stop resuscitation can only be made by a healthcare professional.

UNRESPONSIVE INFANT UNDER ONE YEAR

The following pages describe techniques that may be used for the resuscitation of an unresponsive infant under one year. For a child over the age of one year, use the child resuscitation procedure (pp.74–81).

Treat the infant from the same side for all the stages of resuscitation: opening the airway, checking breathing and giving rescue breaths and chest compressions (cardiopulmonary resuscitation, or CPR). Work through all of the steps in rapid succession. Your first priority is to check that the airway is open and clear. If the infant is not breathing, commence CPR (pp.84–85). If they are breathing normally, check for conditions affecting circulation and hold them in the recovery position (opposite). Call 999/112 for emergency help immediately if an infant with a known heart condition is unresponsive.

HOW TO CHECK THE RESPONSE

Gently tap or flick the sole of the infant's foot and call their name to see if they respond. Never shake an infant.

IF THERE IS A RESPONSE

1 **Use the primary survey** (pp.46–47) to identify the most serious injury and treat conditions in order of priority.

2 **Summon help if needed** – take the infant with you to make the call. Monitor and record vital signs (pp.54–55) until help arrives.

IF THERE IS NO RESPONSE

Shout for help, then lay the infant on their back on a firm surface and open the airway. Go to *How to open the airway* (below).

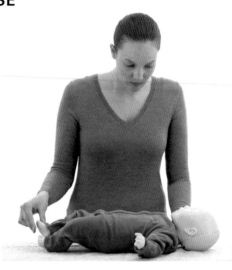

HOW TO OPEN THE AIRWAY

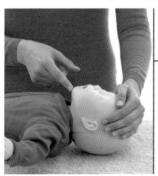

1 **Place one hand** on the infant's forehead and very gently tilt the head back.

2 **Place one fingertip** of your other hand on the point of the infant's chin. Gently lift the point of the chin. Do not push on the soft tissues under the chin since this may block the airway.

3 **Now check to see** if the infant is breathing. Go to *How to check breathing* (opposite).

HOW TO CHECK BREATHING

Keep the airway open and look, listen and feel for normal breathing – look for chest movement, listen for sounds of breathing and feel for breaths on your cheek. Do this for no more than 10 seconds.

IF THE INFANT IS BREATHING

1 **Use the primary survey** (pp.46–47) to identify the most serious injury and treat conditions in order of priority.

2 **Hold the infant** in the recovery position. Monitor and record vital signs (pp.54–55) regularly until help arrives.
Go to *How to hold an infant in the recovery position* (below).

IF THE INFANT IS NOT BREATHING

1 **Ask a helper to** call 999/112 for emergency help. If you are on your own, perform CPR for one minute before making the call yourself. Use your mobile set to speaker phone to make the call or take the infant with you to the telephone if necessary.

2 **Begin CPR** with FIVE initial rescue breaths. Go to *How to give CPR* (pp.84–85).

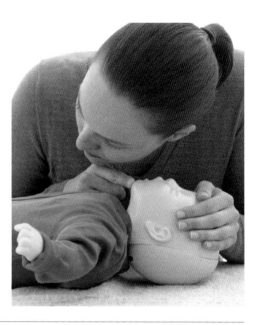

HOW TO HOLD AN INFANT IN THE RECOVERY POSITION

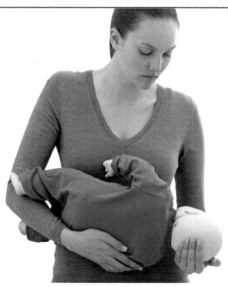

1 **Cradle the infant in your arms** with their head tilted downwards. This position prevents them from choking on their tongue or inhaling vomit.

2 **Monitor and record** the infant's vital signs (pp.54–55) until help arrives.

continued ››

« UNRESPONSIVE INFANT UNDER ONE YEAR

HOW TO GIVE CPR

WHAT TO DO

1 **Place the infant on their back** on a firm surface, at about waist height in front of you, or on the floor. Make sure that the airway is still open by keeping one hand on the infant's forehead and a fingertip of the other hand under the tip of the chin.

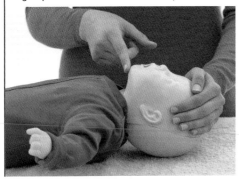

3 **Take a breath.** Place your lips around the infant's mouth and nose to form an airtight seal. If this is not possible, close the infant's mouth and make a seal around the nose only. Blow gently and steadily into the infant's nose for one second; the chest should rise.

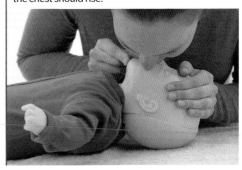

2 **Pick out any visible obstructions** from mouth and nose. Do not sweep the mouth with your finger feeling for obstructions.

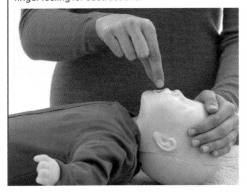

4 **Maintaining head tilt and chin lift,** take your mouth off the infant's mouth and see if their chest falls. If the chest rises visibly as you blow and falls fully when you lift your mouth, you have given a rescue breath. Each complete rescue breath should take one second. Give FIVE rescue breaths.

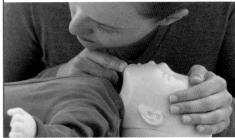

CAUTION

If you cannot achieve rescue breaths:

- Re-check the head tilt and chin lift.
- Re-check the infant's mouth and nose and remove obvious obstructions. Do not do a finger sweep.
- Check that you have a firm seal around the mouth and nose.

- Make no more than FIVE attempts to achieve rescue breaths, before commencing chest compressions.

If the infant vomits during CPR, roll them away from you onto their side to allow the vomit to drain. Resume CPR as soon as possible.

5 Place two fingertips of your lower hand on the centre of the infant's chest. Press down vertically on the infant's breastbone and depress the chest by at least one-third of its depth. Release the pressure without removing your fingers from the breastbone. Allow the chest to come back up fully (recoil) before giving the next compression. The time taken for compression and release should be about the same. Repeat to give 30 compressions at a rate of 100–120 times per minute.

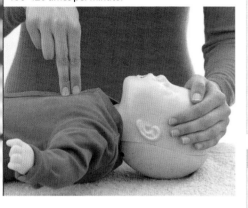

6 Return to the infant's head, open the airway and give TWO further rescue breaths.

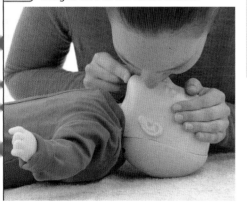

7 If you are on your own, alternate 30 chest compressions with TWO rescue breaths (30:2) for one minute then stop to call 999 / 112 for emergency help. Continue CPR until: emergency help arrives and takes over; the infant shows signs of becoming responsive – such as coughing, opening their eyes, crying or moving – and starts to breathe normally; or you become too exhausted to continue.

HAND POSITION

Place your fingers on the breastbone as indicated here. Make sure that you do not apply pressure over the ribs, the lower tip of the infant's breastbone or the upper abdomen.

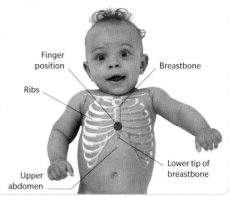

Finger position
Breastbone
Ribs
Lower tip of breastbone
Upper abdomen

CHEST-COMPRESSION-ONLY CPR

While it is better to give a combination of rescue breaths and chest compressions, if you have not had formal training in CPR, you are unwilling or unable to give rescue breaths, or guidelines advise against giving rescue breaths, you can give chest compressions only. The emergency services will give instructions for chest-compression-only CPR. Put your mobile device on speaker phone so you can deliver first aid and talk to the ambulance call handler.

CAUTION

- With more than one rescuer, change every 1–2 minutes with minimal interruption to compressions.

HOW TO USE AN AED

When the heart stops, a cardiac arrest has occurred. The most common cause is an abnormal rhythm of the heart, known as ventricular fibrillation. This abnormal rhythm can occur when the heart muscle is damaged as a result of a heart attack or when insufficient oxygen reaches the heart. A machine called an AED (automated external defibrillator) can be used on adults and children over the age of one year to correct the heart rhythm by giving an electric shock. AEDs can be used safely and effectively without prior training. They are available in many public places, including shopping centres, railway stations and airports – the logo opposite will be visible on the outside of the case. The machine analyses the casualty's heart rhythm and visual prompts or voice prompts describe the action to take at each stage. In most situations when an AED is called for, you will have already started CPR. When the AED is brought, continue with CPR while the pads are being attached to the casualty.

WHAT TO DO

1 **Switch on the AED** and take the pads out of the sealed pack. Remove or cut through clothing and wipe away sweat from the chest if necessary.

2 **Attach the pads to the casualty's chest** in the positions indicated. Remove the backing paper or film from the first pad and place it on the casualty's upper right side, just below the collarbone.

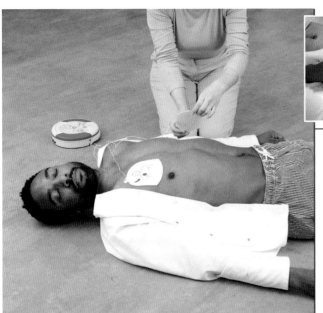

3 **Place the second pad** on the left side of the casualty's chest, just below their armpit (inset above). Follow the manufacturer's instructions on the pad for the exact position and alignment.

4 **The AED will start analysing** the heart rhythm. Ensure that no-one is touching the casualty. Follow the voice and/or visual prompts given by the machine (opposite).

SEQUENCE OF AED INSTRUCTIONS

The AED will start to give you a series of visual and verbal prompts as soon as it is switched on. There are several different AED models available, each of which has different voice prompts.

Do not stop chest compressions while the pads are being applied. You should follow the prompts given by the machine that you have until advanced care arrives.

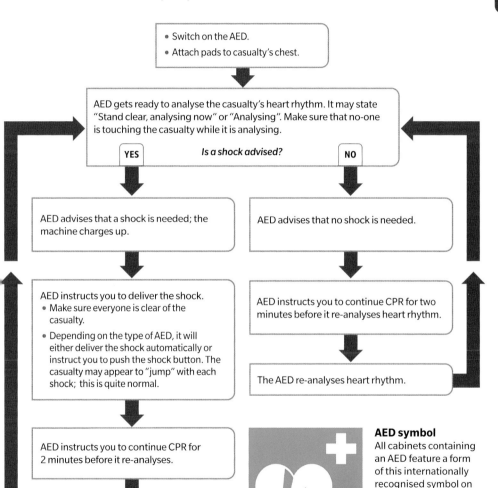

- Switch on the AED.
- Attach pads to casualty's chest.

AED gets ready to analyse the casualty's heart rhythm. It may state "Stand clear, analysing now" or "Analysing". Make sure that no-one is touching the casualty while it is analysing.

YES — *Is a shock advised?* — **NO**

AED advises that a shock is needed; the machine charges up.

AED advises that no shock is needed.

AED instructs you to deliver the shock.
- Make sure everyone is clear of the casualty.
- Depending on the type of AED, it will either deliver the shock automatically or instruct you to push the shock button. The casualty may appear to "jump" with each shock; this is quite normal.

AED instructs you to continue CPR for two minutes before it re-analyses heart rhythm.

The AED re-analyses heart rhythm.

AED instructs you to continue CPR for 2 minutes before it re-analyses.

The AED re-analyses heart rhythm.
- If the casualty shows signs of becoming responsive – such as coughing, opening their eyes, speaking or moving purposefully – and starts to breathe normally, leave them in position and do not remove the AED pads. Monitor the casualty and await the arrival of the emergency services.

AED symbol
All cabinets containing an AED feature a form of this internationally recognised symbol on the front. The standard one is green, as here, but some organisations use other colours.

HOW TO USE AN AED

CONSIDERATIONS WHEN USING AN AED

CAUTION

• Never use an AED on an infant under one year.

The use of an AED is occasionally complicated by underlying medical conditions, external factors, clothing or the cause of the cardiac arrest. Safety of all concerned should always be your first consideration.

CLOTHING AND JEWELLERY
Any clothing or jewellery that could interfere with pads should be removed or cut away where possible. Normal amounts of chest hair are not a problem, but if hair prevents good contact between the skin and the pads, it should be shaved off. Ensure any metal is removed from the area where the pads will be attached. Remove clothing containing metal, such as an underwired bra.

EXTERNAL FACTORS
Water or excessive sweat on the chest can reduce the effectiveness of the shock so the chest should be dry. If a casualty is rescued from water (pp.36–37), dry the chest before applying the AED pads.

If the casualty is unresponsive following an electric shock, start CPR immediately the contact with electricity is broken. The electric current may cause muscle paralysis, which can make rescue breaths and chest compressions more difficult to perform; however, it will not affect the use of the AED.

MEDICAL CONDITIONS
Some casualties with heart conditions have a pacemaker or an implantable cardioverter defibrillator (ICD). This should not stop you using an AED. However, if you can see or feel a device under the chest skin, do not place the pad directly over it. If a casualty has a patch such as a glyceryl trinitrate (GTN) patch on the chest, remove it before you apply the AED.

PREGNANT CASUALTIES
There are no contra-indications to using an AED during pregnancy; however, the increased breast size may present some problems. Therefore, to place the AED pads correctly, you may need to move one or both breasts. This must be carried out with respect and dignity.

POSITIONING AED PADS ON CHILDREN

Standard adult AEDs can be used on children over the age of eight years. For children between the ages of one and eight, use a paediatric AED or a standard machine and paediatric pads. If neither is available, then a standard AED and pads can be used.

CAUTION
- Never use an AED on an infant under one year.

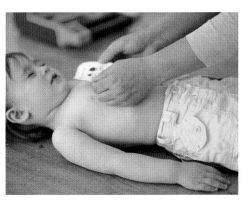

Positioning paediatric AED pads
Place one pad in the centre of the child's back. Then position the second pad over the centre of the child's chest. Make sure both pads are vertical. Connect the pads to the AED and proceed as described on p.87.

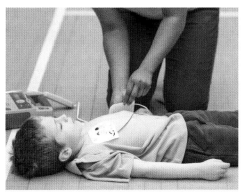

Using AED pads on a larger child
Place the pads on the child's chest as for an adult – one on the child's upper right side, just below their collarbone, and the second pad on the child's left side, just below the armpit. Follow the manufacturer's instructions on the pad for the exact position and alignment.

HANDING OVER TO THE EMERGENCY SERVICES

When the emergency services arrive continue to resuscitate the casualty until they take over from you. They need to know:

- **Casualty's present status;** for example, unresponsive and not breathing.
- **Number of shocks you have delivered.**
- **When the casualty collapsed** and the length of time they have been unresponsive.
- **Any relevant history known.**

If the casualty recovers at any point, leave the AED pads attached to their chest. Ensure that any used materials from the AED cabinet are disposed of as clinical waste (p.242). Inform the relevant person what has been taken out of the cabinet as it will need to be replaced.

05 RESPIRATORY PROBLEMS

Oxygen is essential to life. Every time we breathe in, air containing oxygen enters the lungs. This oxygen is then transferred to the blood, to be transported around the body. Breathing and the exchange of oxygen and carbon dioxide (a waste product from body tissues) are described as respiration. The structures within the body that enable us to breathe – the air passages and the lungs – together make up the respiratory system, and work with the heart and circulatory system.

Respiration can be compromised in several different ways. The air passages may be blocked causing choking or suffocation, the exchange of oxygen and carbon dioxide in the lungs may be affected by the inhalation of smoke or fumes, lung function may be impaired by chest injury, or the breathing mechanism may be affected by conditions such as asthma. Anxiety can also cause breathing difficulties. Problems with respiration can be life threatening and need urgent first aid and hospital treatment.

AIMS AND OBJECTIVES

- To assess the casualty's condition
- To identify and remove the cause of the problem and provide fresh air
- To comfort and reassure the casualty
- To maintain an open airway, check breathing and be prepared to resuscitate if necessary
- To obtain medical help if necessary. Call 999 / 112 for emergency help if you suspect a serious illness or injury

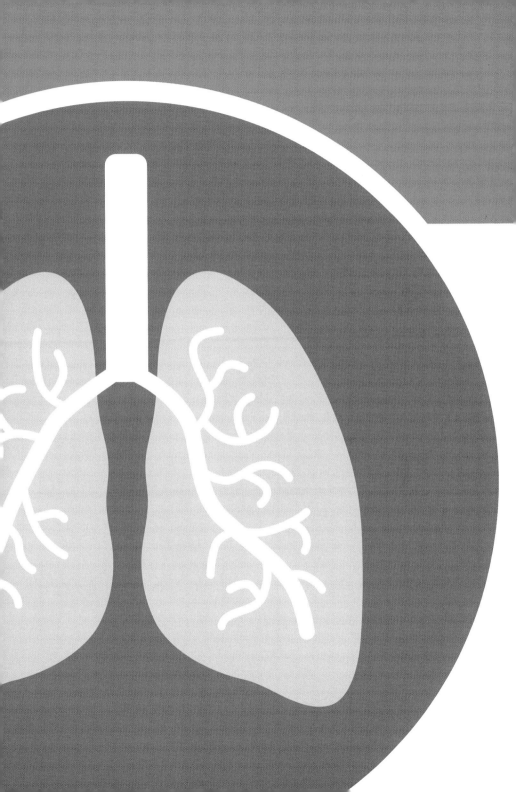

THE RESPIRATORY SYSTEM

This system comprises the mouth, nose, windpipe (trachea), lungs and pulmonary blood vessels (the blood vessels of the lungs). The process of breathing and the exchange of gases (oxygen and carbon dioxide) both in the lungs and in cells throughout the body is known as respiration.

We breathe in air containing oxygen to take oxygen into the lungs; we breathe out to expel the waste gas, carbon dioxide, a by-product of respiration. When we breathe, air is drawn through the nose and mouth into the airway and the lungs. In the lungs, oxygen is passed from air sacs (alveoli) into the pulmonary capillaries. At the same time, carbon dioxide is released from the capillaries into the alveoli. This carbon dioxide is then expelled as we breathe out. On average a man's lungs can hold approximately 6 litres (10 pints) of air and a woman's can hold about 4 litres (7 pints) of air.

Structure of the respiratory system

The lungs form the central part of the respiratory system. Together with the circulatory system, they perform the vital function of gas exchange in order to distribute oxygen around the body and remove carbon dioxide.

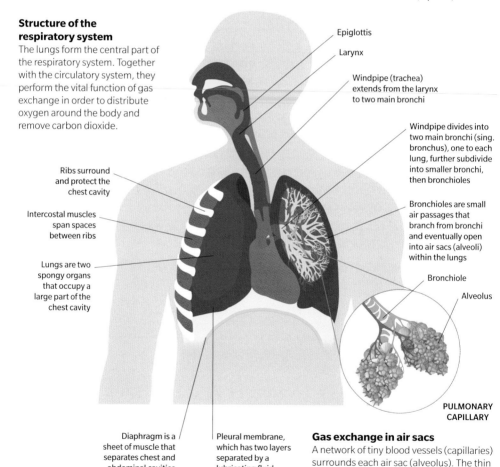

Epiglottis

Larynx

Windpipe (trachea) extends from the larynx to two main bronchi

Windpipe divides into two main bronchi (sing. bronchus), one to each lung, further subdivide into smaller bronchi, then bronchioles

Ribs surround and protect the chest cavity

Intercostal muscles span spaces between ribs

Bronchioles are small air passages that branch from bronchi and eventually open into air sacs (alveoli) within the lungs

Lungs are two spongy organs that occupy a large part of the chest cavity

Bronchiole

Alveolus

PULMONARY CAPILLARY

Diaphragm is a sheet of muscle that separates chest and abdominal cavities

Pleural membrane, which has two layers separated by a lubricating fluid, surrounds and protects each of the lungs

Gas exchange in air sacs

A network of tiny blood vessels (capillaries) surrounds each air sac (alveolus). The thin walls of both structures allow oxygen to diffuse into the blood and carbon dioxide to leave it.

HOW BREATHING WORKS

The breathing process consists of the actions of breathing in (inspiration) and breathing out (expiration), followed by a pause. Pressure differences between the lungs and the air outside the body determine whether air is drawn in or expelled. When the air pressure in the lungs is lower than outside, air is drawn in; when pressure is higher, air is expelled. The pressure within the lungs is altered by the movements of the two main sets of muscles involved in breathing: the intercostal muscles and the diaphragm.

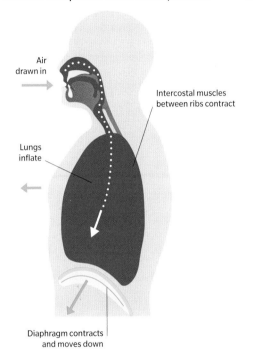

Air drawn in

Intercostal muscles between ribs contract

Lungs inflate

Diaphragm contracts and moves down

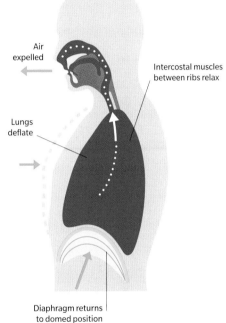

Air expelled

Intercostal muscles between ribs relax

Lungs deflate

Diaphragm returns to domed position

Breathing in
The intercostal muscles (the muscles between the ribs) and the diaphragm contract, causing the ribs to move up and out, the chest cavity to expand, and the lungs to expand to fill the space. As a result, the pressure inside the lungs is reduced, and air is drawn into the lungs.

Breathing out
The intercostal muscles relax, and the ribcage returns to its resting position, while the diaphragm relaxes and resumes its domed shape. As a result, the chest cavity becomes smaller, and pressure inside the lungs increases. Air flows out of the lungs to be exhaled.

HOW BREATHING IS CONTROLLED

Breathing is regulated by a group of nerve cells in the brain called the respiratory centre. This centre responds to changes in the level of carbon dioxide in the blood. When the carbon dioxide level in the body rises, the respiratory centre reacts by stimulating the intercostal muscles and the diaphragm to contract, and a breath occurs. Our breathing rate can be altered consciously under normal conditions or in response to abnormal levels of carbon dioxide, low levels of oxygen, or with stress, exercise, injury or illness.

HYPOXIA

RECOGNITION

In moderate and severe hypoxia, there will be:

- Rapid breathing
- Breathing that is distressed or gasping
- Difficulty speaking
- Grey-blue skin (cyanosis). At first, this is more obvious in the extremities, such as lips, nailbeds and earlobes, but as the hypoxia worsens cyanosis affects the rest of the body
- Anxiety
- Restlessness
- Headache
- Nausea and possibly vomiting
- Cessation of breathing if the hypoxia is not quickly reversed

This condition arises when there is insufficient oxygen in the body tissues. There are a number of causes of hypoxia, ranging from suffocation, choking or poisoning to impaired lung or brain function. The condition is accompanied by a variety of symptoms, depending on the degree of hypoxia. If not treated quickly, hypoxia is potentially fatal because a sufficient level of oxygen is vital for the normal function of all the body organs and tissues, especially the brain.

In a healthy person, the amount of oxygen in the air is more than adequate for the body tissues to function normally. However, in an injured or ill person, a reduction in oxygen reaching the tissues results in deterioration of body function.

Mild hypoxia reduces a casualty's ability to think clearly, but the body normally responds to this by increasing the rate and depth of breathing (p.93). However, if the oxygen supply to the brain cells is cut off for as little as 3–4 minutes, the brain cells will begin to die. All the conditions covered in this chapter can result in hypoxia.

YOUR AIMS

- To identify the cause, restore normal breathing and arrange removal to hospital if needed

INJURIES OR CONDITIONS CAUSING LOW BLOOD OXYGEN (HYPOXIA)

INJURY OR CONDITION	CAUSES
Insufficient oxygen in inspired air	● Suffocation by smoke or gas ● Changes in atmospheric pressure, for example, at high altitude or in a depressurised aircraft
Airway obstruction	● Blocking or swelling of the airway ● Hanging or strangulation ● Something covering the mouth or nose ● Asthma ● Choking ● Anaphylaxis
Conditions affecting the chest wall	● Crushing, for example, by a fall of earth or sand or pressure from a crowd ● Chest wall injury with multiple rib fractures or constricting burns
Impaired lung function	● Lung injury ● Collapsed lung ● Lung infections, such as pneumonia
Damage to the brain or nerves that control respiration	● A head injury or stroke that damages the breathing centre in the brain ● Some forms of poisioning ● Paralysis of nerves controlling the muscles of breathing, as in spinal cord injury
Impaired oxygen uptake by the tissues	● Carbon monoxide or cyanide poisioning ● Shock

SEE ALSO Anaphylactic shock **p.227** | Asthma **p.104** | Burns to the airway **p.179** | Croup **p.105** | Drowning **p.102** | Hanging and strangulation **p.99** | Inhalation of fumes **pp.100–101** | Penetrating chest wound **pp.106–107** | Stroke **pp.214–2**

AIRWAY OBSTRUCTION

The airway may be obstructed externally or internally, for example, by an object that is stuck at the back of the throat (pp.96–98). The main causes of obstruction are:

- **Inhalation** of an object, such as food.
- **Blockage** by the tongue, blood or vomit while a casualty is unresponsive (p.61).
- **Internal swelling** of the throat occurring with burns, scalds, stings or anaphylaxis.
- **Injuries** to the face or jaw.
- **An asthma attack** in which the small airways in the lungs constrict (p.104).
- **External pressure** on the neck, as in hanging or strangulation.
- **Foods** such as peanuts, which can swell up when in contact with body fluids, and grapes can pose a particular danger in young children because they can completely block the airway.

Airway obstruction requires prompt action; be prepared to give chest compressions and rescue breaths if the casualty stops breathing (The unresponsive casualty, pp.56–89).

The information on this page is appropriate for all causes of airway obstruction, but if you need detailed instructions for specific situations, refer to the relevant pages given below.

CAUTION

- If the casualty is unresponsive, open the airway and check breathing (The unresponsive casualty, pp.56–89).

RECOGNITION

- Features of hypoxia (opposite) – grey-blue tinge to the lips, earlobes and nailbeds (cyanosis)
- Difficulty speaking and breathing
- Noisy breathing
- Red, puffy face
- Signs of distress – casualty may point to the throat or grasp neck
- Flaring of the nostrils
- A persistent cough

YOUR AIMS

- To remove the obstruction
- To restore normal breathing
- To arrange removal to hospital

WHAT TO DO

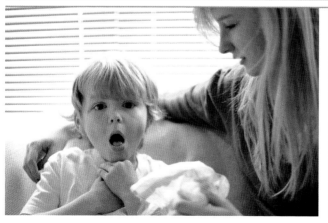

1 **Remove the obstruction** if it is external or visible in the mouth.

2 **If the casualty is responsive** and breathing normally, reassure them, but keep them under observation.

3 **Even if the casualty appears** to have made a complete recovery, call 999/112 for emergency help. Monitor and record the casualty's vital signs (pp.54–55) until help arrives.

SEE ALSO Asthma **p.104** | Burns to the airway **p.179** | Choking adult **p.96** | Choking child **p.97**
Choking infant **p.98** | Drowning **p.102** | Hanging and strangulation **p.99** | Inhalation of fumes **pp.100–101**

CHOKING ADULT

A foreign object that is stuck in the throat may block it and cause muscular spasm. If blockage of the airway is mild, the casualty should be able to clear it; if it is severe, they will be unable to speak, cough or breathe, and will eventually become unresponsive. If they are unresponsive the throat muscles may relax and the airway may open enough to do rescue breathing. Be prepared to begin rescue breaths and chest compressions.

RECOGNITION

Ask the casualty: "Are you choking?"

Mild obstruction:

- Casualty able to speak, cough and breathe

Severe obstruction:

- Casualty unable to speak, cough or breathe, and eventually becomes unresponsive

YOUR AIMS

- To remove the obstruction
- To arrange urgent removal to hospital if necessary

WHAT TO DO

1 **If a casualty is breathing,** encourage them to keep coughing. Remove any obvious obstruction from the mouth.

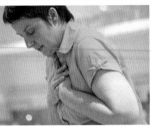

2 **If the casualty cannot speak** or stops coughing or breathing, carry out back blows. Support the upper body with one hand, and help them to lean well forward. Give up to five sharp blows between their shoulder blades with the heel of your hand. Stop if the obstruction clears. Check the mouth.

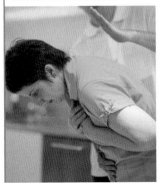

3 **If back blows fail** to clear the obstruction, try abdominal thrusts. Stand behind the casualty and put both arms around the upper part of their abdomen. Make sure that they are still bending well forwards. Clench your fist and place it between the navel and the bottom of the breastbone. Grasp your fist firmly with your other hand. Pull sharply inwards and upwards up to five times.

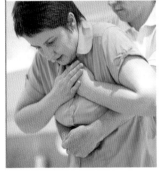

4 **Check the casualty's mouth.** If the obstruction has not cleared, **call 999/112 for** emergency help.

5 Repeat steps 2 and 3 – rechecking the mouth after each step – until help arrives or the casualty becomes unresponsive (see CAUTION, above, left).

CHOKING CHILD ONE YEAR AND OVER

Young children especially are prone to choking. A child may choke on food, or may put small objects into their mouth and cause a blockage of the airway.

If a child is choking, you need to act quickly. If they become unresponsive, the throat muscles may relax and the airway may open enough to do rescue breathing. Be prepared to begin rescue breaths and chest compressions.

WHAT TO DO

1 **If the child is breathing,** encourage them to cough; this may clear the obstruction. Remove any obvious obstruction from their mouth.

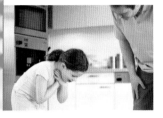

2 **If the child cannot speak,** or stops coughing or breathing, carry out back blows. Bend them well forward and give up to five blows between their shoulder blades using the heel of your hand. Check the mouth, but do not sweep the mouth with your finger.

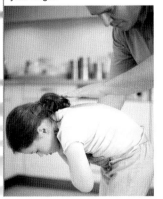

3 **If the back blows fail,** try abdominal thrusts. Put your arms around the child's upper abdomen. Make sure that they are bending well forward. Place your fist between the navel and the bottom of the breastbone, and grasp it with your other hand. Pull sharply inwards and upwards up to five times. Stop if the obstruction clears.

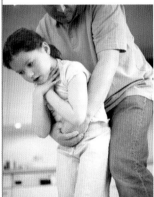

4 **Check the mouth.** If the obstruction has not cleared, call 999 / 112 for emergency help.

5 **Repeat steps 2 and 3 –** rechecking the mouth after each step – until help arrives or the child becomes unresponsive (see CAUTION, above, right).

RECOGNITION

Ask the child: "Are you choking?"

Mild obstruction:

- Child able to speak, cough and breathe

Severe obstruction:

- Child unable to speak, cough or breathe, and eventually becomes unresponsive

YOUR AIMS

- To remove the obstruction
- To arrange urgent removal to hospital if necessary

SEE ALSO Unresponsive child **pp.74–81**

CHOKING INFANT UNDER ONE YEAR

An infant is more likely to choke on food or small objects than an adult. The infant will rapidly become distressed, and you need to act quickly to clear any obstruction. If the infant becomes unresponsive, the throat muscles may relax and the airway may open enough to do rescue breathing. Be prepared to begin rescue breaths and chest compressions.

RECOGNITION

Mild obstruction:

- Infant able to cough, but has difficulty crying or making any other noise

Severe obstruction:

- Unable to make any noise or breathe, and eventually becomes unresponsive

YOUR AIMS

- To remove the obstruction
- To arrange urgent removal to hospital if necessary

WHAT TO DO

1 **If the infant is unable to cry,** cough or breathe, lay them face down along your forearm and thigh and support the head. Give up to five back blows between the shoulder blades, with the heel of your hand.

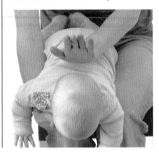

2 **Turn the infant over** so that they are face up along your other leg and check the mouth. Remove any obvious obstructions with your fingertips. Do not sweep the mouth with your finger as this may push the object further down the throat.

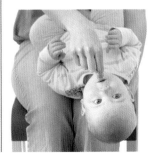

3 **If back blows fail** to clear the obstruction, try chest thrusts. These are similar to chest compressions, but sharper in nature and delivered at a slower rate. Lay the infant face up on your leg, with your arm along the infant's back and support their head with your hand. Place two fingers of your other hand on the lower part of the breastbone one finger's breadth below the infant's nipple line and push downwards. Give up to five chest thrusts.

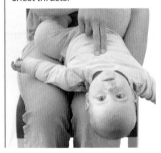

4 **Check the mouth.** If the obstruction still has not cleared, **call 999/112 for emergency help;** take the infant with you if necessary.

5 **Repeat steps 1 to 3 –** rechecking the mouth after each step – until help arrives or the infant becomes unresponsive (see CAUTION, above left).

HANGING AND STRANGULATION

If pressure is exerted on the outside of the neck, the airway is squeezed and the flow of air to the lungs is cut off. The main causes of such pressure are:

- **Hanging** – suspension of the body by a noose around the neck.
- **Strangulation** – constriction or squeezing around the neck or throat.

Sometimes, hanging or strangulation may occur accidentally – for example, by ties or clothing becoming caught in machinery. Hanging may cause a broken neck; for this reason, a casualty in this situation must be handled extremely carefully.

WHAT TO DO

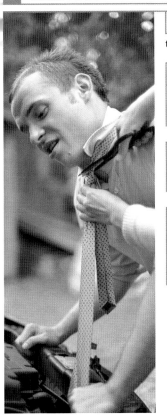

1 **Quickly remove** any constriction from around the casualty's neck.

2 **If the casualty is hanging,** support the body while you relieve the constriction. Be aware that the body will be very heavy if they are unresponsive.

3 **If the casualty is responsive,** help them to lie down while supporting their head and neck.

4 **Call 999/112 for emergency help,** even if they appear to recover fully. Monitor and record the casualty's vital signs (pp.54–55) until help arrives.

RECOGNITION

- A constricting article around the neck
- Marks around the casualty's neck
- Rapid, difficult breathing; impaired consciousness; grey-blue skin (cyanosis)
- Congestion of the face, with prominent veins and, possibly, tiny red spots on the face or on the whites of the eyes

YOUR AIMS

- To restore adequate breathing
- To arrange urgent removal to hospital

INHALATION OF FUMES

The inhalation of smoke, gases (such as carbon monoxide) or toxic vapours can be lethal. A casualty who has inhaled fumes is likely to have low levels of oxygen in their body tissues (Hypoxia, p.94) and therefore needs urgent medical attention.

Do not attempt to rescue a casualty if it is likely to put your own life at risk. Fumes that have built up in a confined space will quickly overcome anyone who is not wearing protective equipment, whether it is you or the casualty.

SMOKE INHALATION

Any person who has been enclosed in a confined space during a fire should be assumed to have inhaled smoke. Smoke from burning plastics, foam padding and synthetic wall coverings is likely to contain poisonous fumes. Casualties who have suffered from fume inhalation should also be examined for other injuries that could result from the fire, such as external burns, or burns to the airway.

INHALATION OF CARBON MONOXIDE

Carbon monoxide is a poisonous gas, but it is hard to detect as it has no taste or smell. The gas acts directly on red blood cells, preventing them from carrying oxygen to the body tissues. If carbon monoxide is inhaled in large quantities – for example, from smoke or vehicle exhaust fumes in a confined space – it can very quickly prove fatal. However, lengthy exposure to even a small amount of carbon monoxide – for example, due to a leakage of fumes from a defective heater or flue – may also prove fatal.

EFFECTS OF FUME INHALATION

FUMES	POSSIBLE SOURCE	EFFECTS
Carbon monoxide	● Exhaust fumes of motor vehicles ● Smoke from most fires ● Back-draughts from blocked chimney flues ● Emissions from defective gas or paraffin heaters, wood burners and pellet (biomass) stoves and poorly maintained boilers ● Disposable or portable barbeques used in a confined space	Prolonged exposure to low levels: ● Headache ● Confusion ● Aggression ● Nausea and vomiting ● Diarrhoea Brief exposure to high levels: ● Grey-blue skin coloration ● Rapid, difficult breathing ● Impaired level of response, leading to unresponsiveness
Smoke	● Fires: smoke is a bigger killer than fire itself. Smoke is low in oxygen (which is used up by the burning of the fire) and may contain toxic fumes from burning materials	● Rapid, noisy and difficult breathing ● Coughing and wheezing ● Burning in the nose or mouth ● Soot around the mouth and nose ● Singeing of nasal hairs and/or eyebrows ● Unresponsiveness
Carbon dioxide	● Tends to accumulate and become dangerously concentrated in deep enclosed spaces, such as coal pits, wells and underground tanks	● Breathlessnes ● Headache ● Confusion ● Unresponsiveness
Solvents and fuels	● Glues ● Cleaning fluids ● Lighter fuels ● Camping gas and propane-fuelled stoves (Solvent abusers may use a plastic bag to concentrate the vapour, especially with glues)	● Headache and vomiting ● Impaired level of response ● Airway obstruction from using a plastic bag or from choking on vomit may result in death ● Solvent abuse is a potential cause of cardiac arrest

WHAT TO DO

1 Call 999/112 for emergency help. Tell the call handler that you suspect fume inhalation.

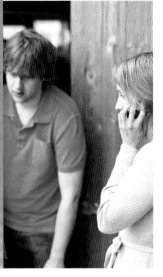

3 Support the casualty and encourage them to breathe normally. If the casualty's clothing is still burning, try to extinguish the flames (p.33). Treat any obvious burns (pp.176–179) or other injuries.

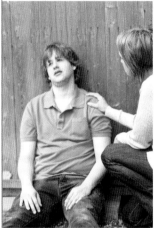

CAUTION

- If the casualty is in a garage filled with vehicle exhaust fumes, open the doors wide and let the gas escape before you enter.
- If the casualty is found unresponsive, open the airway and check breathing (The unresponsive casualty, pp.56–89).

YOUR AIMS

- To restore adequate breathing
- To call 999/112 for emergency help and obtain urgent medical attention

2 If it is necessary to escape from the source of the fumes, help the casualty away from the fumes into fresh air. Do not enter the fume-filled area yourself.

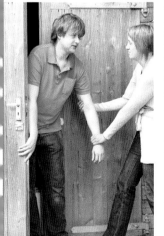

4 Stay with the casualty until emergency services arrive. Monitor and record the casualty's vital signs (pp.54–55) until help arrives.

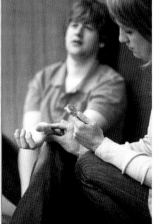

DROWNING

Drowning causes breathing impairment as a result of submersion or immersion in a liquid. Drowning begins when a casualty is unable to breathe because the nose, mouth and air passages are submerged below the surface of a liquid. Any incident involving immersion when there is no problem with breathing is not defined as drowning but as a rescue (p.36).

A casualty rescued from a drowning incident must be assessed using the primary survey (pp.46–47) to establish whether or not CPR is required. If the casualty is unresponsive and not breathing, give five initial rescue breaths before you start chest compressions, then continue with CPR at a rate of 30 chest compressions to two rescue breaths. Always call 999/112 for the emergency services.

YOUR AIMS

- To restore breathing
- To arrange urgent removal to hospital

WHAT TO DO

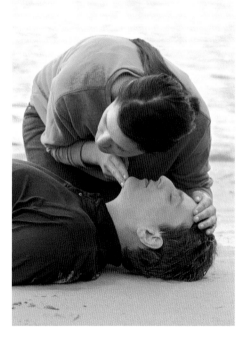

1 When the casualty is rescued from liquid (p.37), start the primary survey. Check the level of response, open the airway and check breathing.

2 If the casualty is unresponsive and not breathing normally, shout for help and call 999/112 for emergency help or ask someone to make the call and request an AED.

3 Check that the airway is open and give FIVE initial rescue breaths. Follow this with 30 chest compressions, then TWO rescue breaths. Continue CPR at a rate of 30:2 until help arrives; the casualty shows signs of becoming responsive – is coughing, opening their eyes, speaking, or moving purposefully – and starts breathing normally; or you are too exhausted to continue.

4 If an AED is available attach it while continuing CPR (pp.86–89).

5 If the casualty starts to breathe normally, treat for hypothermia (pp.188–189) – cover them with warm clothes and blankets. If possible replace wet clothes with dry ones. Monitor and record their vital signs (pp.54–55) until help arrives.

HYPERVENTILATION

This is commonly a manifestation of acute anxiety and may accompany a panic attack. It may occur in individuals who have recently experienced an emotional upset or those with a history of panic attacks.

The unnaturally fast or deep breathing of hyperventilation causes an increased loss of carbon dioxide from the blood, which leads to chemical changes within the blood. These changes result in symptoms such as dizziness and trembling, as well as tingling in the hands. As breathing returns to normal, these symptoms will gradually subside.

WHAT TO DO

1 When speaking to the casualty be kind and reassuring. If possible, lead the casualty away to a quiet place where they may be able to regain control of their breathing more easily. If this is not possible, ask any bystanders to leave.

RECOGNITION

- Unnaturally fast or deep breathing
- Fast pulse rate
- Apprehension

There may also be:

- Dizziness or faintness
- Trembling, sweating and dry mouth, or marked tingling in the hands
- Tingling and cramps in the hands and feet and around the mouth

YOUR AIMS

- To remove the casualty from the cause of distress
- To reassure the casualty and calm them down

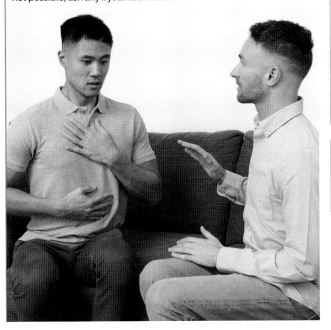

2 Encourage the casualty to seek medical advice on preventing and controlling panic attacks in the future.

SEE ALSO Mental health crisis **p.224** | **103**

ASTHMA

CAUTION

- If this is a first attack and/or the casualty has no medication call 999/112 for emergency help immediately.
- If the casualty becomes unresponsive, open the airway and check breathing (The unresponsive casualty pp.56–89).

RECOGNITION

- Difficulty breathing
- Wheezing
- Difficulty speaking, leading to short sentences and whispering
- Coughing
- Distress and anxiety
- Features of hypoxia (p.94), such as a grey-blue tinge to the lips, earlobes and nailbeds (cyanosis)
- Exhaustion in a severe attack. If the attack worsens the casualty may stop breathing and become unresponsive

YOUR AIMS

- To ease breathing
- To obtain medical help if necessary

In an asthma attack, the muscles of the air passages in the lungs go into spasm. As a result, the airways become narrowed, which makes breathing difficult.

Sometimes, there is a recognised trigger for an attack, such as an allergy, a cold, a particular drug or cigarette smoke. At other times, there is no obvious trigger. Many sufferers have attacks that come on suddenly.

People with asthma usually deal with their own attacks by using a "reliever" inhaler at the first sign of an attack. Most reliever inhalers have blue caps. Preventer inhalers have brown or white caps. They are used to help prevent attacks and should not be used during an asthma attack.

WHAT TO DO

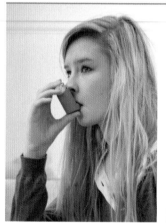

1 Keep calm and reassure the casualty. Sit the casualty down in the position they find most comfortable. Get them to take their usual dose of their reliever inhaler, using a spacer if they have one. Ask them to breathe slowly and deeply.

2 A mild attack should ease within a few minutes. If it does not, the casualty may take 1–2 puffs from their inhaler every 30–60 seconds for up to 10 puffs. If they have a personal asthma plan they should follow this and seek medical advice if necessary.

3 Call 999/112 for emergency help if the attack is severe and one of the following occurs: the inhaler has no effect; the casualty is getting worse; breathlessness makes talking difficult; they are becoming exhausted.

4 Monitor and record the casualty's vital signs (pp.54–55) until help arrives. If there will be a delay of more than 15 minutes repeat step 2.

SPECIAL CASE USING A SPACER DEVICE

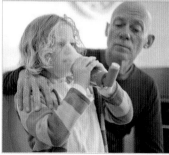

A spacer device can be fitted to an asthma inhaler to help a casualty breathe in the medication more effectively. They are especially useful when giving medication to young children.

CROUP

An attack of **breathing difficulty** in young children is known as croup. It is caused by inflammation in the windpipe and larynx. Croup can be alarming but it usually passes without lasting harm. Attacks of croup usually occur at night and can be made worse if the child is crying and distressed.

If an attack of croup persists, or is severe, and accompanied by fever, **call 999/112 for emergency help.** There is a small risk that the child is suffering from a rare, croup-like condition called epiglottitis, in which the epiglottis (p.92), a small, flap-like structure in the throat, becomes infected and swollen and may block the airway. The child then needs urgent medical attention.

CAUTION

- Do not put your fingers down the child's throat. This can cause the throat muscles to go into spasm and block the airway.

- Do not allow the child to inhale steam or take them into a steamy room – there is no medical benefit and there is a risk of scalding.

WHAT TO DO

1 Sit your child on your knee, supporting their back. Calmly reassure them. Try not to panic; this will only alarm the child, which is likely to make the attack worse.

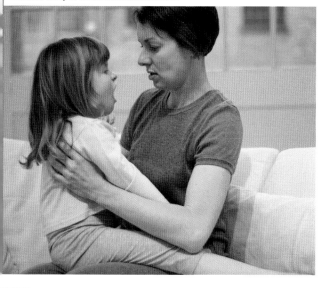

2 **Seek medical help** or, if the croup is severe, call **999/112 for emergency help.** Monitor and record the child's vital signs (pp.54–55) until help arrives.

RECOGNITION

- Distressed breathing in a young child

There may also be:
- A short, barking cough
- A rasping noise, especially on breathing in (stridor)
- Croaky voice
- Blue-grey skin (cyanosis)
- In severe cases, the child uses muscles around the nose, neck and upper arms in trying to breathe

Suspect epiglottitis if:
- A child is in respiratory distress and not improving
- The child has a high temperature

YOUR AIMS

- To comfort and support the child
- To obtain medical help if necessary

PENETRATING CHEST WOUND

RECOGNITION

- Difficult and painful breathing, possibly rapid, shallow and uneven
- Casualty feels an acute sense of alarm
- Features of hypoxia (p.94), including grey-blue skin coloration (cyanosis)

There may also be:

- Coughed-up frothy, red blood
- A crackling feeling of the skin around the wound site, caused by air collecting in the tissues
- Blood bubbling from the wound
- Sound of air being sucked into the chest as casualty breathes in
- Veins in the neck becoming prominent

The heart and lungs, and the major blood vessels around them, lie in the chest, protected by the breastbone and the 12 pairs of ribs that make up the ribcage. The ribcage extends far enough downwards to protect organs such as the liver and spleen in the upper part of the abdomen.

If a sharp object penetrates the chest wall, there may be severe damage to the organs in the chest and the upper abdomen and this will lead to shock (pp.114–115). The lungs are particularly susceptible to injury, either by being damaged themselves or from wounds that perforate the two-layered membrane (pleura) that surrounds and protects each one. Air can then enter between the membranes and exert pressure on the lung, and the lung may collapse – a condition called pneumothorax.

Pressure around the affected lung may build up to such an extent that it affects the uninjured lung. As a result, the casualty becomes increasingly breathless. This build-up of pressure may prevent the heart from refilling with blood properly, impairing the circulation and causing shock – a condition known as a tension pneumothorax.

YOUR AIMS

- To maintain breathing
- To minimise shock
- To arrange urgent removal to hospital

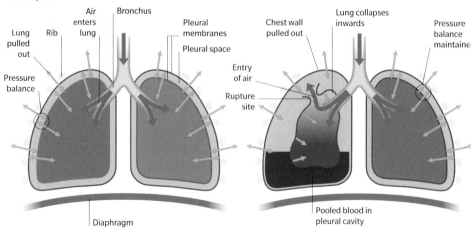

Normal breathing
The lungs inflate by being pulled out as they "suck" onto the chest wall. Pressure is maintained within the fluid-filled pleural space.

Collapsed (right) lung
Air from the right lung enters the surrounding pleural space and changes the pressure balance. The lung shrinks away from the chest wall.

WHAT TO DO

1 Help the casualty to sit down and encourage them to lean towards their injured side. Expose the wound and if it is not bleeding leave it uncovered.

2 If the wound is obviously bleeding, apply direct pressure over a sterile wound dressing or clean pad to control bleeding. The casualty may be able to do this themselves.

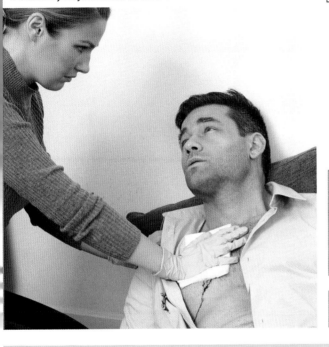

3 Call 999/112 for emergency help. While waiting for help, continue to support the casualty in the same position as long as they remain responsive. If necessary, secure the dressing with hypoallergenic tape.

4 Monitor and record the casualty's vital signs (pp.54–55) until help arrives.

SPECIAL CASE IF THE CASUALTY IS UNRESPONSIVE

If the casualty is, or becomes, unresponsive, open the airway and check breathing (The unresponsive casualty, pp.56–89). If you need to place a breathing casualty in the recovery position, roll them on to their injured side to help the healthy lung to work effectively (p.66).

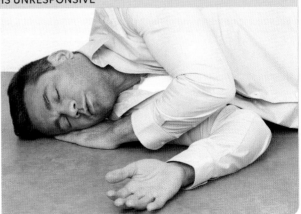

06 WOUNDS AND BLEEDING

The heart and blood vessels are collectively known as the circulatory (cardiovascular) system. This system keeps the body supplied with blood, which carries oxygen and nutrients to all body tissues. The function of the circulatory system may be disrupted by severe internal or external bleeding or fluid loss, for example from burns (pp.176–181). The techniques described in this section show how you can help to maintain an adequate blood supply to the heart and brain following injury that affects the circulatory system.

A break in the skin or the internal body surfaces is known as a wound. Wounds can be daunting, particularly if there is a lot of bleeding, but prompt action reduces the amount of blood loss and minimises shock. Treatments for all types of wound are covered in this chapter.

AIMS AND OBJECTIVES

- To assess the casualty's condition quickly and calmly
- To control blood loss by applying pressure directly over the wound
- To minimise the risk of shock
- To comfort and reassure the casualty
- To call 999 / 112 for emergency help if you suspect a serious injury or illness
- To be aware of your own needs, including the need to protect yourself against blood-borne infections

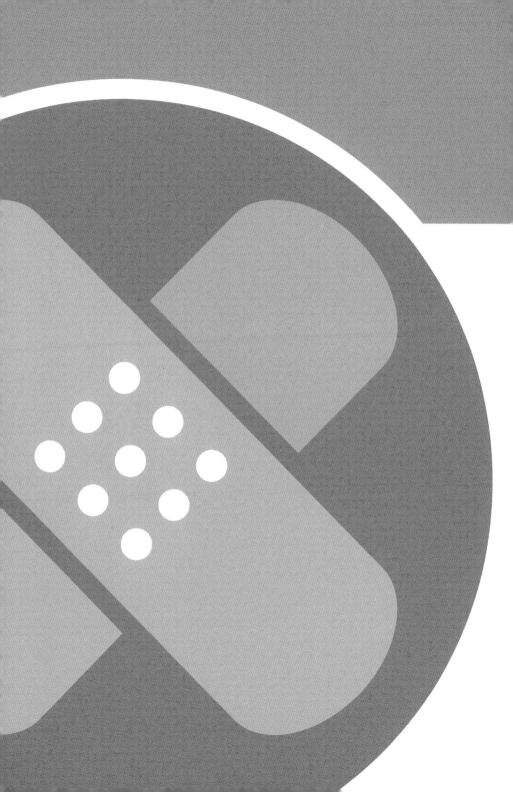

THE HEART AND BLOOD VESSELS

The heart and the blood vessels together make up the circulatory system. These structures supply every part of the body with a constant flow of blood, which carries oxygen and nutrients to the tissues and takes waste products away from them.

Blood is pumped around the body by the rhythmic contractions (beats) of the heart muscle. The blood runs through a network of vessels, divided into three types: arteries, veins and capillaries. The force that is exerted by the blood flow through the main arteries is called blood pressure. This pressure varies with the strength and phase of the heartbeat, the elasticity of the arterial walls and the volume and thickness of the blood.

How blood circulates

Oxygenated blood passes from the lungs to the heart, then travels to body tissues via the arteries. Blood that has given up its oxygen (deoxygenated blood) returns to the heart through the veins.

Carotid artery

Jugular vein

Brachial artery

Brachial vein

Superior vena cava carries deoxygenated blood from upper body to the heart

Aorta carries oxygenated blood to the body tissues

Inferior vena cava carries deoxygenated blood from mid and lower body to the heart

Heart pumps blood around body

Radial artery

Radial vein

Small artery (arteriole)

Femoral artery

Femoral vein

Capillary

Small vein (venule)

Capillary networks

A network of fine thin-walled blood vessels (capillaries) links arteries and veins within body tissues. Oxygen and nutrients pass from the blood into the tissues and waste products pass from the tissues back into the blood, through the capillary walls.

Aorta

Pulmonary artery

Superior vena cava

Coronary artery

Heart muscle

The heart

This muscular organ pumps blood around the body and then to the lungs to pick up oxygen. Coronary blood vessels supply the heart muscle with oxygen and nutrients.

KEY

■ Vessels carrying oxygenated blood
■ Vessels carrying deoxygenated blood

HOW THE HEART FUNCTIONS

The heart pumps blood by muscular contractions called heartbeats, which are controlled by electrical impulses generated in the heart. Each beat has three phases: diastole, when the heart relaxes and blood enters the atria (collecting chambers); atrial systole, when the blood is squeezed from the atria into the ventricles; and ventricular systole, when blood leaves the heart.

In diastole, the heart relaxes. Oxygenated blood from the lungs flows via the pulmonary veins into the left atrium. Blood that has given up its oxygen to body tissues (deoxygenated blood) flows from the venae cavae (large veins that enter the heart) into the right atrium. In atrial systole, the two atria contract and the valves between the atria and the ventricles (pumping chambers) open so that blood flows into the ventricles.

During ventricular systole, the heart's ventricles contract. The thick-walled left ventricle forces blood into the aorta (main artery), which carries it to the rest of the body. The right ventricle pumps blood into the pulmonary arteries, which carry it to the lungs to collect more oxygen.

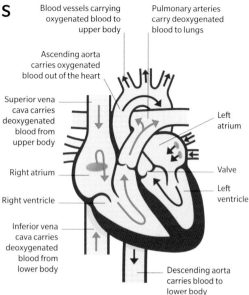

Blood vessels carrying oxygenated blood to upper body

Pulmonary arteries carry deoxygenated blood to lungs

Ascending aorta carries oxygenated blood out of the heart

Superior vena cava carries deoxygenated blood from upper body

Left atrium

Right atrium

Valve

Right ventricle

Left ventricle

Inferior vena cava carries deoxygenated blood from lower body

Descending aorta carries blood to lower body

Blood flow through the heart
The heart's right side pumps deoxygenated blood from the body to the lungs. The left side pumps oxygenated blood to the body via the aorta.

KEY
■ Vessels carrying oxygenated blood
■ Vessels carrying deoxygenated blood

COMPOSITION OF BLOOD

There are about 6 litres (10 pints), or 1 litre per 13 kg of body weight (1 pint per stone), of blood in the average adult body. Blood is made up of a clear yellow fluid (plasma), in which red and white blood cells and platelets are suspended. Red blood cells contain haemoglobin, the red pigment that enables the cells to carry oxygen and gives blood its colour. White blood cells play a key role in defending the body against infection. Platelets help the blood to clot.

Drop of blood
Each drop of blood is more than 50 per cent plasma, which not only contains red and white blood cells and platelets, but also body salts, hormones, fats and sugars.

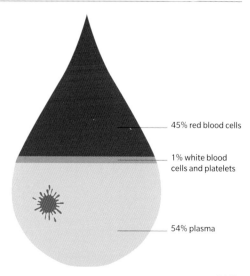

45% red blood cells

1% white blood cells and platelets

54% plasma

BLEEDING AND TYPES OF WOUND

When a blood vessel is damaged, the vessel constricts, and a series of chemical reactions occur to form a blood clot – a "plug" over the damaged area (below). If large blood vessels are torn or severed, uncontrolled blood loss may occur before clotting can take place, and shock (pp.114–115) may develop.

TYPES OF BLEEDING

Bleeding (haemorrhage) is classified by the type of blood vessel that is damaged. Arteries carry oxygenated blood under pressure from the heart. If an artery is damaged, bleeding will be profuse. Blood will spurt out with each heartbeat. If a main artery is severed, the volume of circulating blood will fall rapidly.

Blood from veins, having given up its oxygen into the tissues, is darker red. It is under less pressure than arterial blood, but vein walls can widen greatly and the blood can "pool" inside them (varicose vein). If a large or varicose vein is damaged, blood will flow from the wound profusely and blood volume can fall rapidly.

Bleeding from capillaries occurs with any wound. At first, bleeding may be brisk, but blood loss is usually slight. A blow may rupture capillaries under the skin, causing bleeding into the tissues (bruising).

HOW WOUNDS HEAL

When a blood vessel is severed or damaged, it constricts (narrows) in order to prevent excessive amounts of blood from escaping. Injured tissue cells at the site of the wound, together with specialised blood cells called platelets, then trigger a series of chemical reactions that result in the formation of a substance that creates a mesh. This mesh traps blood cells to make a blood clot. The clot releases a fluid known as serum, which contains antibodies and specialised cells. This serum begins the process of repairing the damaged area.

At first, the blood clot is a jelly-like mass. Fibroblast cells form a plug within the clot. Later, this dries into a crust (scab) that seals and protects the site of the wound until the healing process is complete.

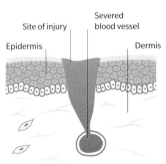

Site of injury | Severed blood vessel
Epidermis | Dermis

Injury
At the site of injury, platelets in the blood arrive to begin formation of a clot. Other cells are attracted to the site to help with repair.

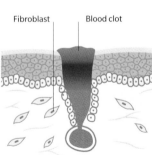

Fibroblast | Blood clot

Clotting
A clot is formed by platelets in the blood and blood-clotting protein. Tissue-forming cells migrate to the damaged area to start repair.

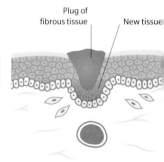

Plug of fibrous tissue | New tissue

Plugging and scabbing
A plug of fibrous tissue forms within the clot. The plug hardens and forms a scab that eventually drops off when the skin beneath it is healed.

TYPES OF WOUND

Wounds can be classified into a number of different types, depending on the object that produces the wound – such as a knife or a bullet – and the manner in which the wound has been inflicted.

Each of these types of wound carries specific risks associated with surrounding tissue damage and infection.

Incised wound

This is caused by a clean surface cut from a sharp-edged object such as a razor. Blood vessels are cut straight across, so bleeding may be profuse. Structures such as tendons or nerves may be damaged.

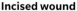
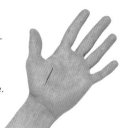

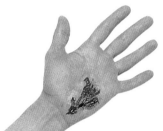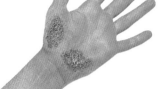

Laceration

Blunt or ripping forces result in tears or lacerations. These wounds may bleed less profusely than incised wounds, but there is likely to be more tissue damage. Lacerations are frequently contaminated with germs, so the risk of infection is high.

Abrasion (graze)

This is a superficial wound in which the topmost layers of skin are scraped off, leaving a raw, tender area. Abrasions are often caused by a sliding fall or a friction burn. They can contain embedded foreign particles that may cause infection.

Contusion (bruise)

A blunt blow can rupture capillaries beneath the skin, causing blood to leak into the tissues. This process results in bruising. Extensive contusion and swelling may indicate deeper damage, such as a fracture or an internal injury.

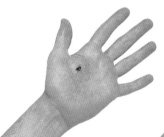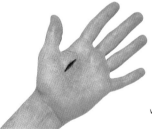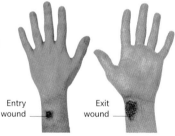

Entry wound

Exit wound

Puncture wound

An injury that results from standing on a nail or being pricked by a needle is known as a puncture wound. It has a small entry site and a deep track of internal damage. Since germs and dirt can be carried far into the body, the infection risk with this kind of wound is high.

Stab wound

This is a deep incision caused by a sharp or bladed instrument, usually a knife, penetrating the body. Stab wounds to the trunk, or abdomen, must always be treated seriously because of the danger of injury to vital organs and the risk of life-threatening internal bleeding.

Gunshot wound

This type of wound is caused by a bullet or missile being driven into or through the body, and results in serious internal injury and clothing and contaminants from the air may be "sucked" into the wound. The entry wound may be small and neat; any exit wound may be large and ragged.

SHOCK

This is a life-threatening condition that occurs when the circulatory system (which distributes oxygen and nutrients to the body tissues and removes waste products) fails and, as a result, vital organs such as the heart and brain are deprived of oxygen. It requires immediate emergency treatment. Shock can be made worse by fear and pain. Minimise the risk of shock developing by reassuring the casualty and making them comfortable.

The most common cause of shock is severe blood loss. If blood loss exceeds 1.2 litres (2 pints), which is about one-fifth of the normal blood volume, shock will develop. This degree of blood loss may result from external bleeding. It may also be caused by: hidden bleeding from internal organs (p.118); blood escaping into a body cavity (p.118); or bleeding from damaged blood vessels due to a closed fracture (pp.138 and 140). Loss of other body fluids can also result in shock. Other conditions that can cause severe fluid loss include diarrhoea, vomiting, bowel obstruction and serious burns.

In addition, shock may occur when there is sufficient blood volume but the heart is unable to pump the blood around the body. This problem can be due to severe heart disease, heart attack or acute heart failure (cardiogenic shock). Other causes of shock include overwhelming infection (septic shock, p.222), severe allergic reaction (anaphylactic shock, p.227) and spinal cord injury (neurogenic shock, pp.159–161).

EFFECTS OF BLOOD OR FLUID LOSS

APPROXIMATE VOLUME	EFFECTS ON THE BODY
0.5 litre (about 1 pint)	● Little or no effect; this is the quantity of blood normally taken in a blood donor session
Up to 2 litres (3½ pints)	● Hormones such as adrenaline are released, quickening the pulse and inducing sweating ● Small blood vessels in non-vital areas, such as the skin, shut down to divert blood and oxygen to the vital organs ● Shock becomes evident
2 litres (3½ pints) or more (over a third of the normal volume in the average adult)	● As blood or fluid loss approaches this level, the pulse at the wrist may become undetectable ● Casualty will gradually become unresponsive ● Breathing will cease and finally the heart will stop

SEE ALSO Anaphylactic shock **p.227** | Internal bleeding **p.118** | Severe burns and scalds **pp.176–177**
 Severe external bleeding **pp.116–117** | Spinal injury **pp.159–161** | The unresponsive casualty **pp.56–89**

WHAT TO DO

1 Treat any possible cause of shock that you can detect, such as severe bleeding (pp.116–117) or serious burns (pp.176–177). Reassure the casualty.

2 Help the casualty to lie down – on a rug or blanket if there is one, as this will protect them from the cold. Raise and support the casualty's legs above the level of their heart to improve blood supply to the vital organs.

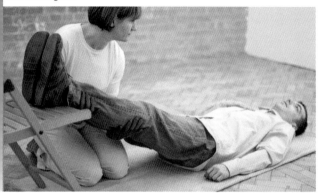

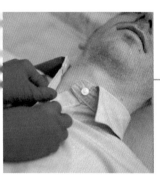

3 Call 999 / 112 for emergency help. Tell the call handler you suspect that the casualty is suffering from shock.

4 Loosen tight clothing to reduce constriction at the casualty's neck, chest and waist.

5 Keep the casualty warm by covering their body and legs with coats or blankets.

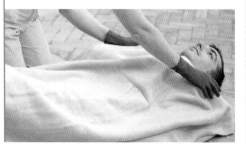

6 Monitor and record the casualty's vital signs (pp.54–55) while you are waiting for help to arrive.

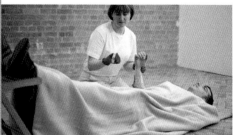

RECOGNITION

Initially there may be:
- A rapid pulse
- Pale, cold, clammy skin
- Sweating

As shock develops:
- Rapid, shallow breathing
- A weak, "thready" pulse. When the pulse at the wrist disappears, about half of the blood volume will have been lost
- Grey-blue skin (cyanosis), especially inside the lips. A fingernail or earlobe, if pressed, will not regain its colour immediately
- Weakness and dizziness
- Nausea, and possibly vomiting
- Thirst

As the brain's oxygen supply weakens:
- Restlessness and aggressive behaviour
- Yawning and gasping for air
- Casualty becomes unresponsive
- Finally, the heart will stop

YOUR AIMS

- To recognise shock
- To treat obvious cause of shock
- To improve the blood supply to the brain, heart and lungs
- To arrange urgent removal to hospital

115

SEVERE EXTERNAL BLEEDING

CAUTION

- Remove or cut away clothing to expose a wound if necessary (p.236).
- If there is an object in the wound, apply pressure on either side of the object (p.123); do not apply any pressure directly over the object.
- If the bleeding is severe, apply a haemostatic dressing (p.239) if there is one available.
- Do not allow the casualty to eat or drink because an anaesthetic may be needed later.
- If the casualty is unresponsive, open the airway and check breathing (The unresponsive casualty, pp.56–89).

YOUR AIMS

- To control bleeding
- To prevent and minimise the effects of shock
- To minimise infection
- To arrange urgent removal to hospital

When bleeding is severe, it can be dramatic and distressing. If bleeding is not controlled shock will develop and the casualty may no longer be responsive.

Bleeding from the mouth or nose may also affect breathing. When treating severe bleeding, check whether there is an object embedded in the wound (p.123); take care not to press directly on an object. Do not remove anything that is embedded in a wound. If bleeding cannot be controlled with direct pressure you may need to apply a tourniquet (opposite).

WHAT TO DO

1 **Apply direct pressure** to the wound with your fingers or the palm of your hand over a sterile wound dressing or clean cloth pad to control the bleeding. If you do not have a sterile dressing or pad, ask the casualty to apply direct pressure themselves; they may need help.

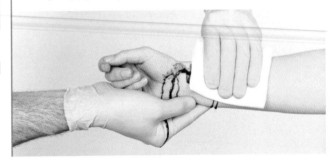

2 **Ask a helper to** call 999/112 for emergency help. Ask the person to give the call handler details of the site of injury and the extent of the bleeding.

3 **Once the bleeding is under control,** secure the dressing or pad with a bandage that is firm enough to maintain pressure, but not so tight that it impairs circulation (p.247). Call 999/112 for emergency help if this has not been done already.

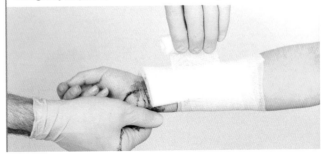

4 As shock is likely to develop (pp.114–115), help the casualty to lie down – on a rug or blanket if there is one, as this will protect them from the cold. Raise and support their legs so that they are above the level of their heart.

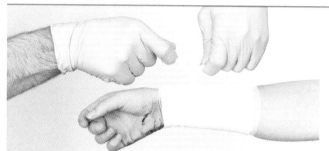

5 If blood loss persists, remove the dressing and reapply direct pressure over a new dressing or pad to control bleeding (see step 1, opposite). Secure the dressing with a bandage once bleeding is controlled; tie the knot over the pad to help maintain pressure.

6 Support the injured part with a sling and/or a bandage. Check the circulation beyond the bandage (p.247) and re-check it every 10 minutes. If the circulation is impaired, loosen the bandage and reapply.

7 Monitor and record the casualty's vital signs (pp.54–55) while waiting for help to arrive.

SPECIAL CASE APPLYING A TOURNIQUET

If you are unable to control bleeding on a limb using the above steps, then you may need to apply a tourniquet. These are specialist pieces of equipment and anyone using them should have had advanced training. Ideally use a manufactured one, and follow the instructions for use. Place it around the limb about 5 cm (2 in) above the injury, but never over a joint. If possible, apply directly on the skin so that it does not slip, and make sure that it does not bunch up or pinch the skin.

If there are no manufactured tourniquets available (and you are trained), you can improvise. Use material that is non-elastic, but wide and long enough that it can be tightened sufficiently – for example, a folded triangular bandage, tie, shirt sleeve or head scarf – and apply the "windlass" technique. Wrap the length of material around the limb as above, and tie a knot. Place a strong, long object, for example a stick, over the first knot and tie a second knot over the top to secure it. Rotate the stick until the bleeding stops, then tie a second fabric strip over it to prevent it moving.

This will be painful for a conscious casualty so pain relief will be required. Make a note of the time the tourniquet was applied and tell the emergency services. Never release the tourniquet yourself – it must only be done by a healthcare professional.

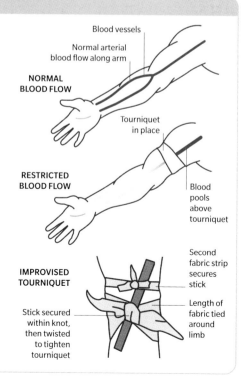

Blood vessels

Normal arterial blood flow along arm

NORMAL BLOOD FLOW

Tourniquet in place

RESTRICTED BLOOD FLOW

Blood pools above tourniquet

IMPROVISED TOURNIQUET

Second fabric strip secures stick

Length of fabric tied around limb

Stick secured within knot, then twisted to tighten tourniquet

INTERNAL BLEEDING

- Initially, pale, cold, clammy skin. If bleeding continues, the skin may turn blue-grey (cyanosis)
- Rapid, weak pulse
- Thirst
- Rapid, shallow breathing
- Confusion, restlessness and irritability
- Possible collapse and casualty may become unresponsive
- Bleeding from body openings (orifices)
- In cases of violent injury, "pattern bruising" – an area of discoloured skin with a shape that matches the pattern of clothes or crushing or restraining objects
- Pain
- Information from casualty that indicates recent injury, illness, or surgery

Bleeding inside body cavities may follow an injury, such as a fracture or a blow from a blunt object, but it can also occur spontaneously – for example, bleeding from a stomach ulcer. The main risk from internal bleeding is shock (pp.114–115). In addition, blood can build up around organs such as the lungs or brain and exert damaging pressure on them.

Suspect internal bleeding if a casualty develops signs of shock without obvious blood loss. Check for any bleeding from body openings (orifices) such as the ear, mouth and nose. There may also be bleeding from the urethra or anus (below).

The signs of bleeding vary depending on the site of the blood loss (below), but the most obvious is a discharge of blood from a body opening. Blood loss from any orifice is significant and can lead to shock. In addition, bleeding from some orifices can indicate a serious underlying injury or illness. Follow treatment for shock (pp.114–115).

YOUR AIMS

- To minimise the effects of shock
- To arrange urgent removal to hospital

POSSIBLE SIGNS OF INTERNAL BLEEDING

SITE	APPEARANCE OF BLOOD	CAUSES OF BLOOD LOSS
Mouth	• Bright red, frothy, coughed-up blood	• Bleeding in the lungs
	• Vomited blood, red or dark reddish-brown, resembling coffee grounds	• Bleeding within the digestive system
Ear	• Fresh, bright red blood	• Injury to the inner or outer ear or perforated eardrum
	• Thin, watery blood	• Leakage of fluid from around the brain due to head injury
Nose	• Fresh, bright red blood	• Ruptured blood vessel in the nostril
	• Thin, watery blood	• Leakage of fluid from around the brain due to head injury
Anus	• Fresh, bright red blood	• Piles or injury to the anus or lower intestine
	• Black, tarry, offensive-smelling stool (melaena)	• Disease or injury to the intestine
Urethra	• Red or smoky appearance to urine, occasionally containing clots	• Bleeding from the bladder, kidneys or urethra
Vagina	• Either fresh or dark blood	• Menstruation • Miscarriage • Pregnancy • Recent childbirth • Assault

IMPALEMENT

If someone has been impaled, for example by falling on to railings, never attempt to lift the casualty off the object involved since this may worsen any internal injuries. **Call 999/112 for emergency help** immediately, giving clear details about the incident. They will bring special cutting equipment with them to free the casualty.

CAUTION
- Do not allow the casualty to eat or drink because an anaesthetic may be needed.

YOUR AIM
- To prevent further injury

WHAT TO DO

1 Call 999/112 for emergency help. Send a helper to make the call if possible. Explain the situation clearly to the call handler, so that the correct equipment can be brought.

2 Support the casualty's body weight until the emergency services arrive and take over. Reassure the casualty while you wait for emergency help.

AMPUTATION

Parts of the body such as fingers or toes, a limb, or even an ear, can be partially or completely severed. In many cases, the part can be reattached by microsurgery. The operation will require a general anaesthetic, so do not allow the casualty to eat or drink. It is vital to get the casualty and the amputated part to hospital as soon as possible. Shock is likely, and needs to be treated.

CAUTION
- Do not wash the severed part.
- Do not let the severed part touch the crushed ice when packing it.
- Do not allow the casualty to eat or drink because an anaesthetic may be needed.

YOUR AIMS
- To control bleeding
- To minimise the effects of shock
- To arrange urgent removal to hospital
- To prevent deterioration of the injured part

WHAT TO DO

1 Control blood loss by applying direct pressure over a sterile wound dressing or clean cloth pad (pp.116–117) and raising the injured part above the level of the casualty's heart.

2 Secure the dressing or pad with a bandage, tight enough to maintain pressure but not so tight that it impairs circulation (p.247). Treat the casualty for shock (pp.114–115).

3 Call 999/112 for emergency help. Tell the call handler that amputation is involved. Monitor and record the casualty's vital signs (pp.54–55) while waiting for help to arrive.

4 Wrap the severed part in plastic kitchen film or a plastic bag. Surround this package with gauze or soft fabric and place it in a container full of crushed ice. Mark the container with the time of injury and the casualty's name. Give it to the emergency service personnel.

SEE ALSO Severe external bleeding **pp.116–117** | Shock **pp.114–115**

CRUSH INJURY

Traffic and building site incidents are the most common causes of crush injuries. Other possible causes include explosions, earthquakes and train crashes.

A crush injury may include a fracture, swelling and internal bleeding. The crushing force may also cause impaired circulation, which results in numbness at or below the site of injury.

DANGERS OF PROLONGED CRUSHING

YOUR AIM

- To obtain specialist medical aid urgently, taking any steps possible to treat the casualty

If the casualty is trapped for any length of time, two serious complications may result. First, prolonged crushing may cause extensive damage to body tissue, especially to muscles. Once the pressure is removed, shock may develop rapidly as tissue fluid leaks into the injured area.

Secondly, and more dangerously, toxic substances will build up in damaged muscle tissue around a crush injury. If released suddenly into the circulation, these toxins may cause kidney failure or sudden cardiac arrest (p.59). This process, called "crush syndrome", is extremely serious and can be fatal.

WHAT TO DO

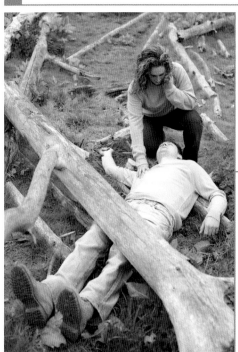

1 If you know the casualty has been crushed for less than 15 minutes and you can release them safely, do this as quickly as possible. Control bleeding, steady and support any suspected fracture (pp.138–140) and treat the casualty for shock (pp.114–115).

2 If the casualty has been crushed for more than 15 minutes, or you cannot move the cause of injury, leave them in the position found. Offer comfort and reassurance.

3 Call 999/112 for emergency help, giving clear details of the incident to the call handler.

4 Monitor and record the casualty's vital signs (pp.54–55) while waiting for help to arrive.

CUTS AND GRAZES

Bleeding from small cuts and grazes is normally easily controlled by direct pressure and elevation. An adhesive dressing is generally all that is required, and the wound will heal by itself in a few days. Medical help need only be sought if: bleeding does not stop; there is a foreign object embedded in the cut (p.123); there is a particular risk of infection, from a human or animal bite (p.205) or a puncture by a dirty object; an old wound shows signs of becoming infected (p.122).

CAUTION

Ask the casualty about tetanus immunisation. Seek medical advice if they:

- Have a dirty wound.
- Have never been immunised.
- Are uncertain about the number or timings of immunisations.

WHAT TO DO

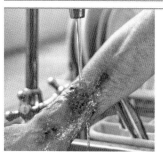

1 If the wound is dirty, clean it by rinsing under running water, or use alcohol-free wipes. Pat the wound dry using a gauze swab and cover it with a pad of sterile gauze. Avoid touching the wound with your hands. Support the injured part if possible.

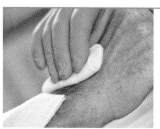

2 Clean the area around the wound with soap and water. Wipe away from the wound and use a clean swab for each stroke. Pat dry. Remove the gauze covering and apply a sterile wound dressing. If there is a particular risk of infection, advise the casualty to seek medical advice.

YOUR AIMS

- To control bleeding
- To minimise the risk of infection

SPECIAL CASE TETANUS

This is a dangerous infection caused by a bacterium that lives in soil. If the bacterium enters a wound, it may multiply in the damaged tissues and release a toxin that spreads through the nervous system, causing muscle spasms and paralysis. Tetanus can be prevented by immunisation, which is normally given during childhood. This may need to be repeated in adulthood.

BRUISING

Caused by bleeding into the skin or into tissues beneath the skin, a bruise can develop rapidly or emerge a few days after injury. Bruising can also indicate deep injury. Elderly people and those taking anticoagulant (anti-clotting) medication can bruise easily.

YOUR AIM

- To reduce blood flow to the injury, and so minimise swelling

WHAT TO DO

1 Raise and support the injury in a comfortable position for the casualty.

2 Place a cold compress (p.245) over the bruise. Leave in place for 20 minutes.

SEE ALSO Foreign object in a wound **p.123** | Infected wound **p.122** | Internal bleeding **p.118**

BLISTERS

Blisters occur when the skin is repeatedly rubbed against another surface or when it is exposed to heat (p.175). The damaged area of skin leaks tissue fluid that collects under the top layer of the skin, forming a blister.

WHAT TO DO

1 **Wash the area** with clean water and rinse. Gently pat the area and surrounding skin dry thoroughly with a sterile gauze pad. If it is not possible to wash the area, keep it as clean as possible.

2 **Cover a blister** caused by friction with an adhesive dressing; make sure the pad of the plaster is larger than the blister. Ideally use a special blister plaster since they have a cushioned pad that provides extra protection and comfort.

INFECTED WOUND

RECOGNITION

• Increasing pain and soreness at the site of the wound

• Swelling, redness and a feeling of heat around the injury

• Pus within, or oozing from, the wound

• Swelling and tenderness of the glands in the neck, armpit or groin

• Faint red trails on the skin that lead to the glands in the neck, armpit or groin

If infection is advanced:

• Signs of fever, such as sweating, thirst, shivering and lethargy

YOUR AIMS

• To prevent further infection

• To obtain medical advice if necessary

Any open wound can become contaminated with micro-organisms (germs). The germs may come from the source of the injury, from the environment, from breath, from the fingers handling the wound or from particles of clothing embedded in it (as may occur in gunshot wounds). Bleeding may flush some dirt away; remaining germs may be destroyed by the white blood cells. However, if dirt or dead tissue remains in a wound, infection may spread through the body. There is also a risk of tetanus infection (p.121).

Any wound that does not begin to heal within 48 hours is likely to be infected. A casualty with a wound that is at high risk of infection may need treatment with antibiotics and/or tetanus immunisation (p.121).

WHAT TO DO

1 **Cover the wound with a sterile dressing** or large clean cloth pad, and bandage it in place.

2 **Raise and support the injured part** with a sling and/or bandages. This helps to reduce the swelling around the injury.

3 **Advise the casualty to seek medical advice.** If infection is advanced (with signs of fever, such as sweating, shivering and lethargy), take or send the casualty to hospital.

FOREIGN OBJECT IN A WOUND

It is important to remove foreign objects, such as small pieces of glass or grit, from a wound before beginning treatment. If left in a wound, they may cause infection or delay healing. The best way to remove superficial pieces of glass or grit from the skin is to pick them out with tweezers. Alternatively, rinse loose pieces off with cold water. Do not try to remove pieces that are firmly embedded in the wound because you may damage the surrounding tissue and aggravate bleeding. Instead, cover the object with a dressing and bandage around it.

CAUTION

Ask the casualty about tetanus immunisation. Seek medical advice if they:

- Have a dirty wound.
- Have never been immunised.
- Are uncertain about the number or timings of immunisations.

YOUR AIMS

- To control bleeding without pressing the object further into the wound
- To minimise the risk of infection
- To arrange transport to hospital if necessary

WHAT TO DO

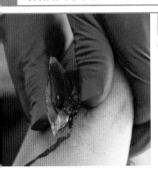

1 **Control bleeding** by applying pressure on either side of the object.

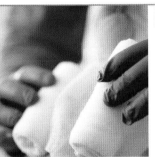

2 **Drape a piece of gauze** over the wound and object. Build up padding on either side of the object (rolled bandages make good padding) until it is higher than the object. Padding should be high enough for you to be able to bandage over the top of object without pressing it further into the wound.

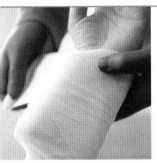

3 **When the padding is high enough** bandage over and around the object and padding making sure you do not press the object into the wound. Hold the padding in place until the bandaging is complete. Arrange to take or send the casualty to hospital.

SPECIAL CASE
BANDAGING AROUND A LARGER OBJECT

If you cannot build padding high enough to bandage over the top of an object, drape a clean piece of gauze loosely over it. Place padding on either side of the object and bandage above and below the object.

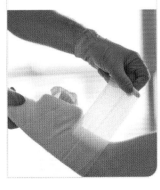

SEE ALSO Cuts and grazes p.121 | Embedded fish hook p.197 | Severe external bleeding pp.116–117 | Splinter p.196

SCALP AND HEAD WOUNDS

YOUR AIMS

- To control bleeding
- To arrange transport to hospital

The scalp has many small blood vessels running close to the skin surface, so any cut can result in profuse bleeding, which often makes a scalp wound appear worse than it is.

In some cases, however, a scalp wound may form part of a more serious underlying head injury, such as a skull fracture, or may be associated with a neck injury. For these reasons, you should examine a casualty with a scalp wound very carefully, particularly if it is possible that signs of a serious head injury are being masked by alcohol or drug intoxication. If you are in any doubt, follow the treatment for head injury (pp.146–147). In addition, bear in mind the possibility of a neck (spinal) injury.

WHAT TO DO

1 If there are any displaced flaps of skin at the injury site, carefully replace them over the wound. Reassure the casualty.

2 Cover the wound with a sterile wound dressing or a clean cloth pad. Apply firm, direct pressure on the pad to help control bleeding to reduce blood loss, and minimise the risk of shock.

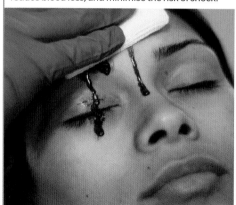

3 Keep the pad in place with a roller bandage to secure it and maintain pressure.

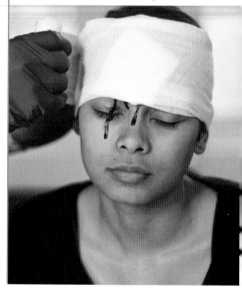

4 Help the casualty to lie down with their head and shoulders slightly raised. If they feel faint or dizzy or show any signs of shock, call 999/112 for emergency help. Monitor and record the casualty's vital signs (pp.54–55) while waiting for help to arrive.

EYE WOUND

The eye can be bruised or cut by direct blows or by sharp, chipped fragments of metal, grit and glass.

All eye injuries are potentially serious because of the risk to the casualty's vision. Even superficial grazes to the surface (cornea) of the eye can lead to scarring or infection, with the possibility of permanent deterioration of vision.

CAUTION

- Do not touch or attempt to remove anything that is sticking to, or embedded in, the eyeball or on the coloured part (iris) of the eye.

WHAT TO DO

1 **Help the casualty to lie on their back.** Hold their head to keep it as still as possible. Tell the casualty to keep both eyes still; movement of the "good" eye will cause movement of the injured one, which may damage it further.

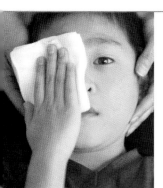

2 **Give the casualty a sterile** dressing or a clean cloth pad to hold over the affected eye. If it will take some time to obtain medical help, secure the pad in place with a bandage.

3 **Arrange to take or send** the casualty to hospital.

RECOGNITION

- Pain in the eye or eyelids
- Visible wound and/or bloodshot appearance
- Partial or total loss of vision
- Leakage of blood or clear fluid from a wound

YOUR AIMS

- To prevent further damage
- To arrange transport to hospital

BLEEDING FROM THE EAR

This may be due to a burst (perforated) eardrum, an ear infection, a blow to the side of the head or an explosion. Symptoms include sharp pain, earache, deafness and possible dizziness. The presence of blood or blood-stained watery fluid may indicate a more serious, underlying head injury (pp.146–147).

CAUTION

- If you suspect a head injury (pp.146–147), support the casualty's head in the position you found them and call 999/112 for emergency help.

WHAT TO DO

1 **Help the casualty into a half-sitting** position, with their head tilted towards the injured side to allow blood to drain from the ear.

2 **Hold a sterile wound dressing** or a clean cloth pad lightly in place on the ear. Do not plug the ear. Send or take the casualty to hospital.

YOUR AIM

- To arrange transport to hospital

SEE ALSO Foreign object in the ear **p.199** | Head injury **pp.146–147**

NOSEBLEED

YOUR AIMS

- To maintain an open airway
- To control bleeding

Bleeding from the nose most commonly occurs when tiny blood vessels inside the nostrils are ruptured, either by a blow to the nose, or as a result of sneezing, picking or blowing the nose. Nosebleeds may also occur as a result of high blood pressure and anti-coagulant (anti-clotting) medication.

A nosebleed can be serious if the casualty loses a lot of blood. In addition, if bleeding follows a head injury, the blood may appear thin and watery. The latter is a very serious sign because it indicates that the skull is fractured and fluid is leaking from around the brain.

WHAT TO DO

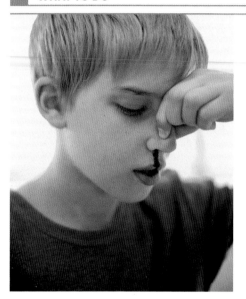

1 **Tell the casualty to sit down** and tilt their head forward to allow the blood to drain from the nostrils. Ask them to breathe through their mouth (this will also have a calming effect) and to pinch the soft part of their nose for up to 10 minutes. Reassure and help them if necessary.

2 **Advise the casualty not to speak, swallow, cough, spit or sniff** since this may disturb blood clots that have formed in the nose. Give them a clean cloth or tissue to mop up any dribbling.

3 **After 10 minutes,** tell the casualty to release the pressure. If the bleeding has not stopped, tell them to reapply the pressure for two further periods of 10 minutes.

4 **Once the bleeding has stopped,** and with the casualty still leaning forwards, clean around their nose with lukewarm water. Advise them to rest quietly for a few hours. Tell them to avoid exertion and, in particular, not to blow their nose, because this could disturb any clots.

5 **If bleeding stops and then restarts,** help the casualty to reapply pressure.

6 **If the nosebleed is severe,** or if it lasts longer than 30 minutes, arrange to take or send the casualty to hospital.

SPECIAL CASE FOR A YOUNG CHILD

A child may be worried by a nosebleed. Tell them to lean forward, and then pinch the nose for them, reassure them and give them a bowl to spit or dribble into.

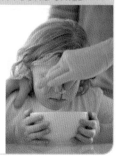

KNOCKED-OUT ADULT TOOTH

If a secondary (adult) tooth is knocked out, it should be replaced in its socket as soon as possible. Alternatively, wrap it in plastic kitchen film or place it in a small container of cow's milk to prevent it from drying out. In all circumstances a casualty should see a dentist as soon as possible as they may be able reimplant it.

WHAT TO DO

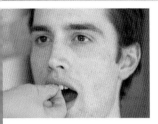

2 If the tooth cannot be replaced, rinse it for 10 seconds in cold water and wrap it in plastic film. If cold water is not available, place the tooth in a container of cow's milk – not water or saline.

1 Pick up the tooth by its crown, and rinse it under cold running water for 10 seconds. Push the tooth gently into the socket and cover it with a piece of gauze. Ask the casualty to gently close their mouth over it.

3 Send the casualty to a dentist so that the tooth can be reimplanted.

SPECIAL CASE
BLEEDING TOOTH SOCKET

To control bleeding from a tooth socket, give the casualty a gauze pad thick enough to prevent the teeth meeting. Ask them to put the pad in the tooth socket, then to bite down on it.

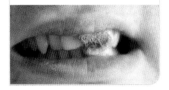

BLEEDING FROM THE MOUTH

Cuts to the tongue, lips or lining of the mouth range from minor injuries to more serious wounds. The cause is often the casualty's own teeth or a dental extraction. Bleeding from the mouth may be profuse and can be alarming. There is a risk that blood could also be inhaled into the lungs, causing breathing problems.

WHAT TO DO

1 Ask the casualty to sit down, with their head forwards and tilted slightly to the injured side, to allow blood to drain from their mouth. Place a sterile gauze pad over the wound. Ask the casualty to squeeze the pad between their finger and thumb and press on the wound for 10 minutes.

2 If bleeding persists, replace the pad. Tell the casualty to let the blood dribble out; if they swallow it, it may induce vomiting. Do not wash the mouth out because this may disturb a clot. Advise the casualty to avoid drinking anything hot for 12 hours.

YOUR AIMS

- To control bleeding
- To safeguard the airway by preventing any inhalation of blood

FINGER WOUND

YOUR AIMS

- To control bleeding
- To assess whether or not the wound needs a medical assessment

Injuries to the fingers are common and can vary from small cuts and grazes to wounds with underlying damage to bones, tendons and ligaments. Injuries to the nails are the most common. All finger wounds need good management as the hand is a finely coordinated part of the body that must function correctly for many everyday activities.

A cut to a finger may go through the skin only or it can cut through blood vessels, nerves and tendons that lie just under the skin. There will be bleeding, which can be profuse, and possibly bruising, deformity or loss of movement or sensation if the underlying structures are damaged.

WHAT TO DO

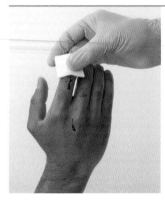

1 **Press a sterile dressing** or clean cloth pad on the wound and apply direct pressure to control bleeding.

2 **Raise and support** the injured hand and maintain pressure on the wound until the bleeding stops.

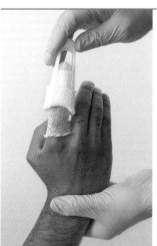

3 **When the bleeding has stopped,** cover the wound to protect it. Use an adhesive dressing or, for a larger wound, apply a dressing pad and secure it with a tubular gauze bandage or a finger bandage roll (pp.240 and 252).

4 **Seek medical help** if necessary. If you need to take the casualty to hospital, support the injured arm in an elevation sling (p.256).

WOUND TO THE PALM

The palm of the hand has a good blood supply, which is why a wound there may cause profuse bleeding. A deep wound to the palm may sever tendons and nerves in the hand and result in loss of feeling or movement in the fingers.

Bandaging the fist can be an effective way to control bleeding. If, however, a casualty has a foreign object embedded in a palm wound, it will be impossible for them to clench the fist. In such cases, treat the injury using the method described on p.123.

YOUR AIMS

- To control bleeding and the effects of shock
- To minimise the risk of infection
- To arrange transport to hospital

WHAT TO DO

1 Press a sterile wound dressing or clean pad firmly into the palm, and ask the casualty to clench their fist or to grasp the fist with the other hand.

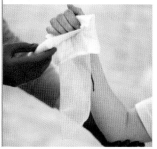

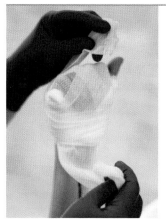

2 Raise and support the hand. Bandage the casualty's fingers so that they are clenched over the pad; leave the thumb free so that you can check circulation. Tie the ends of the bandage over the top of the fingers to help maintain pressure.

3 Support the arm in an elevation sling (p.256). Take or send the casualty to hospital. Check the circulation in the thumb (p.247), and re-check it every 10 minutes. Remove the bandage, and reapply if needed.

WOUND AT A JOINT CREASE

Large blood vessels pass across the inside of the elbow and back of the knee. If severed, these vessels will bleed profusely. The steps given below help to control bleeding and shock (pp.114–115). Take care to ensure that there is adequate circulation to the part of the limb beyond the bandage.

YOUR AIMS

- To control bleeding
- To prevent and minimise the effects of shock
- To arrange transport to hospital

WHAT TO DO

1 Press a sterile dressing or clean cloth pad on the injury and apply direct pressure to control bleeding. Raise and support the injured limb.

2 Secure the dressing with a bandage tied firmly enough to maintain pressure. If possible, help the casualty to lie down with their legs raised. Take or send the casualty to hospital.

3 Check the circulation (p.247) in the lower part of the limb beyond the bandage, and re-check it every 10 minutes. If necessary, remove the bandage, and apply more loosely.

SEE ALSO Foreign object in a wound **p.123** | Shock **pp.114–115**

ABDOMINAL WOUND

YOUR AIMS

- To minimise shock
- To arrange urgent removal to hospital

A stab wound, gunshot or crush injury to the abdomen may cause a serious wound. Organs and large blood vessels can be punctured, lacerated or ruptured. There may be external bleeding, protruding abdominal contents and internal injury and bleeding, so this is an emergency.

WHAT TO DO

1 Help the casualty to lie down on a firm surface, on a blanket if available. Loosen any tight clothing, such as a belt or a shirt.

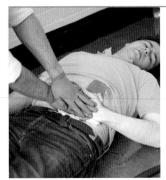

2 Cover the injury with a sterile wound dressing or clean pad and hold it firmly in place; the casualty may be able to help. Raise and support the casualty's knees to ease strain on the injury.

3 Call 999/112 for emergency help. Treat the casualty for shock (pp.114–115. Monitor and record the casualty's vital signs (pp.54–55) while waiting for help to arrive.

VAGINAL BLEEDING

YOUR AIMS

- To make the person comfortable and reassure them
- To arrange removal to hospital if necessary

Be sensitive to the person's feelings. The bleeding is most likely to be menstrual bleeding, but it can also indicate a more serious condition such as miscarriage, pregnancy, recent termination of pregnancy, childbirth or injury as a result of sexual assault. If the bleeding is severe, shock may develop.

If a person has been sexually assaulted, it is vital to preserve the evidence if possible. Gently advise them to refrain from washing or using the toilet until a forensic examination has been performed. If they wish to remove their clothing, keep it intact in a clean plastic bag if possible. Be aware that the person may be feeling vulnerable and may prefer to be treated by a person of the same gender.

1 Allow the casualty privacy and give them a sanitary towel. Make them as comfortable as possible in whichever position they prefer.

2 If the casualty has period pains, they may take the recommended dose of paracetamol or their own preferred painkillers.

BLEEDING VARICOSE VEIN

Veins contain one-way valves that keep the blood flowing towards the heart. If these valves fail, blood collects (pools) behind them and makes the veins swell. This problem, called varicose veins, usually develops in the legs.

A varicose vein has taut, thin walls and is often raised, typically producing knobbly skin over the affected area. The vein can burst following a gentle knock, and this may result in profuse bleeding. Shock will quickly develop if bleeding is not controlled.

YOUR AIMS

- To control bleeding
- To minimise shock
- To arrange urgent removal to hospital

WHAT TO DO

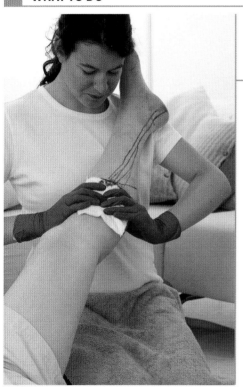

1 Help the casualty to lie down on their back. Raise and support the injured leg as high as possible immediately; this reduces the amount of bleeding.

2 Rest the injured leg on your shoulder or on a chair. Apply firm, direct pressure on the injury, using a sterile dressing or a clean cloth pad, until the blood loss is under control. If necessary, carefully cut away clothing to expose the site of the bleeding.

3 Remove tight-fitting garments such as elastic-topped stockings or long socks that extend above the wound because they may cause the bleeding to continue.

4 Keeping the leg raised, put another soft pad over the dressing. Bandage it firmly enough to exert even pressure, but not so tightly that the circulation in the limb is impaired (p.247).

5 Call 999/112 for emergency help. Keep the injured leg raised and supported until the ambulance arrives. Monitor and record the casualty's vital signs (pp.54–55) regularly until help arrives. In addition, check the circulation in the limb beyond the bandage (p.247) and re-check it every 10 minutes.

07 BONE, JOINT AND MUSCLE INJURIES

The skeleton is the supporting framework around which the body is constructed. It is jointed in many places, and muscles attached to the bones enable us to move. Most of our movements are controlled at will and coordinated by impulses that travel from the brain via the nerves to every muscle and joint in the body.

It is difficult for a first aider to distinguish between different bone, joint and muscle injuries, so this chapter begins with an overview of how bones, muscles and joints function and how injuries affect them. First aid treatments for most injuries, from serious fractures to sprains, strains and dislocations, are included in this section.

First aid for head and spinal injuries is also covered in this chapter. There is anatomical information about the nervous system that explains how and why these injuries can be made worse by potential damage to the brain and spinal cord.

AIMS AND OBJECTIVES

- To assess the casualty's condition quickly and calmly
- To support the injured part of the body
- To minimise shock
- To call 999/112 for emergency help if you suspect a serious injury
- To comfort and reassure the casualty
- To be aware of your own needs

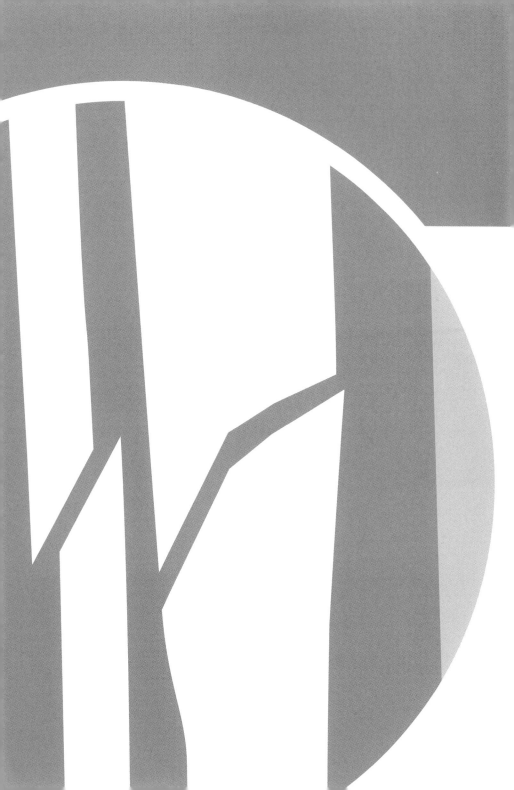

THE SKELETON

The body is built on a framework of bones called the skeleton. This structure supports the muscles, blood vessels and nerves of the body. Many bones of the skeleton also protect important organs such as the brain and heart. At many points on the skeleton, bones articulate with each other by means of joints. These are supported by ligaments and moved by muscles that are attached to the bones by tendons.

The skeleton

There are 206 bones in the skeleton, providing a protective framework for the body. The skull, spine and ribcage protect vital body structures; the pelvis supports the abdominal organs; and the bones and joints of the arms and legs enable the body to move.

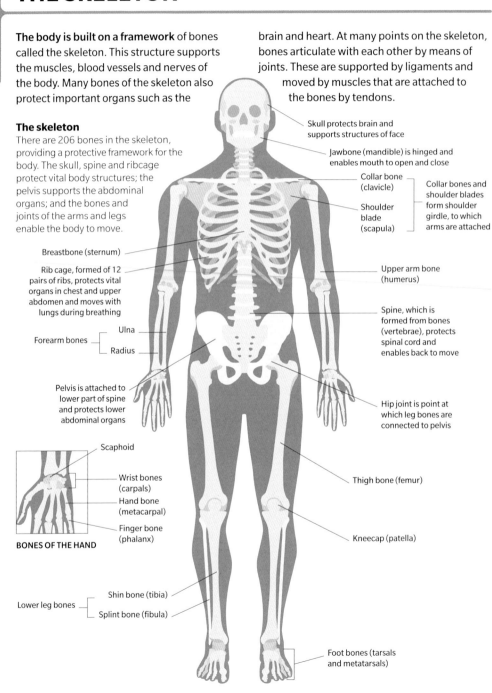

Skull protects brain and supports structures of face

Jawbone (mandible) is hinged and enables mouth to open and close

Collar bone (clavicle)

Shoulder blade (scapula)

Collar bones and shoulder blades form shoulder girdle, to which arms are attached

Breastbone (sternum)

Rib cage, formed of 12 pairs of ribs, protects vital organs in chest and upper abdomen and moves with lungs during breathing

Upper arm bone (humerus)

Forearm bones — Ulna
                 Radius

Spine, which is formed from bones (vertebrae), protects spinal cord and enables back to move

Pelvis is attached to lower part of spine and protects lower abdominal organs

Hip joint is point at which leg bones are connected to pelvis

Scaphoid

Wrist bones (carpals)

Hand bone (metacarpal)

Finger bone (phalanx)

BONES OF THE HAND

Thigh bone (femur)

Kneecap (patella)

Lower leg bones — Shin bone (tibia)
                  Splint bone (fibula)

Foot bones (tarsals and metatarsals)

THE SPINE

Also known as the backbone, or spinal column, the spine has a number of functions. It supports the head, makes the upper body flexible, helps to support the body's weight and protects the spinal cord (p.144). It is made up of a column of 33 bones called vertebrae, which are connected by joints. Between individual vertebrae are discs of fibrous tissue, or intervertebral discs, which help to make the spine flexible and cushion it from jolts. Muscles and ligaments attached to the vertebrae help to stabilise the spine and control the movements of the back.

Spinal column, left
There are five groups of vertebrae: the cervical vertebrae support the head and neck; the thoracic vertebrae form an anchor for the ribs; the lumbar vertebrae help to support the body's weight and give stability; the sacrum supports the pelvis; and the coccyx forms the end of the spine.

Structures that make the spine flexible, below
The joints connecting the vertebrae, and the discs between them, allow the spine to move. There is only limited movement between adjacent vertebrae, but together the bones, discs and ligaments allow a range of movements in the spine as a whole.

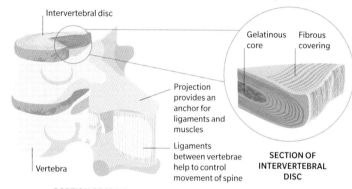

Cervical spine (7 bones)

Thoracic spine (12 bones)

Lumbar spine (5 bones)

Sacrum (5 fused bones)

Coccyx (4 fused bones)

Intervertebral disc

Gelatinous core

Fibrous covering

Projection provides an anchor for ligaments and muscles

Ligaments between vertebrae help to control movement of spine

Vertebra

PORTION OF SPINE

SECTION OF INTERVERTEBRAL DISC

THE SKULL

This bony structure protects the brain and the top of the spinal cord. It also supports the eyes and other facial structures. The skull is made up of several bones, most of which are fused at joints called sutures. Within the bone are air spaces (sinuses), which lighten the skull. The bones covering the brain form a dome called the cranium. Several other bones form the eye sockets, nose, cheeks and jaw.

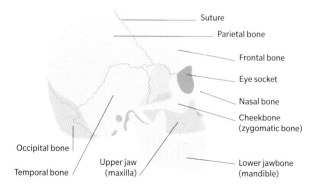

Suture

Parietal bone

Frontal bone

Eye socket

Nasal bone

Cheekbone (zygomatic bone)

Lower jawbone (mandible)

Occipital bone

Upper jaw (maxilla)

Temporal bone

Structures of the skull
This illustration shows the cranium and the main bones of the face. The lower jawbone (mandible) is the only bone in the skull that moves.

BONES, MUSCLES AND JOINTS

Bone is a living tissue containing calcium and phosphorus: minerals that make it hard, rigid and strong. From birth to early adulthood, bones grow by laying down calcium on the outside. They can also generate new tissue after injury.

Age and certain diseases can weaken bones, making them brittle and susceptible to breaking or crumbling, either under stress or spontaneously. Inherited problems, or bone disorders such as rickets, cancer and infections, can cause bones to become distorted and weakened. Damage to the bones during adolescence can also shorten a bone or impair movement. In older people, a disorder called osteoporosis can cause bones to lose density, making them brittle and prone to breaking.

Parts of a bone
Each bone is covered by a membrane (periosteum) that contains nerves and blood vessels. Under this membrane is a layer of compact, dense bone; at the core is spongy bone. In some bones, there is a cavity at the centre containing soft tissue called bone marrow.

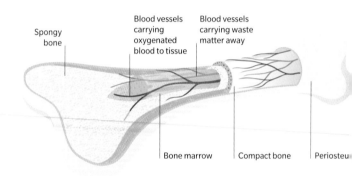

Spongy bone

Blood vessels carrying oxygenated blood to tissue

Blood vessels carrying waste matter away

Bone marrow

Compact bone

Periosteu

THE MUSCLES

Muscles cause various parts of the body to move. Skeletal (voluntary) muscles control movement and posture. They are attached to bones by bands of strong, fibrous tissue (tendons), and many operate in groups.

As one group of muscles contracts, its paired group relaxes. Involuntary muscles operate the internal organs, such as the heart, and work constantly, even while we are asleep. They are controlled by the autonomic nerves (p.145).

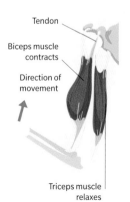

Tendon

Biceps muscle contracts

Direction of movement

Triceps muscle relaxes

Bending the arm
The biceps muscle, at the front of the upper arm, shortens (contracts), pulling the bones of the forearm upwards to bend the arm. At the same time, the triceps muscle relaxes and lengthens.

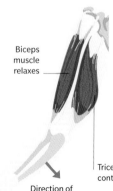

Biceps muscle relaxes

Direction of movement

Triceps muscle contracts

Straightening the arm
The triceps muscle, at the back of the upper arm, shortens (contracts) to pull down the bones of the forearm. The biceps muscle, at the front of the arm, relaxes.

THE JOINTS

A joint is where one bone meets another. In a few joints (immovable joints), the bone edges fit together or are fused. Immovable joints are found in the skull and pelvis. Most joints, however, are movable, and the bone ends are joined by fibrous tissue called ligaments, which form a capsule around the joint. The capsule lining (synovial membrane) produces fluid to lubricate the joint; the ends of the bones are also protected by smooth cartilage.

Muscles that move joints are attached to the bones by tendons. The degree and type of movement depends on the way the ends of the bones fit together, the strength of the ligaments that support the joints and the arrangement of the muscles.

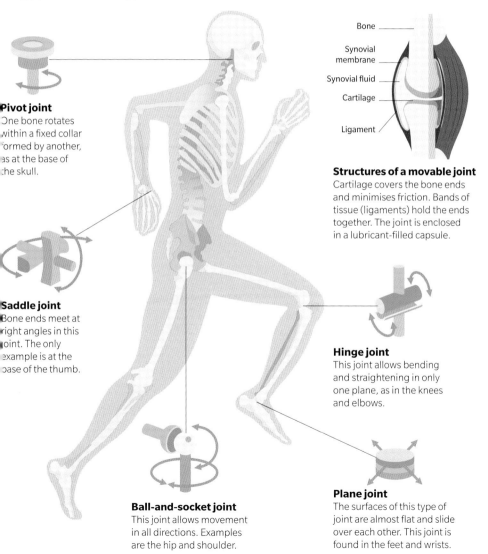

Pivot joint
One bone rotates within a fixed collar formed by another, as at the base of the skull.

Bone

Synovial membrane

Synovial fluid

Cartilage

Ligament

Structures of a movable joint
Cartilage covers the bone ends and minimises friction. Bands of tissue (ligaments) hold the ends together. The joint is enclosed in a lubricant-filled capsule.

Saddle joint
Bone ends meet at right angles in this joint. The only example is at the base of the thumb.

Hinge joint
This joint allows bending and straightening in only one plane, as in the knees and elbows.

Ball-and-socket joint
This joint allows movement in all directions. Examples are the hip and shoulder.

Plane joint
The surfaces of this type of joint are almost flat and slide over each other. This joint is found in the feet and wrists.

FRACTURES

A **break or crack in a bone** is called a fracture. Considerable force is needed to break a bone, unless it is diseased or old. However, bones that are still growing are supple and may split, bend or crack like a twig (greenstick fracture). A bone may break at the point where a heavy blow is received (direct force). Fractures may also result from a twist or a wrench (indirect force).

TYPES OF INJURY

Fractures can be closed, where the skin around a break remains intact, or open, in which one of the broken bone ends pierces the skin surface, or there is a wound at the fracture site (p.140). The latter carry a high risk of becoming infected.

A fracture can be described as stable when the broken bone ends do not move because they are not completely broken or they are impacted. Such injuries are common at the wrist, shoulder, ankle and hip. Usually, these fractures can be gently handled without further damage. In an unstable fracture, the broken bone ends can easily move. In a closed fracture the bones may be displaced (unstable), and there is a risk that they may damage blood vessels, nerves and organs around the injury, which can result in internal bleeding and the casualty may develop shock (pp.114–115). Unstable injuries can occur if the bone is broken and/or the ligaments are torn (ruptured). They should be handled carefully to prevent further damage.

WHAT TO DO FOR A CLOSED FRACTURE

1 **Advise the casualty to keep still.** Support the joints above and below the injured area with your hands, or ask a helper to do this, until it is immobilised with a sling or bandages.

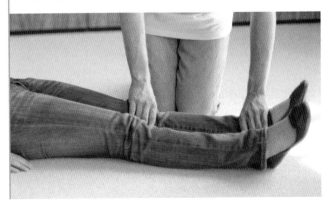

2 **Place padding around the injury** for extra support. Take or send the casualty to hospital. If they have an arm injury they may be transported by car; **call 999/112 for emergency help** for a leg injury.

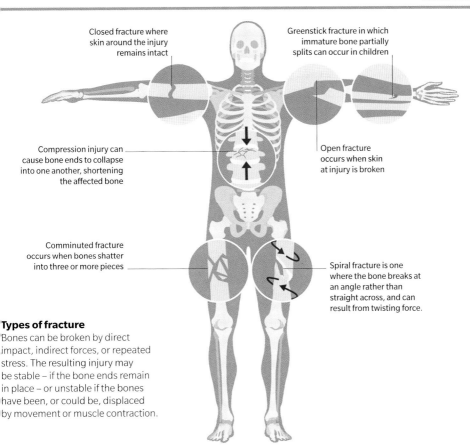

Closed fracture where skin around the injury remains intact

Greenstick fracture in which immature bone partially splits can occur in children

Compression injury can cause bone ends to collapse into one another, shortening the affected bone

Open fracture occurs when skin at injury is broken

Comminuted fracture occurs when bones shatter into three or more pieces

Spiral fracture is one where the bone breaks at an angle rather than straight across, and can result from twisting force.

Types of fracture

Bones can be broken by direct impact, indirect forces, or repeated stress. The resulting injury may be stable – if the bone ends remain in place – or unstable if the bones have been, or could be, displaced by movement or muscle contraction.

3 **For firmer support** and/or if removal to hospital is likely to be delayed, secure the injured part to an unaffected part of the body. For upper limb fractures, immobilise the arm with a sling (pp.255–257). For lower limb fractures, move the uninjured leg to the injured one and secure with broad- and narrow-fold bandages (p.253). Always tie the knots against the uninjured side.

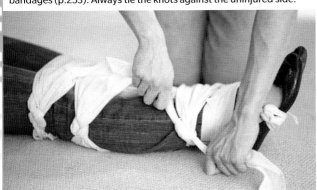

CAUTION

- Do not move the casualty until the injured part is secured and supported, unless they are in immediate danger.
- Do not allow the casualty to eat or drink because an anaesthetic may be needed.

4 **Check the circulation** beyond a bandage or sling (p.247) and re-check it every 10 minutes. If circulation is impaired loosen them and reapply. Treat for shock if necessary (pp.114–115), but if a leg is injured do not raise the legs. Monitor and record vital signs (pp.54–55) while waiting for help.

SEE ALSO Crush injury **p.120** | Internal bleeding **p.118** | Shock **pp.114–115** >> | **139**

⟪ FRACTURES

CAUTION

- Do not move the casualty until the injured part is secured and supported, unless they are in immediate danger.
- Do not allow the casualty to eat or drink because an anaesthetic may be needed.
- Do not press directly on a protruding bone end.

YOUR AIMS

- To prevent blood loss, movement and infection at the site of injury
- To arrange removal to hospital, with comfortable support during transport

SPECIAL CASE
PROTRUDING BONE

If a bone end is protruding, build up pads of clean, soft material around the bone, until you can bandage over it without pressing on the injury.

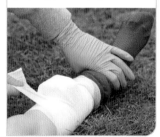

WHAT TO DO FOR AN OPEN FRACTURE

1 **Support the joints above and below the injury;** ask bystanders to do this if possible. Cover the wound with a sterile dressing or large, clean pad. Apply pressure around the injury to control bleeding (pp.116–117); be careful not to press on a protruding bone.

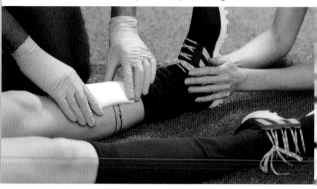

2 **Bandage the dressing in place.** Ask your helpers to raise the limb slightly so you can pass the bandage under the limb. Secure the ends of the bandage, keeping the knot or pin away from the site of the injury (inset). Check the circulation beyond the bandage (p.247) and re-check it every 10 minutes.

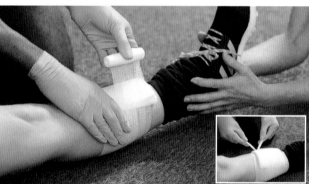

3 **Place padding around the injury** as for a closed fracture (pp.138–139). Take or send the casualty to hospital. A casualty with an arm injury may be transported by car; **call 999/112 for emergency help** for a leg injury. If the journey will be delayed, secure the injured limb to an unaffected part of the body (p.139).

4 **Treat the casualty for shock** (pp.114–115) if necessary. If a leg is injured do not raise the legs. Monitor and record vital signs (pp.54–55) while waiting for help to arrive.

DISLOCATED JOINT

This is a joint injury in which the bones are partially or completely pulled out of their normal position. Dislocation can be caused by a strong force that wrenches the bone into an abnormal position, or by violent muscle contraction. This very painful injury most often affects the shoulder, knee, jaw or joints in the thumbs or fingers. Dislocations may be associated with torn ligaments (pp.142–43), or with damage to the synovial membrane that lines the joint capsule (p.137).

Joint dislocation can have serious consequences. If vertebrae are dislocated, the spinal cord can be damaged. Dislocation of the shoulder or hip may damage the large nerves that supply the limbs and result in paralysis. A dislocation of any joint may also fracture the bones involved. It is difficult to distinguish a dislocation from a closed fracture (p.138). If you are in any doubt, treat the injury as a fracture.

RECOGNITION

- "Sickening", severe pain
- Inability to move the joint
- Swelling and bruising around the affected joint
- Shortening, bending or deformity of the area

YOUR AIMS

- To prevent movement at the injury site
- To arrange removal to hospital, with comfortable support during transport

WHAT TO DO

1 **Advise the casualty to keep still.** If, for example, they have a dislocated shoulder, help them to support the injured arm in the position they find most comfortable.

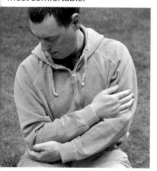

2 **Immobilise the injured arm** with a sling (pp.255–257) or use padding and/or broad-fold bandages (p.253) for a leg injury, whichever is most comfortable.

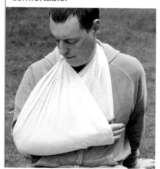

3 **For extra support** for an injured arm, secure the limb to the chest by tying a broad-fold bandage (p.253) right around the chest and the sling.

4 **Arrange to take or send** the casualty to hospital. Treat for shock if necessary (pp.114–115) ; if a leg is injured do not raise the legs. Monitor and record the vital signs (pp.54–55) while waiting for help.

5 **Check the circulation** beyond a bandage or sling (p.247) and re-check it every 10 minutes; loosen and reapply if necessary.

STRAINS AND SPRAINS

The softer structures around bones and joints – the ligaments that hold the bones together at a joint and the muscles and tendons which move the bones – can be injured in many ways. Injuries to these soft tissues are commonly called strains and sprains. They occur when the tissues are overstretched and partially or completely torn (ruptured) by violent or sudden movements. For this reason, strains and sprains are frequently associated with sporting activities.

Strains and sprains should be treated initially using the following principles:

- Rest the injured part.
- Place a cold compress such as an ice pack or a cold pad (p.245) on the injury.
- Provide comfortable support and elevate the injured part.

This may be sufficient to relieve the symptoms, but if you are in any doubt as to the severity of the injury, treat it as a fracture (pp.138–140).

TYPES OF INJURY

Muscles and tendons may be strained, ruptured or bruised. A strain occurs when the muscle is overstretched; it may be partially torn, often at the junction between the muscle and the tendon that joins it to a bone. In a rupture, a muscle or tendon is torn completely; this may occur in the main bulk of the muscle or in the tendon. Deep bruising can be extensive in parts of the body where there is a large bulk of muscle. Injuries in these areas are usually accompanied by bleeding into the surrounding tissues, which can lead to pain, swelling and bruising.

A sprain occurs when ligaments – the fibrous cords that connect bones at a joint – are torn, partially or completely. The ankle is the most commonly affected part of the body. Sprains are often caused by a sudden or unexpected wrenching motion that pulls the bones in the joint too far apart and tears the surrounding tissues.

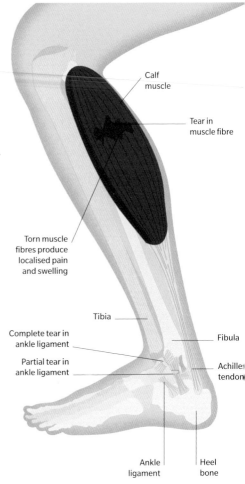

Calf muscle

Tear in muscle fibre

Torn muscle fibres produce localised pain and swelling

Tibia

Complete tear in ankle ligament

Partial tear in ankle ligament

Fibula

Achilles tendon

Ankle ligament

Heel bone

Muscle and tendon strain
A sprain is the stretching or tearing of a ligament, while a strain is the stretching or tearing of a muscle or a tendon, which connects the muscle to bone. Muscle strains and ligament sprains occur when falling or twisting causes tissues to stretch or tear. This leads to painful spasms, swelling, and can result in temporary stiffness and reduced mobility.

WHAT TO DO

1 Help the casualty to sit or lie down. Support the injured part in a comfortable position, preferably raised.

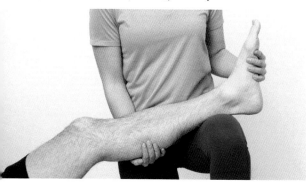

RECOGNITION

There may be:
- Pain and tenderness
- Difficulty in moving the injured part, especially if it is a joint
- Swelling and bruising in the area

YOUR AIMS

- To reduce swelling and pain
- To obtain medical help if necessary

2 **Cool the area** by applying a cold compress, such as an ice pack or cold pad (p.245), to the injury. This helps to reduce swelling, bruising and pain.

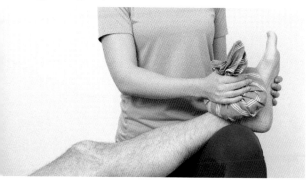

3 **Support the injured part in a raised position** to help minimise bruising and swelling in the area. Leave the cold compress in place over the injury for no more than 20 minutes.

4 **If the pain is severe,** or the casualty is unable to use the injured part, arrange to take or send them to hospital. Otherwise, advise the casualty to rest the injury and to seek medical advice if necessary.

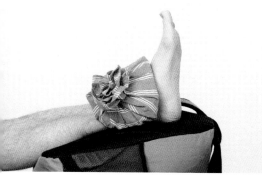

THE BRAIN AND NERVES

The nervous system is the body's information-gathering, storage and control system. It consists of a central processing unit – the brain – and a network of nerve cells and fibres.

There are two main parts to the nervous system: the central nervous system, consisting of the brain and spinal cord, and the peripheral nervous system, which consists of all the nerves that connect the brain and the spinal cord to the rest of the body. In addition, the autonomic (involuntary) nervous system controls body functions such as digestion, heart rate and breathing. The central nervous system receives and analyses information from all parts of the body. The nerves carry messages, in the form of high-speed electrical impulses, between the brain and the rest of the nervous system.

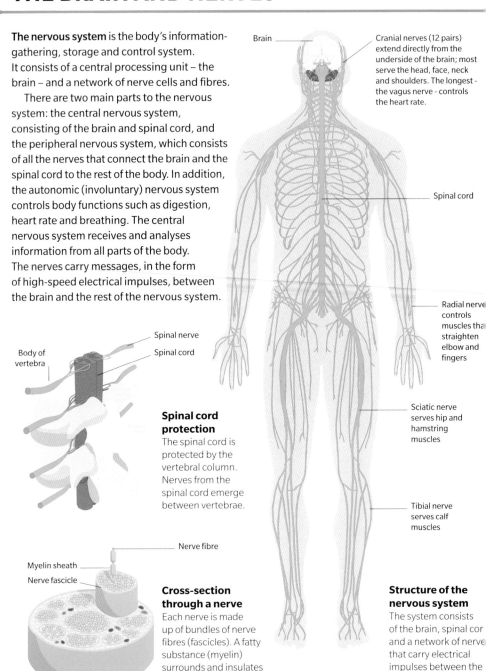

Brain

Cranial nerves (12 pairs) extend directly from the underside of the brain; most serve the head, face, neck and shoulders. The longest - the vagus nerve - controls the heart rate.

Spinal cord

Radial nerve controls muscles that straighten elbow and fingers

Sciatic nerve serves hip and hamstring muscles

Tibial nerve serves calf muscles

Spinal nerve

Spinal cord

Body of vertebra

Spinal cord protection
The spinal cord is protected by the vertebral column. Nerves from the spinal cord emerge between vertebrae.

Nerve fibre

Myelin sheath

Nerve fascicle

Cross-section through a nerve
Each nerve is made up of bundles of nerve fibres (fascicles). A fatty substance (myelin) surrounds and insulates larger nerve fibres.

Structure of the nervous system
The system consists of the brain, spinal cord and a network of nerves that carry electrical impulses between the brain and the body.

THE BRAIN AND SPINAL CORD

Together the brain and spinal cord make up the central nervous system (CNS). This system contains billions of interconnected nerve cells (neurons) and is enclosed by three membranes called meninges. A clear fluid called cerebrospinal fluid flows around the brain and spinal cord. It functions as a shock absorber, provides oxygen and nutrients and removes waste products.

The brain has three main structures: the cerebrum, which is concerned with thought, sensation and conscious movement; the cerebellum, which coordinates movement, balance and posture; and the brain stem, which controls basic functions such as breathing. The main function of the spinal cord is to convey signals between the brain and the peripheral nervous system (below).

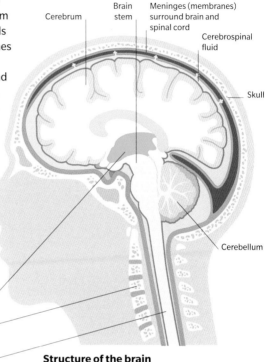

Cerebrum

Brain stem

Meninges (membranes) surround brain and spinal cord

Cerebrospinal fluid

Skull

Cerebellum

Mid-brain

Vertebral column protects delicate spinal cord

Spinal cord extends from brain stem to lower end of spine

Structure of the brain
The brain is enclosed within the skull. It has three main parts: the cerebrum, which has an outer layer called the cortex; the cerebellum; and the brain stem.

PERIPHERAL NERVES

The peripheral nervous system consists of two sets of paired nerves – the cranial and spinal nerves – which connect the CNS to the body.

The cranial nerves emerge in 12 pairs from the underside of the brain. The 31 pairs of spinal nerves branch off at intervals from the spinal cord, passing into the rest of the body. Nerves comprise bundles of nerve fibres that can relay both incoming (sensory) and outgoing (motor) signals.

AUTONOMIC NERVES

Some of the cranial nerves, and several small spinal nerves, work together as the autonomic nervous system. This system is concerned with vital body functions such as heart rate and breathing. The system's two parts – the sympathetic and parasympathetic systems – counterbalance each other. The sympathetic nerves prepare the body for action by releasing hormones that raise the heart rate and reduce the blood flow to the skin and intestines. The parasympathetic nerves release hormones with the opposite, calming, effect.

HEAD INJURY

ASSESSING THE LEVEL OF RESPONSE

Assess a casualty's level of response at regular intervals. Make a note of your findings at each assessment, paying particular attention to any change – the casualty's condition may improve or deteriorate while you are looking after them.

- **Is the casualty alert?** Are their eyes open and do they respond to questions?
- **Does the casualty respond to your voice?** Can the casualty answer simple questions and obey commands?
- **Does the casualty respond to pain?** Do they open their eyes, move or groan if you pinch their earlobe?
- **Is the casualty not responding** to any stimulus?

Head injuries are common. They are potentially serious because they can lead to damage to the brain. There may also be injuries to the spine in the neck, scalp wounds and/or a skull fracture.

If a casualty has sustained a minor injury such as a bruise or scalp wound, they are likely to be responding normally. If they have suffered a more serious blow to the head, such as in a sporting impact, responsiveness may be temporarily impaired.

The brain lies inside the skull, cushioned by fluid and can therefore be shaken by a blow to the head. This is called concussion and it may result in a temporary period of unresponsiveness. The casualty may be confused, but this lasts only a short time and is followed by a full recovery.

If a casualty has suffered a severe blow to the head, this may cause bleeding and swelling inside the skull that can press on the brain (compression). This is a serious condition. The pressure can rise immediately after the impact or it may develop a few hours or even days later. The severity of the head injury is related to the mechanism of injury and its impact on the casualty's head. A serious head injury is likely after a high-speed motor collision or a fall from a height.

Causes of head injury

The brain can be literally "shaken" inside the skull with concussion (below). Injury that results in bleeding can cause pressure to build up inside the skull and damage the tissues of the brain (below right).

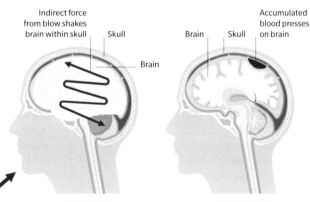

Indirect force from blow shakes brain within skull · Skull · Brain

Accumulated blood presses on brain · Brain · Skull

Direction of force

CONCUSSION

COMPRESSION

WHAT TO DO

1 Sit the casualty down. Gently place a cold compress (p.245) against the injury and ask the casualty to hold it in place. Carry out an assessment of the casualty's level of response (box, opposite). Treat a scalp wound by applying direct pressure to the wound (p.124).

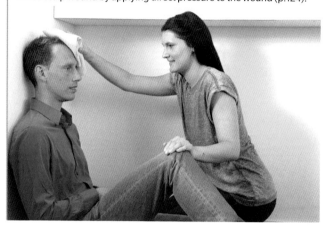

2 Regularly monitor and record the casualty's vital signs (pp.54–55). Watch especially for any changes in their level of response.

3 When the casualty has recovered, ask a responsible person to look after them.

4 If a casualty's injury is the result of a sporting incident, do not allow them to return to the sport until they have been fully assessed by a medical practitioner.

5 Advise the casualty to seek medical help if they develop signs and symptoms of a worsening head injury (see CAUTION, opposite), or if ANY of the following apply:
They are over 65 years of age.
They have had previous brain surgery.
They are taking anti-coagulant (anti-clotting) medication.
The head injury is accompanied by drug or alcohol intoxication.
There is no responsible person to look after them.

SPECIAL CASE SEVERE HEAD INJURY

Call 999 / 112 for emergency help – tell the call handler that you suspect head injury. Maintain an open and clear airway, leaving the casualty in the position you found them – try not to move them because of the additional risk of spinal injury (pp.160–161). If this is not possible, use the jaw-thrust method to open the airway (p.160). Regularly monitor and record vital signs (pp.54–55) while waiting for help to arrive; watch especially for changes in the level of response.

SEE ALSO Facial injury **p.148** | Scalp and head wounds **p.124** | The unresponsive casualty **pp.56–89** | **147**

RECOGNITION

There may be:
- Brief period of impaired response or unresponsiveness
- Scalp wound
- Dizziness or nausea
- Loss of memory of events at the time of, or immediately preceding the injury
- Mild generalised headache
- Confusion

For severe head injury there may also be:
- History of a severe blow to the head
- Deteriorating level of response
- Loss of responsiveness
- Leakage of blood or blood-stained watery fluid from the ear or nose
- Unequal pupil size

YOUR AIMS

- To place the casualty in the care of a responsible person
- To obtain medical help if necessary; for serious head injury arrange urgent removal to hospital

FACIAL INJURY

CAUTION

- Never place a bandage around the lower part of the face or lower jaw in case the casualty vomits or has difficulty breathing.
- Do not allow the casualty to eat or drink because an anaesthetic may be needed.
- If the casualty becomes unresponsive, open the airway and check breathing (The unresponsive casualty, pp.56–89).
- If an unresponsive casualty is breathing, place them in the recovery position (pp.66–67) with their injured side downwards so that blood or other body fluids can drain away. Place soft padding under the head. Be aware of the risk of neck (spinal) injury.

Fractures of facial bones are usually due to hard impacts. Serious facial fractures may appear frightening. There may be distortion of the eye sockets, general swelling and bruising, as well as bleeding from displaced tissues or from the nose and mouth. The main danger with any facial fracture is that blood, saliva or swollen tissue may obstruct the casualty's airway and cause breathing difficulties.

When you are examining a casualty with a facial injury, assume that there is damage to the skull, brain or neck. There is also a danger that you may misinterpret the symptoms of a facial fracture as a black eye.

WHAT TO DO

1 Help the casualty to sit down and make sure the airway is open and clear.

2 Ask the casualty to spit out any blood, displaced teeth or dentures from their mouth. Keep any teeth to send to hospital with them (p.127).

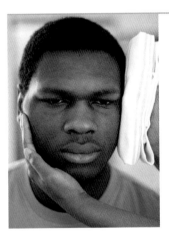

3 Gently place a cold compress (p.245) against the casualty's face to help reduce pain and minimise swelling; they may be able to hold it in place themselves. Treat for shock (pp.114–115) if necessary.

4 Call 999 / 112 for emergency help.

5 Monitor and record the casualty's vital signs (pp.54–55) while waiting for help to arrive.

RECOGNITION

There may be:

- Pain around the affected area; if the jaw is injured, difficulty speaking, chewing or swallowing
- Difficulty breathing
- Swelling and distortion of the face
- Bruising and/or a black eye
- Blood or bloodstained watery fluid leaking from the nose or ear

YOUR AIMS

- To keep the airway open
- To minimise pain and swelling
- To arrange urgent removal to hospital

SEE ALSO Head injury **pp.146–147** | Knocked-out adult tooth **p.127** | Shock **pp.114–115** | Spinal injury **pp.159–161**
The unresponsive casualty **pp.56–89**

LOWER JAW INJURY

Jaw fractures are usually the result of direct force, such as a heavy blow to the chin. In some situations, a blow to one side of the jaw produces indirect force, which causes a fracture on the other side of the face. A fall on to the point of the chin can fracture the jaw on both sides. The lower jaw may also be dislocated by a blow to the face, or is sometimes dislocated by yawning.

If the face is seriously injured, with the jaw fractured in more than one place, treat as for a facial injury (opposite).

RECOGNITION

There may be:

- Difficulty speaking, swallowing and moving the jaw
- Pain and nausea when moving the jaw
- Displaced or loose teeth and dribbling from the mouth
- Swelling and bruising inside and outside the mouth

WHAT TO DO

1 If the casualty is not seriously injured, help them to sit with their head forward to allow fluids to drain from their mouth. Encourage them to spit out any loose teeth, and keep them to send to hospital with the casualty (p.127).

2 Give the casualty a soft pad to hold firmly against their jaw in order to support it.

3 Arrange to take or send the casualty to hospital. Keep their jaw supported throughout.

YOUR AIMS

- To protect the airway
- To arrange transport to hospital

CHEEKBONE AND NOSE INJURY

Fractures of the cheekbone and nose are usually the result of direct blows to the face. Swollen facial tissues are likely to cause discomfort, and the air passages in the nose may become blocked, making breathing difficult. These injuries should always be examined in hospital.

CAUTION

- If there is blood or bloodstained watery fluid leaking from the casualty's nose, treat the casualty as for a head injury (pp.146–147).
- Do not allow the casualty to eat or drink because an anaesthetic may be needed.

WHAT TO DO

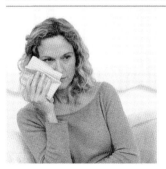

1 Gently place a cold compress (p.245) against the injured area to help reduce pain and minimise swelling. The casualty may be able to hold the compress in place themselves.

2 If the casualty has a nosebleed, try to pinch the nose to stop the bleeding (p.126). Arrange to take or send the casualty to hospital.

RECOGNITION

There may be:

- Pain, swelling and bruising
- Obvious wound or bleeding from the nose or mouth

YOUR AIMS

- To minimise pain and swelling
- To arrange transport to hospital

COLLAR BONE INJURY

RECOGNITION

There may be:

- Pain and tenderness, increased by movement
- Swelling and deformity of the shoulder
- Attempts by the casualty to relax muscles and relieve pain; they may support their injured arm at the elbow, and incline their head towards their injured side

The collar bones (clavicles) form "struts" between the shoulder blades and the top of the breastbone to help support the arms. It is rare for a collar bone to be broken by a direct blow. Usually, a fracture results from an indirect force transmitted from an impact at the shoulder or passing along the arm, for example, from a fall onto an outstretched arm.

Collar bone fractures often occur in young people as a result of sports activities. The broken ends of the collar bone may be displaced, causing swelling and bleeding in the surrounding tissues as well as distortion of the shoulder.

YOUR AIMS

- To immobilise the injured shoulder and arm
- To arrange transport to hospital

WHAT TO DO

1 Help the casualty to sit down. Gently place the injured arm across their body in the position that they find most comfortable. Ask the casualty to support the elbow on the injured side with their other hand, or help them to do it.

2 Support the arm on the affected side with an arm sling (p.255). Make sure the knot is clear of the site of injury.

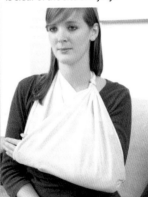

3 For extra support, secure the arm to the chest by tying a broad-fold bandage (p.253) around the chest and the sling. Once the arm is supported the casualty will be more comfortable.

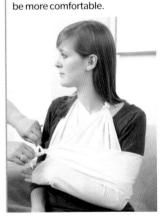

4 Arrange to take or send the casualty to hospital in the position they find most comfortable.

SHOULDER INJURY

A fall on to the shoulder or an outstretched arm, or a wrenching force may pull the head of the upper arm bone (humerus) out of the joint socket – dislocation of the shoulder. At the same time, ligaments around the shoulder joint may be torn. This injury can be extremely painful. Some people experience repeated dislocations and may need surgery to strengthen the shoulder.

A fall onto the point of the shoulder may damage the ligaments bracing the collar bone at the shoulder. Other shoulder injuries include damage to the joint capsule and to the tendons around the shoulder; these injuries tend to be common in older people. To treat a shoulder sprain, follow the procedure described for strains and sprains – rest the affected part, cool the injury with a cold compress (p.245), provide comfortable support and elevate the injured area (pp.142–143).

CAUTION

- Do not attempt to replace a dislocated bone into its socket.
- Do not allow the casualty to eat or drink because an anaesthetic may be needed.

RECOGNITION

There may be:

- Severe pain, increased by movement; the pain may make the casualty reluctant to move
- Attempts by the casualty to relieve pain by supporting the arm and inclining the head to the injured side
- A flat, angular look to the shoulder

YOUR AIMS

- To support and immobilise the injured limb
- To arrange transport to hospital

WHAT TO DO

1 Help the casualty to sit down. Gently place the arm on the injured side across the body in the position that is most comfortable. Ask the casualty to support the elbow on the injured side, or help them to do it.

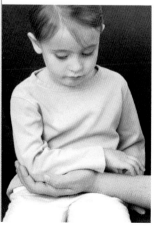

2 Support the arm on the injured side with an arm sling (p.255).

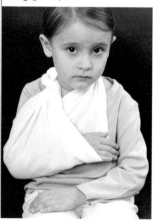

3 For extra support if necessary, secure the arm to the chest by tying a broad-fold bandage (p.253) around the chest and the sling.

4 Arrange to take or send the casualty to hospital in the position they find most comfortable.

UPPER ARM INJURY

CAUTION

- Do not allow the casualty to eat or drink because an anaesthetic may be needed.

The most serious form of upper arm injury is a fracture of the long bone in the upper arm (humerus). The bone may be fractured across the centre by a direct blow. However, it is much more common, especially in elderly people, for the arm bone to break at the shoulder end, usually in a fall.

A fracture at the top of the bone is often a stable injury (pp.138–139), as the broken bone ends stay in place. For this reason, it may not be immediately apparent that the bone is broken, although the arm is likely to be painful. There is a possibility that the casualty will cope with the pain and leave the fracture untreated for some time.

RECOGNITION

There may be:
- Pain, increased by movement
- Tenderness and deformity over the site of a fracture
- Rapid swelling
- Bruising, which may develop more slowly

YOUR AIMS

- To immobilise the arm
- To arrange transport to hospital

WHAT TO DO

1 **Help the casualty to sit** down. Remove all jewellery such as bracelets, rings and watches. Gently place the forearm horizontally across their body in the position that is most comfortable. Ask them to support their elbow if possible.

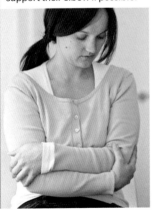

2 **Slide a triangular bandage** in position between the arm and the chest, ready to make an arm sling (p.255). Place soft padding between the injured arm and the body, then support the arm and its padding in an arm sling.

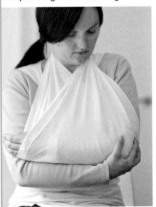

3 **For extra support**, or if the journey to hospital is prolonged, secure the arm by tying a broad-fold bandage (p.253) around the chest and over the sling; make sure that the broad-fold bandage is below the fracture site.

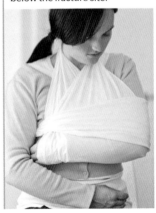

4 **Arrange to take or send** the casualty to hospital.

ELBOW INJURY

Fractures or dislocations at the elbow usually result from a fall on to the hand. Children often fracture the upper arm bone just above the elbow. This is an unstable fracture (p.138), and the bone ends may damage blood vessels. Circulation in the arm needs to be checked regularly. In any elbow injury, the elbow will be stiff and difficult to straighten. Never try to force a casualty to bend it.

WHAT TO DO

1 If the elbow can be bent, treat as for upper arm injury, opposite. Remove all jewellery such as bracelets, rings and watches.

2 If the casualty cannot bend their arm, help them to sit down. Place padding, such as a towel, around the elbow for comfort and support.

3 Secure the arm in the most comfortable position for the casualty using broad-fold bandages. Keep the bandages clear of the fracture site.

RECOGNITION

There may be:
- Pain, increased by movement
- Tenderness over the site of a fracture
- Swelling, bruising and deformity
- Fixed elbow

YOUR AIMS
- To immobilise the arm without further injury to the joint
- To arrange transport to hospital

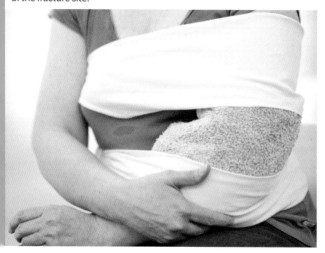

4 Arrange to take or send the casualty to hospital.

5 Check the wrist pulse (p.55) in the injured arm every 10 minutes until they receive medical help. If you cannot feel a pulse, gently undo the bandages and straighten the arm until the pulse returns. Support the arm in this position.

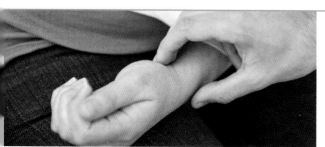

FOREARM AND WRIST INJURIES

RECOGNITION

There may be:

- Pain, increased by movement
- Swelling, bruising and deformity
- Possible bleeding with an open fracture

YOUR AIMS

- To immobilise the arm
- To arrange transport to hospital

The bones of the forearm (radius and ulna) can be fractured by an impact such as a heavy blow or a fall. As the bones have little fleshy covering, the broken ends may pierce the skin, producing an open fracture (p.138 and p.140).

A fall onto an outstretched hand can result in a fracture of the wrist. This is called a Colles fracture and commonly occurs in elderly people.

The wrist joint is rarely dislocated, but is often sprained. It can be difficult to distinguish between a sprain and a fracture, especially if the tiny scaphoid bone (at the base of the thumb) is injured. If you are in any doubt about the injury always treat as a fracture.

WHAT TO DO

1 **Ask the casualty to sit** down. Steady and support the injured forearm and place it across the casualty's body; ask them to support it if they can. Remove any jewellery. Expose and treat any wound.

2 **Slide a triangular bandage** in position between the arm and the chest, ready to make an arm sling (p.255). Surround the forearm in soft padding.

3 **Support the arm** and the padding with an arm sling; make sure the knot is tied on the injured side.

4 **For extra support,** or if the journey to hospital is likely to be prolonged, secure the arm to the body by tying a broad-fold bandage (p.253) over the sling and body. Position the bandage as close to the elbow as you can. Arrange to take or send the casualty to hospital.

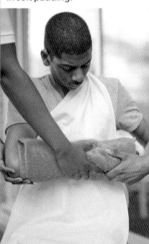

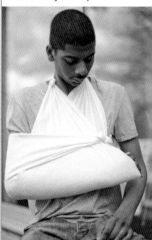

HAND AND FINGER INJURIES

he bones and joints in the hand can suffer various types
f injury, such as fractures, cuts and bruising. Minor fractures are
sually caused by direct force. A fracture of the knuckle often
esults from a punch.

Multiple fractures, affecting many or all of the bones in the
and, are usually caused by crushing injuries. The fractures
nay be open, with severe bleeding and swelling, needing
mmediate first aid treatment. The joints in the fingers or
humb are sometimes dislocated or sprained as a result of
 casualty falling on to their hand.

Always compare the suspected fractured hand with the
ninjured hand because finger fractures result in deformities
hat may not be immediately obvious.

RECOGNITION

There may be:

- Pain, increased by movement
- Swelling, bruising and deformity
- Possible bleeding with an open fracture

YOUR AIMS

- To elevate the hand and immobilise it
- To arrange transport to hospital

WHAT TO DO

1 **Help the casualty to sit** down and ask them to raise and support the affected wrist and hand; help them if necessary. Treat any bleeding and loosely cover the wound with a sterile dressing or large clean pad.

2 **Remove any rings** before the hand begins to swell, and keep the hand raised to minimise swelling. Wrap the casualty's hand in soft padding for extra protection.

3 **Gently support the** affected arm across the casualty's body by placing it in an elevation sling (p.256).

4 **For extra support,** or if the journey to hospital is likely to be prolonged, secure the arm by tying a broad-fold bandage (p.253) around the chest and over the sling; keep it away from the injury. Arrange to take or send the casualty to hospital.

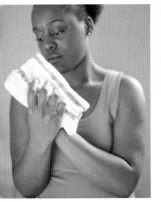

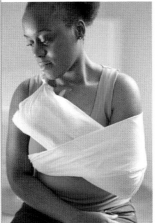

RIB INJURY

One or more ribs can be fractured by direct force to the chest from a blow or a fall, or by a crush injury (p.120). If there is a wound over the fracture, or if a broken rib pierces a lung, the casualty's breathing may be seriously impaired.

An injury to the chest can cause an area of fractured ribs to become detached from the rest of the chest wall, producing what is called a "flail-chest" injury. The detached area moves inwards when the casualty breathes in, and outwards as they breathe out. This "paradoxical" breathing causes severe breathing difficulties.

Fractures of the lower ribs may injure internal organs such as the liver and spleen, and may cause internal bleeding.

RECOGNITION

- Pain at the site of injury
- Pain on taking a deep breath
- Bruising, swelling or a wound at the fracture site
- Shallow breathing
- Paradoxical chest movement
- Signs of internal bleeding (p.118) and shock (pp.114–115)

YOUR AIMS

- To support the chest wall
- To arrange transport to hospital

WHAT TO DO

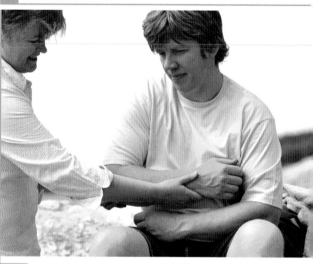

1 Help the casualty to sit down and ask them to support their arm on the injured side. For extra support if necessary, place the arm on the injured side in a sling (pp.255–257).

2 Arrange to take or send the casualty to hospital.

ELVIC INJURY

njuries to the pelvis are usually caused by forces such as a car rash, a fall from a height or by crushing. These incidents can esult in a stable or unstable fracture of the pelvis. An unstable racture can be life-threatening.

A fracture of the pelvic bones may also be complicated by njury to the tissues and organs in the pelvis, such as the bladder nd the urinary passages. The bleeding from large organs and lood vessels in the pelvis may be severe and can lead to shock.

WHAT TO DO

1 **Help the casualty to lie** down on their back with head flat/low to minimise shock. Keep their legs straight and flat.

2 **Place padding** between the bony points of their knees and ankles. Immobilise the legs by bandaging them together with folded triangular bandages (p.253); secure the feet and ankles with a narrow-fold bandage (1) tied in a figure of eight, and the knees with a broad-fold bandage (2).

3 **Call 999/112 for emergency help.** Treat the casualty for shock (pp.114–115). Do not raise their legs.

4 **Monitor and record** the casualty's vital signs (pp.54–55) while waiting for help to arrive.

RECOGNITION

There may be:

- An inability to walk or even stand, although the legs appear uninjured
- Pain and tenderness in the region of the hip, groin or back, which increases with movement
- Difficulty or pain passing urine, and bloodstained clothing
- Signs of shock and internal bleeding

YOUR AIMS

- To minimise the risk of shock
- To arrange urgent removal to hospital

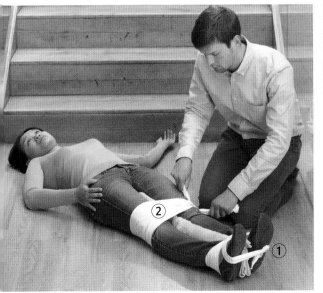

BACK PAIN

Lower back pain is common and most adults may experience it at some point in their lives. It may be acute (sudden onset) or chronic (long term). It is usually caused by age-related degenerative changes or results from minor injury affecting muscles, ligaments, vertebrae, discs or nerves. It may be the result of heavy manual work, a fall or a turning or twisting movement. Serious conditions causing back pain are rare and beyond the scope of first aid.

Most instances are simple backache, often in the lower back, in people aged 20–55 who are otherwise well. In a small number of casualties, the pain may extend down one leg. This is called sciatica and is caused by pressure on the nerve root (a so-called "trapped nerve").

Spine injuries in those under 20 or over 55, or that result from a more serious injury, require investigation and treatment (Spinal injury, opposite and pp.160–161).

RECOGNITION

- Pain in the lower back following lifting or manual work
- Possible pain radiating down the back of one leg with numbness or tingling in the affected leg – sciatica

YOUR AIM

- To relieve pain

WHAT TO DO

1 **Advise the casualty to stay active** to mobilise the injured area. Encourage them to return to normal activity as soon as possible.

2 **An adult casualty may take** the recommended dose of their own painkillers.

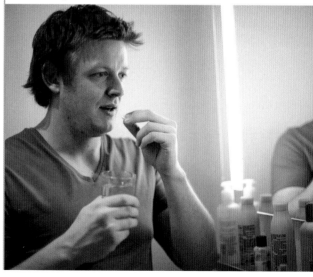

3 **Advise the casualty** to seek medical advice if necessary.

SPINAL INJURY

Injuries to the spine can involve one or more parts of the back and/or neck: the bones (vertebrae), the discs of tissue that separate the vertebrae, the surrounding muscles and ligaments, or the spinal cord and the nerves that branch off from it.

The most serious risk associated with spinal injury is damage to the spinal cord. Such damage can cause loss of power and/or sensation below the injured area. The spinal cord or nerve roots can suffer temporary damage if they are pinched by displaced or dislocated discs, or by fragments of broken bone. If the cord is partly or completely severed, damage may be permanent.

CAUSES OF SPINAL INJURY

The most important indicator is the mechanism of the injury. Suspect spinal injury if abnormal forces have been exerted on the back or neck, and particularly if a casualty complains of any changes in sensation or loss of movement. If the incident involved violent forward or backward bending, or twisting of the spine, you must assume that the casualty has a spinal injury. You must take particular care to avoid unnecessary movement of the head, neck and spine at all times.

Although spinal cord injury may occur without any damage to the vertebrae, spinal fracture greatly increases the risk. The areas that are most vulnerable are the bones in the neck and those in the lower back.

Any of the following incidents should alert you to the possibility of a spinal injury:

- **Falling from a height,** such as a ladder.
- **Falling awkwardly,** for instance, while doing gymnastics or trampolining.
- **Diving into a shallow pool** and hitting the bottom.
- **Falling from a horse or motorbike.**
- **Collapsed rugby scrum.**
- **Sudden deceleration** in a motor vehicle.
- **A heavy object falling across the back.**
- **Injury to the head or the face.**

RECOGNITION

When the vertebrae are damaged, there may be:

- Pain in the neck or back at the injury site. This may be masked by other, more painful, injuries
- Step, irregularity or twist in the normal curve of the spine
- Tenderness and/or bruising in the skin over the spine

When the spinal cord is damaged, there may be:

- Loss of control over limbs – movement may be weak or absent
- Loss of sensation, or abnormal sensations such as burning or tingling; a casualty may tell you that their limbs feel stiff, heavy or clumsy
- Loss of bladder and/or bowel control
- Breathing difficulties

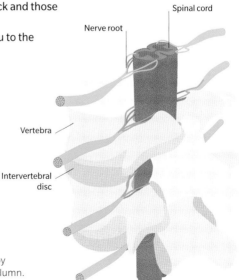

Spinal cord

Nerve root

Vertebra

Intervertebral disc

Spinal cord protection
The spinal cord is protected by the bony vertebral (spinal) column. Nerves branching from the cord emerge between adjacent vertebrae.

continued ≫

SPINAL INJURY

YOUR AIMS

- To prevent further spinal damage
- To arrange urgent removal to hospital

WHAT TO DO FOR A RESPONSIVE CASUALTY

1 **Reassure the casualty.** Advise them not to move, but to maintain the head and neck in a stable position. **Call 999/112 for emergency help**, or ask a helper to do this.

2 **If the casualty cannot maintain a stable head position**, kneel or lie behind their head. Rest your elbows on the ground or on your knees to keep your arms steady. Grasp the sides of the casualty's head. Spread your fingers so that you do not cover their ears – they need to be able to hear you. Steady and support the casualty's head in this neutral position, in which the head, neck and spine are aligned.

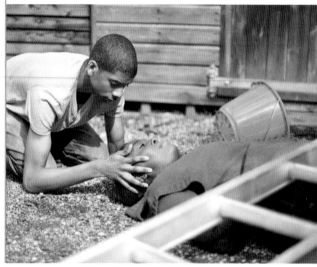

3 Ask a helper to place rolled-up blankets, towels or items of clothing on either side of the casualty's head while you keep their head in the neutral position. Continue to support the casualty's head until emergency services take over, no matter how long this may be.

4 Get your helper to monitor and record vital signs (pp.54–55) while waiting for help to arrive.

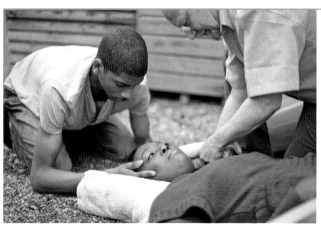

WHAT TO DO FOR AN UNRESPONSIVE CASUALTY

1 **Kneel or lie behind the casualty's head.** Rest your elbows on the ground or on your knees to keep your arms steady. Grasp the sides of the casualty's head and support it so that their head, trunk and legs are in a straight line.

2 **Open the casualty's airway** using the jaw-thrust technique. Place your fingertips at the angles of the casualty's jaw. Gently lift the jaw to open the airway. Take care not to tilt the casualty's neck.

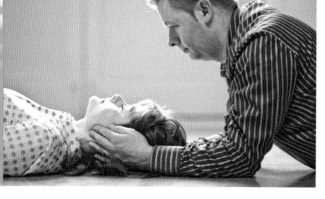

CAUTION

- If the casualty has to be moved and you have help, use the log-roll technique (below).
- If you are alone and you need to leave the casualty to call for emergency help, and the casualty is unable to maintain an open airway, you should place them in the recovery position (pp.66–67) before you leave them.

YOUR AIMS

- To maintain an open airway
- To begin CPR if necessary
- To prevent further spinal damage
- To arrange urgent removal to hospital

3 **Check the casualty's breathing.** If they are breathing, continue to support their head. **Call 999/112 for emergency help** or ask a helper to do this.

4 **If the casualty is not breathing,** begin CPR (pp.68–69). If you need to turn the casualty, use the log-roll technique (below).

5 **Monitor and record** the casualty's vital signs (pp.54–55) while waiting for help to arrive.

SPECIAL CASE LOG-ROLL TECHNIQUE

This technique should be used to turn a casualty with a spinal injury. While you support the casualty's head and neck, ask your helpers to straighten the limbs gently. Position three people along one side to pull the casualty towards them, and two on the other to guide them forwards. The person at the legs should place their hands under the furthest leg, while the middle helper supports the leg and hip. Direct your helpers to roll the casualty, keeping their head, trunk and legs in a straight line at all times – the upper leg should be supported in a slightly raised position to keep the spine straight.

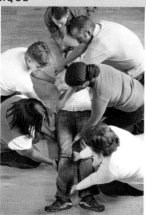

POSITIONING FIRST AIDERS

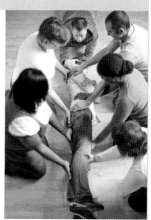

TURNING CASUALTY

HIP AND THIGH INJURIES

The most severe injury of the thigh bone (femur) is a fracture. It takes a considerable force, such as a car crash or a fall from a height, to fracture the shaft of the femur. This is a serious injury because the broken bone ends can pierce major blood vessels, causing severe blood loss, and shock may result.

Fracture of the neck of the femur is common in elderly people, particularly women, whose bones become less dense and more brittle with age (osteoporosis). When the bone ends are impacted this can be a stable injury and a casualty may be able to walk for some time before the fracture is identified. Less commonly, the hip joint can become dislocated, particularly in those who have had hip replacement surgery.

RECOGNITION

There may be:

- Pain at the site of the injury
- An inability to walk
- Signs of shock
- Shortening of the leg and turning outwards of the knee and foot

YOUR AIMS

- To immobilise the limb
- To arrange urgent removal to hospital

SPECIAL CASE PREPARING A CASUALTY FOR A DELAYED OUTDOOR RESCUE

If the injury occurs while you are outdoors in a remote rural location, for example, hill walking, there may be a lengthy wait for the emergency services to arrive and helicopter evacuation may be necessary. Call 999/112 for emergency help and remain with the casualty. Protect the casualty from the cold to prevent hypothermia (pp.190–191). If possible, place a layer of dry insulating material such as heather, bracken or spare, preferably waterproof, clothing beneath them; do not use your clothing. Immobilise the leg by securing to the uninjured one as described opposite. Cover the casualty with blankets or spare outer garments (not yours) – make sure to cover their head – and wrap them in a foil or plastic survival bag if available. Monitor the casualty's vital signs (pp.54–55) while waiting for help to arrive.

It may be of benefit to incorporate a splint such as a walking pole or stick or a fence post that extends from the hip to the foot for additional support. Place the splint on the outer side of the injured limb. Insert padding between the casualty's legs and between the splint and the injured leg. Secure both to the uninjured leg with bandages as opposite.

WHAT TO DO

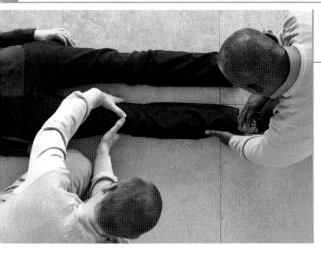

1 Help the casualty to lie down and make them as comfortable as possible.

2 Support the injured leg at the knee and ankle. If possible, ask someone else to help you.

3 Call 999/112 for emergency help. If the ambulance is expected to arrive quickly, keep the leg supported in the same position until the emergency services arrive.

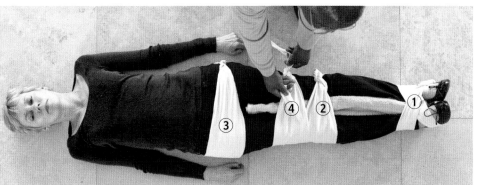

4 If the ambulance is not expected to arrive quickly, immobilise the leg by securing it to the uninjured one. Gently bring the uninjured leg alongside the injured one. Position a narrow-fold bandage (p.253) at the ankles and feet (1), then a broad-fold one at the knees (2). Add additional bandages above (3) and below (4) the fracture site. Place soft padding between the legs to prevent the bony parts from rubbing. Secure the bandages on the uninjured side.

5 Check the circulation beyond the bandages (p.247) and re-check it every 10 minutes; loosen and reapply bandages if necessary. Take any steps possible to treat the casualty for shock (pp.114–115): insulate the casualty from the cold with blankets or clothing, but do not raise the casualty's legs. Monitor and record the casualty's vital signs (pp.54–55) while waiting for help to arrive.

LOWER LEG INJURIES

Injuries to the lower leg include fractures of the shin bone (tibia) and the splint bone (fibula), as well as damage to the soft tissues (muscles, ligaments and tendons).

Fractures of the tibia are usually due to a heavy blow (for example, from the bumper of a moving vehicle). In addition, as there is little flesh over the tibia, a fracture is more likely to be accompanied by a wound – open fracture (p.140). The fibula can also be broken by the twisting forces that sprain an ankle.

RECOGNITION

There may be:

- Localised pain
- Swelling, bruising and deformity of the leg
- An open wound
- Inability to stand on the injured leg

YOUR AIMS

- To immobilise the leg
- To arrange transport to hospital

WHAT TO DO

1 **Help the casualty to lie down** and make them comfortable. Steady and support the injured leg by hand at the knee and ankle to prevent any movement. If there is a wound, carefully expose it and treat the bleeding. Place a dressing over the wound to protect it.

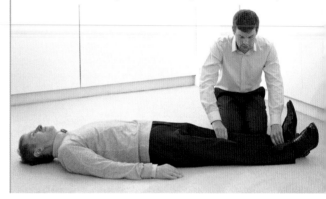

2 **Call 999/112 for emergency help.** Maintain support until the ambulance arrives. Treat for shock if necessary (pp.114–115). Do not raise the legs even if shock is present.

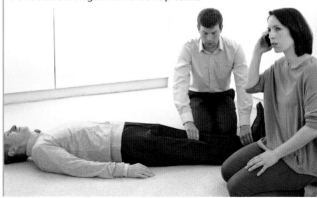

3 If the ambulance is delayed, support the injured leg by splinting it to the other leg. Bring the uninjured leg alongside the injured one and slide bandages under both legs. Position a narrow-fold bandage (p.253) at the feet and ankles (1), then broad-fold bandages at the knees (2) and above and below the fracture site (3 and 4). Insert padding between the lower legs. Tie a figure-of-eight bandage around the feet and ankles, then secure the other bandages; tie knots on the uninjured side.

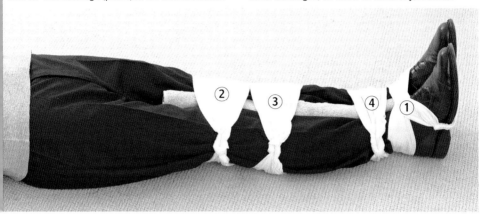

4 If the casualty's journey to hospital is likely to be long and uncomfortable, place additional soft padding on the outside of the injured leg, from the knee to the foot. Secure the legs with broad-fold bandages as above. Treat the casualty for shock (pp.114–115) if necessary, but do not raise their legs.

SPECIAL CASE IF THE FRACTURE IS NEAR THE ANKLE

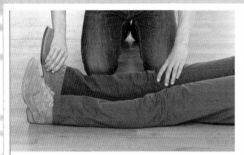

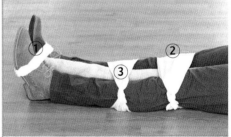

1 Steady and support the injured leg by hand at the knee and foot (not over the fracture site) to prevent any movement. If there is a wound, treat the bleeding and place a dressing over the wound to protect it. Call 999/112 for emergency help. Maintain support until the ambulance arrives. Treat the casualty for shock if necessary (pp.114–115). Do not raise the legs even if shock is present.

2 If the ambulance is delayed, splint the injured leg to the other leg – ask a helper to maintain support while you secure bandages. Bring the uninjured leg to the injured one. Position a narrow-fold bandage (p.253) at the feet. Slide two broad-fold bandages under both knees; leave one at the knee (2) and slide the other down to just above the fracture site (3). Insert padding between the lower legs, then tie the feet together (1). Secure the other two bandages (2 then 3). Tie all knots on the uninjured side.

KNEE INJURY

RECOGNITION

There may be:

- Pain on attempting to move the knee
- Swelling at the knee joint

YOUR AIMS

- To protect the knee in the most comfortable position for the casualty
- To arrange urgent removal to hospital

The knee is the hinge joint between the thigh bone (femur) and shin bone (tibia). It is capable of bending, straightening and, in the bent position, slight rotation.

The knee joint is supported by strong muscles and ligaments and is protected at the front by a disc of bone called the kneecap (patella). Discs of cartilage protect the end surfaces of the major bones. Direct blows, violent twists or sprains can damage these structures. Possible knee injuries include fracture of the patella, sprains and damage to the cartilage.

A knee injury may make it impossible for the casualty to bend or straighten the joint, and you should ensure that the casualty does not try to walk on the injured leg. Bleeding or fluid in the knee joint may cause marked swelling around the knee.

WHAT TO DO

1 **Help the casualty to lie down,** preferably on a blanket to insulate them from the floor or ground. Place soft padding, such as pillows, blankets or coats, under the injured knee to support it in the most comfortable position.

2 **Wrap soft padding around the joint.** Secure the padding with a roller bandage (pp.248–251) that extends from the middle of the casualty's lower leg to mid-thigh.

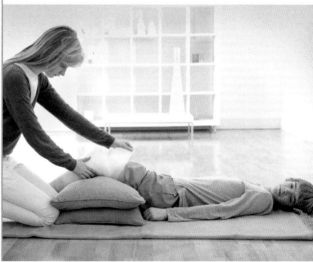

3 **Call 999/112 for emergency help.** The casualty needs to remain in the position they find most comfortable and should be transported to hospital by ambulance.

ANKLE INJURY

A sprain is the most common ankle injury. It is usually caused by a twist to the ankle and can be treated using the procedure described for strains and sprains (pp.142–143):
● Rest the affected part.
● Cool the injury with a cold compress (p.245).
● Provide comfortable support.
● Elevate the injury.
If the casualty cannot bear any weight on the injured leg or there is severe pain, swelling and/or deformity at the ankle, suspect a break and treat it as a fracture of the lower leg near the ankle (p.165). Be aware too, however, that a casualty may have a fracture but still be able to walk and move their toes. If you are in any doubt about an ankle injury, treat it as a fracture.

RECOGNITION

● Pain, increased either by movement or by putting weight on the foot
● Swelling at the site of injury

WHAT TO DO

1 **Support the ankle** in the most comfortable position for the casualty, preferably raised.

YOUR AIMS

● To relieve pain and swelling
● To obtain medical aid if necessary

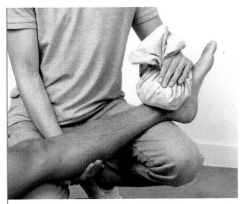

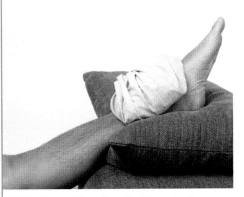

2 **Apply a cold compress,** such as an ice pack or a cold pad (p.245), to the site to reduce swelling and bruising.

3 **Support the injured limb in a raised position.** Leave the cold compress in place for no longer than 20 minutes. If the pain is severe, or the casualty is unable to walk on the injured leg, arrange to take or send them to hospital. Advise the casualty to rest the ankle and seek medical advice if necessary.

SEE ALSO Lower leg injuries **pp.164–165** | Strains and sprains **pp.142–143**

FOOT AND TOE INJURIES

The bones and joints in the foot can suffer various types of injury, such as fractures, cuts and bruising. Minor fractures are usually caused by direct force. Always compare the injured foot with the uninjured foot, especially toes, because fractures can result in deformities that may not be immediately obvious. Multiple fractures, affecting many or all of the bones in the foot, are usually caused by crushing injuries. These fractures may be open, with severe bleeding and swelling, needing immediate first aid treatment. Foot and toe injuries must be treated in hospital.

RECOGNITION

- Difficulty in walking
- Stiffness of movement
- Bruising and swelling
- Deformity

YOUR AIMS

- To minimise swelling
- To arrange transport to hospital

WHAT TO DO

1 **Help the casualty to lie down,** and carefully steady and support the injured leg. If there is a wound, carefully expose it and treat the bleeding. Place a dressing over the wound to protect it.

2 **Remove any foot jewellery** before the area begins to swell.

3 **Apply a cold compress,** such as an ice pack or a cold pad (p.245). This will also help to relieve swelling and reduce pain. Leave the cold compress in place for no longer than 20 minutes.

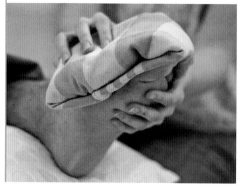

4 **Place padding** around the casualty's foot and secure it with a bandage.

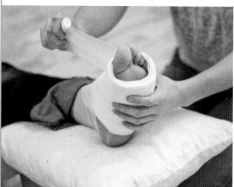

5 **Arrange to take or send the casualty** to hospital. If they are not being taken by ambulance, try to ensure that the injured foot remains elevated during travel. Check the circulation beyond the bandage (p.247), and re-check it every 10 minutes. If the circulation is impaired, loosen the bandage and reapply.

CRAMP

This condition is a sudden painful spasm in one or more muscles. Cramp commonly occurs during sleep. It can also develop after strenuous exercise, due to a build-up of chemical waste products in the muscles, or to excessive loss of salts and fluids from the body through sweating or dehydration. Cramp can often be relieved by stretching and massaging the affected muscles.

YOUR AIM
- To relieve the spasm and pain

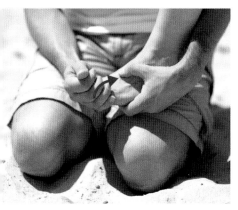

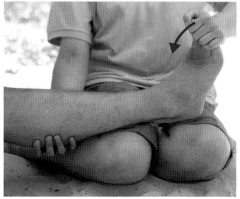

Cramp in the foot
Help the to casualty stand with their weight on the front of their foot (or rest the foot on your knee) to stretch the affected muscles. Once the spasm has passed, massage the affected part of the foot with your fingers.

Cramp in the calf muscles
Help the casualty straighten their knee, while supporting their foot. Flex the affected foot upwards towards the casualty's shin to stretch the calf muscles, then massage the affected area on the back of the calf.

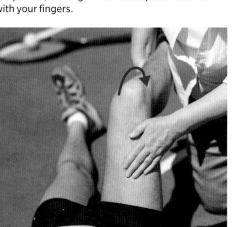

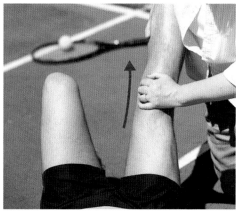

Cramp in the front of the thigh
Help the casualty to lie down. Bend the knee to stretch the affected muscles. Massage the muscles once the spasm has passed.

Cramp in the back of the thigh
Help the casualty to lie down. Raise the leg and straighten the knee to stretch the muscles. Massage the area once the spasm has passed.

SEE ALSO Dehydration p.184

08 EFFECTS OF HEAT AND COLD

This chapter deals with the effects of injuries and illnesses caused by environmental factors such as extremes of heat and cold. The skin protects the body and helps to maintain body temperature within a normal range. It can be damaged by fire, hot liquids or caustic substances. This chapter contains advice on how to assess and deliver first aid for burns, whether minor or severe.

The effects of temperature extremes can also impair skin and other body functions. Injuries may be localised – such as frostbite or sunburn – or generalised, as in heat exhaustion or hypothermia. Young children and the elderly are most susceptible to problems caused by extremes of temperature.

AIMS AND OBJECTIVES

- To assess the casualty's condition quickly and calmly
- To comfort and reassure the casualty
- To call 999 / 112 for emergency help if you suspect a serious illness or injury
- To be aware of your own needs

For burns:
- To protect yourself and the casualty from danger
- To assess the burn, prevent further damage and relieve symptoms

For extremes of temperature:
- To protect the casualty from heat or cold
- To restore normal body temperature

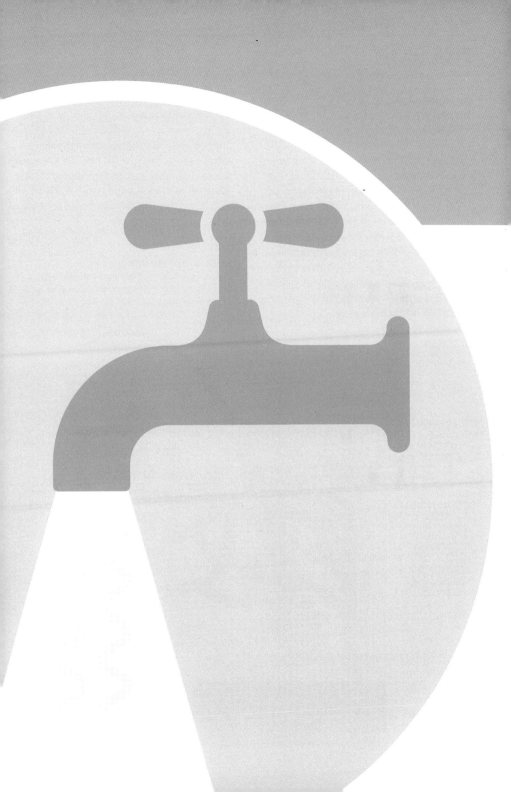

THE SKIN

The largest organ of the body, the skin plays key roles in protecting the body from injury and infection and in maintaining the body at a constant temperature.

The skin consists of two layers of tissue – an outer layer (epidermis) and an inner layer (dermis) – which lie on a layer of fatty tissue (subcutaneous fat). The top part of the epidermis is made up of dead, flattened skin cells, which are constantly shed and replaced by new cells made in the lower part of this layer. The epidermis is protected by an oily substance called sebum – secreted from glands called sebaceous glands – which keeps the skin supple and waterproof.

The lower layer of the skin, the dermis, contains the blood vessels, nerves, muscles, sebaceous glands, sweat glands and hair roots (follicles). The ends of sensory nerves within the dermis register sensations from the body's surface, such as heat, cold, pain and even the slightest touch. Blood vessels supply the skin with nutrients and help to regulate body temperature by preserving or releasing heat (opposite).

Structure of the skin
The skin is made up of two layers: the thin, outer epidermis and the thicker dermis beneath it. Most of the structures of the skin, such as blood vessels, nerves and hair roots, are contained within the dermis.

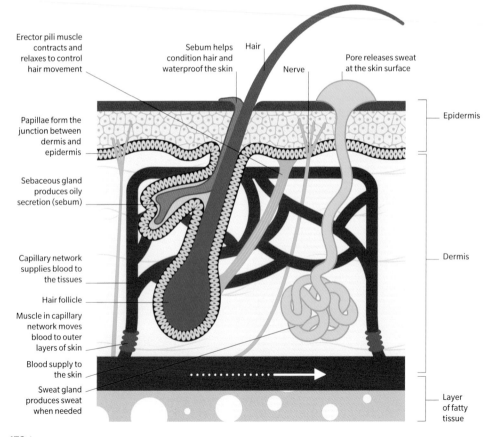

Erector pili muscle contracts and relaxes to control hair movement

Sebum helps condition hair and waterproof the skin

Hair

Nerve

Pore releases sweat at the skin surface

Epidermis

Papillae form the junction between dermis and epidermis

Sebaceous gland produces oily secretion (sebum)

Capillary network supplies blood to the tissues

Hair follicle

Muscle in capillary network moves blood to outer layers of skin

Blood supply to the skin

Sweat gland produces sweat when needed

Dermis

Layer of fatty tissue

MAINTAINING BODY TEMPERATURE

One of the major functions of the skin is to help maintain the body temperature within its optimum range of 36–37°C (97–99°F). A region of the brain called the hypothalamus regulates body temperature. If the temperature of blood passing through this thermostat falls or rises to a level outside the optimum range, mechanisms are activated to either warm or cool the body.

HOW THE BODY KEEPS WARM

When the body becomes too cold, changes take place to prevent heat from escaping. Blood vessels at the body surface narrow (constrict) to keep warm blood in the main part (core) of the body. The activity of the sweat glands is reduced, and hairs stand on end to "trap" warm air close to the skin. In addition to the mechanisms that prevent heat loss, other body systems act to produce more warmth. The rate of metabolism is increased. Heat is also generated by muscle activity, which may be either voluntary (for example, during physical exercise) or, in cold conditions, involuntary (shivering).

HOW THE BODY LOSES HEAT

In hot conditions, the body activates a number of mechanisms to encourage heat loss and thus prevent the body temperature from becoming too high. Blood vessels that lie in or just under the skin widen (dilate). As a result, blood flow to the body surface increases and more heat is lost. In addition, the sweat glands become more active and secrete more sweat. This sweat then cools the skin as it evaporates.

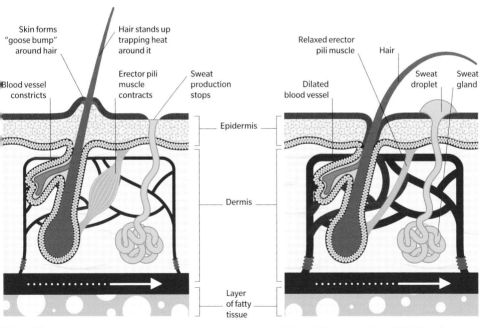

How skin responds to low body temperature

Skin forms "goose bump" around hair — Hair stands up trapping heat around it — Erector pili muscle contracts — Sweat production stops — Blood vessel constricts — Epidermis — Dermis — Layer of fatty tissue

Relaxed erector pili muscle — Hair — Sweat droplet — Sweat gland — Dilated blood vessel

How skin responds to low body temperature

Blood vessels narrow (constrict) to reduce blood flow to the skin. The erector pili muscles contract, making the hairs stand upright and trap warm air close to the skin.

How skin responds to high body temperature

Blood vessels widen (dilate), making the skin appear flushed, and heat is lost. Sweat glands become active and produce sweat droplets, which evaporate to cool the skin.

ASSESSING A BURN

When skin is damaged by burning, it can no longer function effectively as a natural barrier against infection. In addition, body fluid may be lost because tiny blood vessels in the skin leak tissue fluid (serum). This fluid either collects under the skin to form blisters or it leaks through the surface. There may be related injuries, and significant fluid loss and infection may develop later.

WHAT TO ASSESS

It is particularly important to consider the circumstances in which the burn has occurred; whether or not the airway is likely to have been affected; and the extent, location and depth of the burn.

There are many possible causes of burns (see below). By establishing the cause of the burn, you may be able to identify any other potential problems that could result. For example, a fire in an enclosed space is likely to have produced poisonous carbon monoxide gas, or other toxic fumes may have been released if burning material was involved. If the casualty's airway has been affected, they may have difficulty breathing and will need urgent medical attention and admission to hospital.

The extent of the burn will also indicate whether or not shock is likely to develop. Shock a life-threatening condition that occurs whenever there is a serious loss of body fluids (pp.112–113). In a burn that covers a large area of the body, fluid loss will be significant and the risk of shock high.

If the burn is on a limb, fluid may collect in the tissues around it, causing swelling and pain. This build-up of fluid is particularly serious if the limb is being constricted, for example by tight clothing, footwear or jewellery.

Burns allow germs to enter the skin and so carry a serious risk of infection.

TYPES OF BURN AND POSSIBLE CAUSES

TYPE OF BURN	CAUSES
Dry burn	● Flames ● Contact with hot objects, such as domestic appliances or cigarettes ● Friction – for example, rope burns
Scald	● Steam ● Hot liquids, such as tea and coffee, or hot fat
Electrical burn	● Low-voltage current, as used by domestic appliances ● High-voltage currents, as carried in mains overhead cables ● Lightning strikes
Cold injury	● Frostbite ● Contact with freezing metals ● Contact with freezing vapours, such as liquid oxygen or liquid nitrogen
Chemical burn	● Industrial chemicals, including inhaled fumes and corrosive gases ● Domestic chemicals and agents, such as paint stripper, caustic soda, weed killers, bleach, oven cleaner or any other strong acid or alkali chemical
Radiation burn	● Sunburn ● Over-exposure to ultraviolet rays from a sunlamp ● Exposure to a radioactive source, such as an X-ray

DEPTH OF BURNS

Burns are classified according to the depth of skin damage. There are three depths: superficial, partial-thickness and full-thickness. A casualty may suffer burns of one or more depths in a single incident.

A superficial burn involves only the outermost layer of skin, the epidermis. It usually heals well if first aid is given promptly and if blisters do not form. Sunburn is one of the most common types of superficial burn. Other causes include minor domestic incidents.

Partial-thickness burns are very painful. They destroy the epidermis and cause the skin to become red and blistered. They usually heal well, but if they affect more than 20 per cent of the body in an adult or 10 per cent in a child they can be life-threatening.

In full-thickness burns, pain sensation is lost, which can mask the severity of the injury. The skin may look waxy, pale or charred and needs urgent medical attention. There are likely to be areas of partial and superficial burns around them.

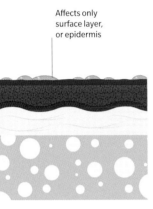

Affects only surface layer, or epidermis

Damage occurs in epidermis and dermis

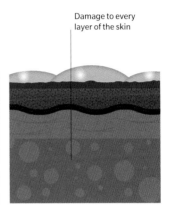

Fluid-filled blisters form on skin surface

Damage to every layer of the skin

Superficial burn
This type of burn involves only the outermost layer of skin. Superficial burns are characterised by redness, swelling and tenderness.

Partial-thickness burn
This affects the dermis and the epidermis, and the skin becomes red and raw. Blisters form over the skin due to fluid released from the damaged tissues beneath.

Full-thickness burn
With this type of burn, all the layers of the skin are affected; there may be some damage to nerves, fat tissue, muscles and blood vessels.

BURNS THAT NEED HOSPITAL TREATMENT

If the casualty is a child, seek medical advice or take the child to hospital, however small the burn appears. For adults, medical attention should be sought for any serious burn. Such burns include:
- All full-thickness burns.
- All burns involving the face, hands, feet or genital area.
- All burns that extend right around an arm or a leg.

- All partial-thickness burns larger than one per cent of the body surface (an area the size of the palm of the casualty's hand).
- All superficial burns larger than five per cent of the casualty's body surface (equivalent to five palm areas).
- All electrical and chemical burns.
- Burns with a mixed pattern of varying depths.

If you are unsure about the severity of any burn, seek medical advice.

SEVERE BURNS AND SCALDS

RECOGNITION

There may be:

- Areas of superficial, partial and/or full-thickness burns
- Pain
- Difficulty breathing
- Features of shock (pp.114–115)

YOUR AIMS

- To stop the burning as soon as possible and relieve pain
- To maintain an open airway
- To treat associated injuries and minimise the risk of infection and shock
- To arrange urgent removal to hospital
- To gather information for the emergency services

Take great care when treating burns. The longer the burning continues, the more severe the injury will be, and the longer it will take to heal. If the casualty has been injured in a fire, assume that smoke or hot air has also affected their airways (p.179).

Your priority is to cool the burn as soon as possible (which stops the burning process and relieves the pain) and continue cooling for at least 20 minutes, or until the pain is relieved. A casualty with a severe burn or scald injury will almost certainly be suffering from shock because of the fluid loss and will need urgent hospital treatment.

The possibility of non-accidental injury must always be considered, no matter what the age of the casualty. Keep an accurate record of what has happened and any treatment you have given. If you have to remove or cut away clothing, keep it in case of future investigation.

WHAT TO DO

1 **Start cooling the injury as soon as possible.** Flood the burn with plenty of cold water, but do not delay the casualty's removal to hospital. Help the casualty to sit or lie down. If possible, try to prevent the burnt area from coming into contact with the ground to keep the burn as clean as possible.

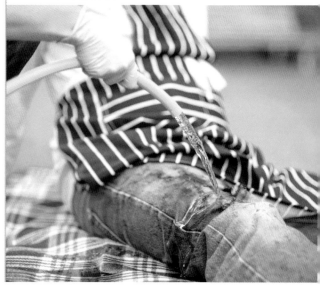

2 Call 999/112 for emergency help. If possible, get someone to do this while you continue cooling the burn.

3 Continue cooling the affected area for at least 20 minutes, or until the pain is relieved. Watch for signs of breathing difficulty. Be aware that overcooling the casualty may lower the body temperature to a dangerous level, causing hypothermia. This is a particular hazard for babies and elderly people.

4 Do not touch or otherwise interfere with the burn. Gently remove any rings, watches, and other jewellery, belts, shoes and burnt or smouldering clothing before the tissues begin to swell. A helper can do this while you are cooling the burn. Do not remove any clothing that is stuck to the burn.

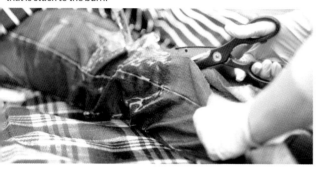

5 When the burn is cooled, cover the injured area with kitchen film to protect it from infection. Discard the first two turns from the roll and then apply it lengthways over the burn. A clean plastic bag can be used to cover a hand or foot; secure it with a bandage or adhesive tape applied over the plastic, not the damaged skin. If there is no plastic film available, use a sterile dressing, or improvise with a folded triangular bandage (p.253), or pad of material.

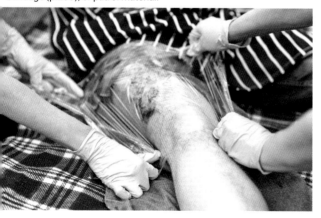

6 Reassure the casualty and cover them to keep them warm. Treat them for shock (pp.114–115) if necessary. Record details of the casualty's injuries. Monitor and record the casualty's vital signs (pp.54–55) while waiting for help to arrive.

MINOR BURNS AND SCALDS

RECOGNITION

- Reddened skin
- Pain in the area of the burn

Later there may be:

- Blistering of the affected skin

YOUR AIMS

- To stop the burning
- To relieve pain and swelling
- To minimise the risk of infection

SPECIAL CASE BLISTERS

Never burst a blister; they usually need no treatment. However, if a blister breaks or is likely to burst, cover it with a non-adhesive sterile dressing that extends well beyond the edges of the blister. Leave the dressing in place until the blister subsides.

Small, superficial burns and scalds are often due to domestic incidents, such as touching a hot iron or oven shelf. Most minor burns can be treated successfully by first aid and will heal naturally. However, you should advise the casualty to seek medical advice if you are at all concerned about the severity of the injury (Assessing a burn, pp.174–175).

After a burn, blisters may form. These thin "bubbles" are caused by tissue fluid (serum) leaking into the burnt area just beneath the skin's surface. You should never break a blister caused by a burn because you risk introducing infection into the wound.

WHAT TO DO

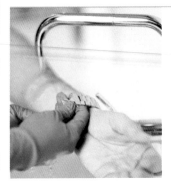

1 **Flood the injured part with cold** water for at least 20 minutes or until the pain is relieved.

2 **Gently remove any rings** and other jewellery, watches, belts or constricting clothing from the injured area before it begins to swell.

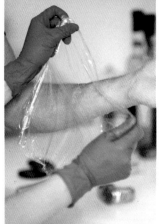

3 **When the burn is cooled,** cover it with kitchen film or place a clean plastic bag over a foot or hand. Apply the kitchen film lengthways over the burn, not around the limb because the tissues swell. If you do not have kitchen film or a plastic bag, use a sterile dressing or clean pad, and bandage loosely in place.

4 **Seek medical advice** if the casualty is a child, or if you are in any doubt about the casualty's condition.

BURNS TO THE AIRWAYS

Any burn to the face, mouth or throat is very serious because the air passages rapidly become swollen. Usually, signs of burning will be evident. Always suspect damage to the airway if a casualty sustains burns in a confined space since they are likely to have inhaled hot air or gases.

There is no specific first aid treatment for an extreme case of burns to the airway; the swelling will rapidly block the airway, and there is a serious risk of hypoxia. Immediate and specialised medical help is required.

WHAT TO DO

1 Call 999/112 for emergency help. Tell the call handler that you suspect burns to the casualty's airway.

2 Take any steps possible to improve the casualty's air supply, such as loosening clothing around their neck.

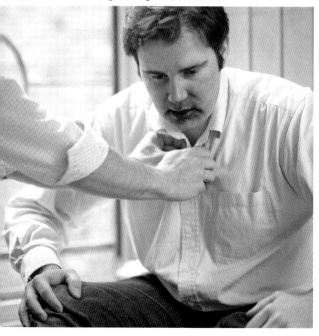

3 Offer the casualty ice or small sips of cold water to reduce swelling and pain.

4 Reassure the casualty. Monitor and record vital signs (pp.54–55) while waiting for emergency help to arrive.

CAUTION

- If the casualty becomes unresponsive, open the airway and check breathing (The unresponsive casualty, pp.56–89).

RECOGNITION

There may be:
- Soot around the nose or mouth
- Singeing of the nasal hairs
- Redness, swelling or actual burning of the tongue
- Damage to the skin around the mouth
- Hoarseness of the voice
- Breathing difficulties

YOUR AIMS

- To maintain an open airway
- To arrange urgent removal to hospital

SEE ALSO Hypoxia p.94 | Shock pp.114–115 | The unresponsive casualty pp.56–89 | **179**

ELECTRICAL BURN

Burns may occur when electricity passes through the body. There may be surface damage along the point of contact, or at the points of entry and exit of the current. In addition, there may also be internal damage between the entry and exit points; the position and direction of wounds will alert you to the likely site and extent of hidden injury, and to the degree of shock that the casualty may suffer.

Burns may be caused by a lightning strike or by a low- or high-voltage electric current. Electric shock can cause cardiac arrest. If the casualty is unresponsive, your priority, once the area is safe, is to open their airway and check their breathing.

RECOGNITION

There may be:

- No response from casualty
- Full-thickness burns, with swelling, scorching and charring
- Burns at points of entry and exit of electricity
- Signs of shock

YOUR AIMS

- To treat the burns and shock
- To arrange urgent removal to hospital

WHAT TO DO

1 **Make sure that contact** with the electrical source is broken before you touch the casualty (pp.34–35).

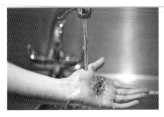

2 **Flood the injury** with cold water (at the entry and exit points if both are present) for at least 20 minutes or until pain is relieved.

3 **Gently remove any jewellery,** watches, belts or constricting clothing from the injured area before it begins to swell. Do not touch the burn.

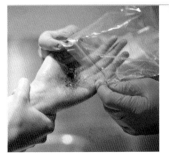

4 **When the burn is cooled,** place a clean plastic bag over a burn on a foot or hand – tape the bag loosely in place (attach tape to the bag, not the skin). Or, cover it with kitchen film – lay the film along the length of the limb not around it. If neither is available, cover the burn with a sterile dressing or a clean pad, and bandage loosely.

5 **Call 999/112 for emergency help.** Reassure the casualty and treat them for shock (pp.114–115). Monitor and record the casulaty's vital signs (pp.54–55) while waiting for medical help to arrive.

SEE ALSO Electrical injury **pp.34–35** | Severe burns and scalds **pp.176–177** | Shock **pp.114–115**
The unresponsive casualty **pp.56–89**

CHEMICAL BURN

Certain chemicals may irritate, burn or penetrate the skin, causing widespread and sometimes fatal damage. Most strong, corrosive chemicals are found in industry, but chemical burns can also occur in the home; for instance from splashed or sprayed dishwasher products (the most common cause of alkali burns in children), oven cleaners, pesticides and paint stripper.

Chemical burns are always serious, and the casualty will need hospital treatment. If possible, note the name or brand of the burning substance. Before treating the casualty, ensure the safety of yourself and others because some chemicals give off poisonous fumes, which can cause breathing difficulties.

CAUTION

- Never attempt to neutralise acid or alkali burns unless trained to do so.
- Do not delay starting treatment by searching for an antidote.
- If the incident occurs in the workplace, notify the safety officer and/or emergency services.

WHAT TO DO

1 Make sure that the area around the casualty is safe. Ventilate the area to disperse fumes. Wear gloves and eye protection to prevent you from coming into contact with the chemical. If it is safe to do so, seal the chemical container. Move the casualty if necessary. If the chemical is in powder form, it can be brushed off the skin.

2 Flood the burn with cold water for at least 20 minutes to disperse the chemical and stop the burning. If the casualty is lying on the ground, make sure that the contaminated water drains away and does not collect underneath them. Pour water away from yourself.

RECOGNITION

There may be:
- Evidence of chemicals in the vicinity
- Intense, stinging pain

Later:
- Discoloration, blistering and peeling of skin
- Swelling of the affected area

YOUR AIMS

- To make the area safe and inform the relevant authority
- To disperse the harmful chemical
- To arrange transport to hospital

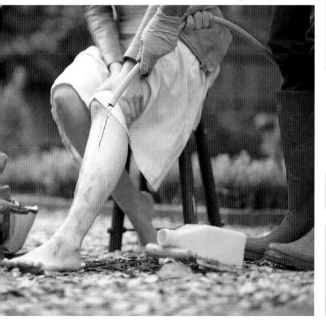

3 Gently remove any contaminated clothing while flooding the injury.

4 Arrange to take or send the casualty to hospital. Monitor and record vital signs (pp.54–55) while waiting for medical help to arrive. Pass the details of the chemical on to medical staff if you can identify it.

SEE ALSO Chemical burn to the eye **p.180** | Inhalation of fumes **pp.100–101**

CHEMICAL BURN TO THE EYE

Chemicals that are splashed or sprayed into the eye can cause serious injury if not treated quickly. Some chemicals damage the surface of the eye, resulting in scarring and even blindness.

Your priority is to wash out (irrigate) the eye so that the chemical is diluted and dispersed. When irrigating the eye, be careful that the contaminated rinsing water does not splash you or the casualty. Before beginning to treat the casualty, put on protective gloves if available and give some to the casualty.

RECOGNITION

There may be:

- Intense pain in the eye
- Inability to open the injured eye
- Redness and swelling around the eye
- Copious watering of the eye
- Evidence of chemical substances or containers in the immediate area

YOUR AIMS

- To disperse the harmful chemical
- To arrange transport to hospital

WHAT TO DO

1 **Put on protective gloves.** If the casualty's eye is shut in a spasm of pain, gently, but firmly, try to pull the eyelids open; the casualty may be able to assist by pulling their lower eye lid down. Hold the casualty's head, affected eye downwards, under gently running cold water for at least 20 minutes. Irrigate the eyelid thoroughly both inside and out, allowing water to drain into the sink.

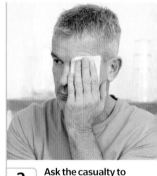

3 **Ask the casualty to remove their gloves** and give them a clean pad to hold against the injured eye; help them if necessary. If medical attention is delayed, bandage the pad loosely in position.

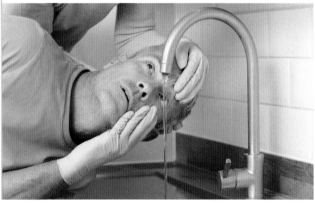

2 **Make sure that contaminated water** does not splash the casualty's uninjured eye or their face. You may find it easier to pour the water over the eye using an eye irrigator or a glass. If the casualty is wearing contact lenses, ask them to remove them if they can.

4 **Arrange to take or send** the casualty to hospital. Identify the chemical if possible and pass on the details to medical staff.

FLASH BURN TO THE EYE

This condition occurs when the surface (cornea) of the eye is damaged by exposure to ultraviolet light, such as prolonged glare from sunlight reflected off snow. Flash burns can also be caused by glare from a welder's torch. Symptoms usually develop gradually, commonly over several hours.

- Intense pain in the affected eye(s)

There may also be:

- A "gritty" feeling in the eye(s)
- Sensitivity to light
- Redness and watering of the eye(s)

WHAT TO DO

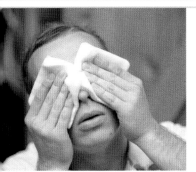

1 **Reassure the casualty**. Ask them to hold an eye pad against each injured eye. If it is likely to take some time to obtain medical attention, lightly bandage the pad(s) in place.

2 **Arrange to take or send** the casualty to hospital.

YOUR AIMS

- To prevent further damage
- To arrange transport to hospital

IRRITANT SPRAY EXPOSURE

There are several types of irritant spray. The most commonly used are CS spray and PAVA spray. Both are used by the police forces for riot control and self-protection, and have been used by unauthorised people as weapons in assault situations. They are both aerosols and have the same effects. The effects usually wear off 15–20 minutes after a person has been exposed to the spray.

CAUTION

- If the casualty suffers from asthma (p.104) the spray may trigger an attack.
- If the casualty's symptoms persist seek medical advice.

WHAT TO DO

1 **Move the casualty outside,** or to a well-ventilated area with a free flow of air, to ensure rapid dispersal of the spray.

2 **Put on gloves and eye protection** if you are handling an affected casualty or contaminated items such as clothing. Advise the casualty to avoid rubbing their eyes and to remove contact lenses – they may need help. Remove clothing and put it in a sealed plastic bag.

3 **If the casualty cannot open their eyes** after 20 minutes flush the face with copious amounts of cold tap water; do not use water any sooner as it can worsen the symptoms. Sterile saline solution can be used to flush out the eyes.

RECOGNITION

There may be:

- Burning sensation and watering of the eyes
- Sneezing and runny nose
- Stinging sensation on the skin with redness and possibly blistering
- Difficulty breathing

YOUR AIM

- To remove the casualty from the spray area

SEE ALSO Allergy **p.226** | Asthma **p.104**

DEHYDRATION

This condition occurs when the amount of fluids lost from the body is not adequately replaced. Dehydration can begin to develop when a person loses as little as one per cent of their bodyweight through fluid loss. A 2 to 6 per cent loss can occur during a typical period of exercise on a warm day; the average daily intake of fluids is 2.5 litres (4 pints). This fluid loss needs to be replaced. In addition to fluid, the body loses essential body salts through sweating.

Dehydration is mainly the result of: excessive sweating during sporting activities, especially in hot weather; prolonged exposure to sun, or hot, humid conditions; sweating through raised body temperature during a fever; and loss of fluid through severe diarrhoea and vomiting. Young children, older people or those involved in prolonged periods of activity are particularly at risk. Severe dehydration can cause muscle cramps through the loss of body salts. If untreated, dehydration can lead to heat exhaustion.

The aim of first aid is to replace the lost water and salts through rehydration. Water is usually sufficient but oral rehydration solutions can help to replace lost salt, so can help rehydrate the casualty more quickly. Do not offer alcoholic or caffeine beverages to rehydrate a casualty.

WHAT TO DO

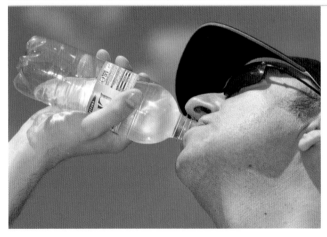

1 **Reassure the casualty.** Help them to sit down. Give them plenty of fluids to drink. Water is usually sufficient, but rehydration powders with water can help with salt replacement and may rehydrate the casualty more quickly.

2 **If the casualty is suffering from cramp,** stretch and massage the affected muscles (p.169). Advise the casualty to rest.

3 **Monitor and record** the casualty's condition. If they continue to be unwell, seek medical advice straightaway.

SUNBURN

Over-exposure to the sun or a sunlamp can result in sunburn. At high altitudes, sunburn can occur even on an overcast summer's day, or in the snow in winter. Some medicines can trigger severe sensitivity to sunlight. Rarely, sunburn can be caused by exposure to radioactivity.

Sunburn can be prevented by staying in the shade, wearing protective clothing and by regularly applying a high factor sunscreen.

Most sunburn is superficial, but in severe cases, the skin is lobster-red and blistered. In addition, the casualty may suffer from heat exhaustion or heatstroke.

CAUTION

- If there is extensive blistering, or other skin damage, seek medical advice.

RECOGNITION

- Reddened skin
- Pain in the area of the burn

Later there may be:

- Blistering of the affected skin

YOUR AIMS

- To move the casualty out of the sun as soon as possible
- To relieve discomfort and pain

WHAT TO DO

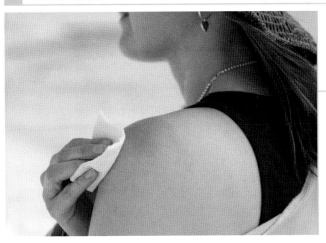

1 Cover the casualty's skin with light clothing or a towel. Help them to move out of the sun into the shade or, if at all possible, indoors.

2 Encourage the casualty to have frequent sips of cold water. Cool the affected skin by dabbing with cold water. If the area is extensive, the casualty may prefer to soak the affected skin in a cold bath for up to 20 minutes.

3 If the burns are mild, after-sun lotion may soothe them. The casualty may take the recommended dose of paracetamol or their own painkillers. A child may have the recommended dose of paracetamol suspension (not aspirin). Advise the casualty to stay inside or in the shade. Seek medical advice if there is blistering or other skin damage.

SEE ALSO Dehydration **opposite** | Heat exhaustion **p.186** | Heatstroke **p.187** | Minor burns and scalds **p.178**

HEAT EXHAUSTION

RECOGNITION

As the condition develops, there may be:

- Headache, dizziness and confusion
- Loss of appetite and nausea
- Sweating, with pale, clammy skin
- Cramps in the arms, legs or abdomen
- Rapid, weakening pulse and breathing

YOUR AIMS

- To cool the casualty down
- To replace lost body fluids and salts
- To obtain medical help if necessary

This disorder is caused by loss of salt and water from the body through excessive sweating. It usually develops gradually and often affects people who are not acclimatised to hot, humid conditions. People who are unwell, especially those with illnesses that cause vomiting and diarrhoea, are more susceptible than others to developing heat exhaustion.

Heat exhaustion can occur when people (especially the elderly or the very young) are exposed to high external temperatures – this is non-exertional heat exhaustion. Excessive physical activity in a hot environment can produce more heat than the body can cope with – exertional heat exhaustion. Both conditions can lead to heatstroke (hyperthermia), opposite, and even death. Some non-prescription drugs such as ecstasy, can affect the body's temperature regulation system. This, combined with dancing in a hot environment, can result in a person becoming overheated and dehydrated, which can also lead to heatstroke.

WHAT TO DO

1 Help the casualty to a cool, shady place. Encourage them to lie down then raise and support their legs.

2 Give them plenty of water to drink. Rehydration powders added to water or isotonic drinks will help with salt replacement.

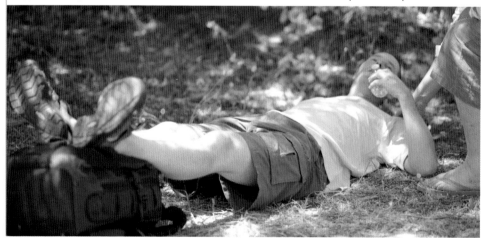

3 Monitor and record the casualty's vital signs (pp.54–55), including temperature. Even if they recover quickly, advise them to seek medical advice.

4 If the casualty's vital signs worsen, call 999/112 for emergency help. Continue to monitor and record their vital signs (pp.54–55) while you are waiting for medical help to arrive.

HEATSTROKE

Also known as hyperthermia, this condition is caused by a failure of the "thermostat" in the brain, which regulates body temperature. The body becomes dangerously overheated, usually due to a high fever or prolonged exposure to heat. Heatstroke can also result from the use of drugs such as ecstasy. In some cases, heatstroke follows heat exhaustion when sweating ceases, and the body then cannot be cooled by the evaporation of sweat.

Heatstroke can develop with little warning. The fastest way to cool a casualty is to immerse them in a bath of cold water. But, as as they may be agitated and uncooperative or may become unresponsive within minutes of feeling unwell, this is not always practicable and can be unsafe.

WHAT TO DO

1 **Quickly move the casualty to a cool place.** Remove as much of their outer clothing as possible. **Call 999 / 112 for emergency help.**

2 **Help the casualty to sit down,** supported with cushions. Wrap them in a cold, wet sheet until their temperature falls to 38°C (100.4°F). Keep the sheet wet by continually pouring cold water over it. If there is no sheet available, fan the casualty, and/or sponge them with cold water.

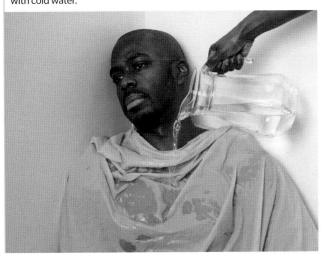

3 **Once the casualty's temperature** appears to have returned to normal, replace the wet sheet with a dry one.

4 **Monitor and record** the casualty's vital signs (pp.54–55), including temperature, while waiting for help to arrive. If the casualty's temperature rises again, repeat the cooling process.

RECOGNITION

There may be:

- Headache, dizziness and discomfort
- Restlessness and confusion
- Hot, flushed and dry skin
- Rapid deterioration in the level of response
- Full, bounding pulse
- Body temperature above 40°C (104°F)

YOUR AIMS

- To lower the casualty's body temperature as quickly as possible
- To arrange urgent removal to hospital

HYPOTHERMIA

RECOGNITION

As hypothermia develops there may be:

- Shivering, and cold, pale, dry skin
- Apathy, disorientation or irrational behaviour
- Lethargy or impaired responsiveness
- Slow and shallow breathing
- Slow and weakening pulse. In extreme cases, the heart may stop

YOUR AIMS

- To prevent the casualty losing more body heat
- To re-warm the casualty
- To obtain emergency help if necessary

This is a condition that develops when the body temperature falls below 35°C (95°F). The effects vary depending on the speed of onset and the level to which the body temperature falls. The blood supply to the superficial blood vessels in the skin shuts down to maintain the function of the vital organs such as the heart and brain. Moderate hypothermia can usually be reversed. Severe hypothermia – when the core body temperature falls below 30°C (86°F) – is often, although not always, fatal. No matter how low the body temperature becomes, persist with life-saving procedures until emergency help arrives because in hypothermia, survival may be possible even after prolonged periods of resuscitation.

WHAT CAUSES HYPOTHERMIA

Hypothermia can be caused by prolonged exposure to cold. Moving air has a much greater cooling effect than still air, so a high "wind-chill factor" in cold weather can substantially increase the risk of a person developing hypothermia. Immersion in cold water can cause death from hypothermia. When surrounded by cold water, the body can cool up to 30 times faster than in dry air, and body temperature falls rapidly.

Hypothermia may also develop indoors in poorly heated houses. Elderly people, infants, homeless people and those who are thin and frail are particularly vulnerable. Lack of activity, chronic illness and fatigue all increase the risk; alcohol and drugs can also exacerbate the condition.

TREATING HYPOTHERMIA WHEN OUTDOORS

1 Take the casualty to a sheltered place as quickly as possible. Shield the casualty from the wind.

2 Remove and replace any wet clothing if possible; do not give them your clothes. Make sure their head is covered.

3 Protect the casualty from the ground. Lay them on a thick layer of dry insulating material, such as pine branches, heather or bracken. Put them in a dry sleeping bag and/or cover them with blankets or newspapers. Wrap them in a plastic or foil survival bag, if available. You can also shelter and warm them with your body.

4 Call 999/112 or send for emergency help. Ideally, two people should go for help and stay together if you are in a remote area. It is important that you do not leave the casualty by themselves; someone must remain with them at all times.

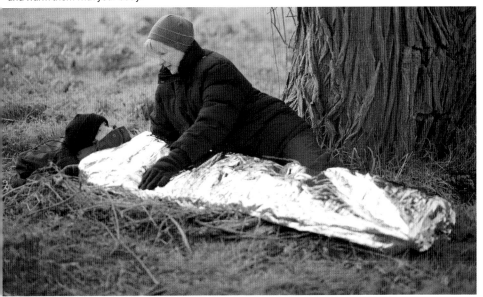

5 To help re-warm a casualty who is fully alert, give them warm non-alcoholic drinks and high-energy foods such as chocolate, if available.

6 Monitor and record the casualty's vital signs (pp.54–55), including temperature, while waiting for emergency help to arrive.

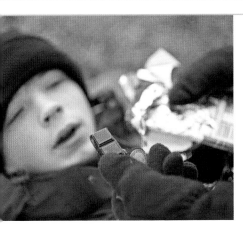

« HYPOTHERMIA

TREATING HYPOTHERMIA WHEN INDOORS

1 The casualty must be re-warmed. Cover the casualty with layers of blankets and warm the room to about 25°C (77°F).

2 Give the casualty a warm non-alcoholic **drink** such as soup and/or high-energy foods such as chocolate to help re-warm them.

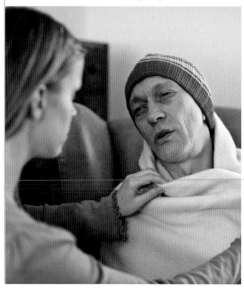 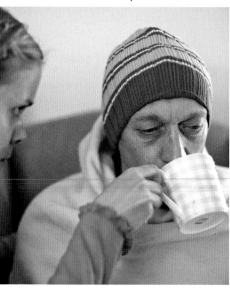

3 Seek medical advice. Be aware that hypothermia may also be disguising the symptoms of a serious underlying illness such as a stroke (pp.214–215), heart attack (p.213) or underactive thyroid gland (hypothyroidism).

4 Monitor and record the casualty's vital signs (pp.54–55), including temperature, as they are rewarmed.

SPECIAL CASE HYPOTHERMIA IN INFANTS

A baby's mechanisms for regulating body temperature are under-developed, so they may develop hypothermia in a cold room. The baby's skin may look healthy but feel cold, and they may be limp, unusually quiet and refusing to feed. Re-warm the baby by wrapping them in blankets and warming the room. You should always seek medical advice if you suspect a baby has hypothermia.

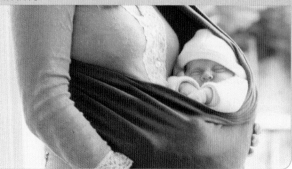

FROSTBITE

With this condition, the tissues of the extremities – usually the fingers and toes – freeze due to low temperatures. In severe cases, this freezing can lead to permanent loss of sensation and, eventually, tissue death and gangrene as the blood vessels and soft tissues become permanently damaged.

Frostbite usually occurs in freezing or cold and windy conditions. People who cannot move around to increase their circulation are particularly susceptible.

In many cases, frostbite is accompanied by hypothermia (pp.188–190), and this should be treated accordingly.

(pp.188–190)

CAUTION

- Do not put the affected part near direct heat.
- Do not attempt to thaw the affected part if there is danger of it refreezing.

RECOGNITION

There may be:

- At first, "pins-and-needles"
- Paleness (pallor) followed by numbness
- Hardening and stiffening of the skin
- A colour change to the skin of the affected area: first white, then mottled and blue. On recovery, the skin may be red, hot, painful and blistered. Where gangrene occurs, the tissue may become black due to loss of blood supply

YOUR AIMS

- To warm the affected area slowly to prevent further tissue damage
- To arrange transport to hospital

WHAT TO DO

1 Advise the casualty to put their hands in their armpits. Move the casualty into warmth before you thaw the affected part further.

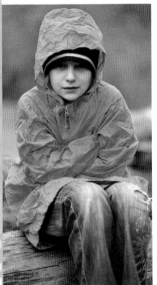

2 Once inside, gently remove gloves, rings and any other constrictions, such as boots. Warm the affected part with your hands, in your lap or continue to warm them in the casualty's armpits. Avoid rubbing the affected area because this can damage skin and other tissues.

3 Place the affected parts in warm water at around 40°C (104°F). Dry carefully, and apply a light dressing of dry gauze bandage.

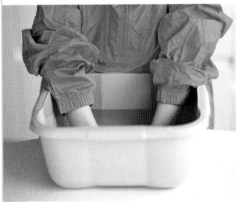

4 Raise the affected limb to reduce swelling. An adult may take the recommended dose of paracetamol or their own painkillers. A child may have the recommended dose of paracetamol suspension (not aspirin). Take or send the casualty to hospital.

09 FOREIGN OBJECTS, POISONING, BITES AND STINGS

Objects that find their way into the body, either through a wound in the skin or via an orifice, are known as "foreign objects". These range from grit in the eye to small objects that young children may push into their noses and ears. These injuries can be distressing but do not usually cause serious problems for the casualty.

Poisoning may result from exposure to, or ingestion of, toxic substances, chemicals and contaminated food. The effects of poisons vary but medical advice will be needed in most cases.

Insect stings and marine stings can often be treated with first aid. However, multiple stings can produce a reaction that requires urgent medical help. Animal and human bites always require medical attention due to the risk of infection.

AIMS AND OBJECTIVES

- To ensure the safety of yourself and the casualty
- To assess the casualty's condition quickly and calmly
- To assess the potential danger of a foreign object
- To identify the poisonous substance
- To comfort and reassure the casualty
- To look for and treat any injuries associated with the condition
- To obtain medical help if necessary. Call 999/112 for emergency help if you suspect a serious illness or injury
- To be aware of your own needs

THE SENSORY ORGANS

THE SKIN

The body is covered and protected by the skin, the largest organ of the body. Skin is made up of two layers: an outer layer called the epidermis, and an inner layer, the dermis. The skin forms a barrier against harmful substances and germs. It is also an important sense organ, containing nerves that ensure the body is sensitive to heat, cold, pain and touch.

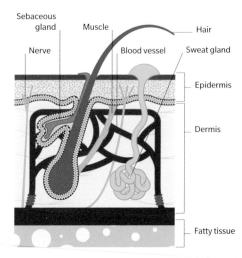

Sebaceous gland — Muscle — Hair — Nerve — Blood vessel — Sweat gland — Epidermis — Dermis — Fatty tissue

Structure of the skin
The skin consists of the thin epidermis and the thicker dermis, which sit on a layer of fatty tissue (subcutaneous fat). Blood vessels, nerves, muscles, sebaceous (oil) glands, sweat glands and hair roots (follicles) lie in the dermis.

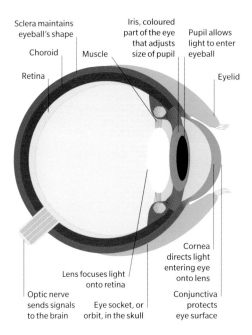

Sclera maintains eyeball's shape — Iris, coloured part of the eye that adjusts size of pupil — Pupil allows light to enter eyeball — Choroid — Muscle — Retina — Eyelid — Cornea directs light entering eye onto lens — Lens focuses light onto retina — Conjunctiva protects eye surface — Optic nerve sends signals to the brain — Eye socket, or orbit, in the skull

Structure of the eye
The eyes are fluid-filled, spherical structures about 2.5 cm (1 in) in diameter. They have focusing parts (cornea and lens), and light- and colour-sensitive cells in the retina.

THE EYES

These complex organs enable us to see the world around us. Each eye consists of a coloured part (iris) with a small opening (pupil) that allows rays of light to enter the eye. The size of the pupil changes according to the amount of light that is entering the eye.

Light rays are focused by the transparent lens onto a "screen" (retina) at the back of the eye. Special cells in the retina convert this information into electrical impulses that then travel, via the optic nerve that leads from the eye, to the part of the brain where the impulses are analysed.

Each eye is protected by a bony socket in the skull (p.135). The eyelids and delicate membranes called conjunctiva protect the front of the eyes.

Tears form a protective film across the front of the conjunctiva, lubricating the surface and flushing away dust and dirt.

THE EARS

As well as being the organs of hearing, the ears also play an important role in balance. The visible part of each ear, the auricle, funnels sounds into the ear canal to vibrate the eardrum. Fine hairs in the ear canal filter out dust, and glands secrete ear wax that traps any other small particles.

The vibrations of the eardrum pass across the middle ear to the hearing apparatus (cochlea) in the inner ear. This structure converts the vibrations into nerve impulses and transmits them to the brain via the auditory nerve. The vestibular apparatus within the inner ear is involved in balance.

Structure of the ear

The ear is divided into three main parts: the outer, middle and inner ear. The eardrum separates the outer and middle ear. The inner ear contains the organs of hearing and balance.

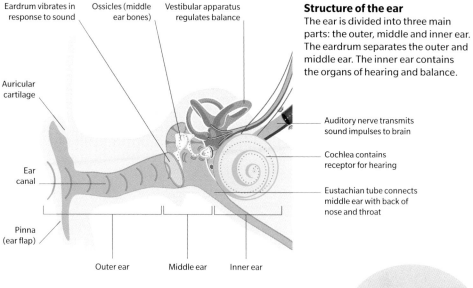

Eardrum vibrates in response to sound

Ossicles (middle ear bones)

Vestibular apparatus regulates balance

Auricular cartilage

Auditory nerve transmits sound impulses to brain

Ear canal

Cochlea contains receptor for hearing

Eustachian tube connects middle ear with back of nose and throat

Pinna (ear flap)

Outer ear   Middle ear   Inner ear

THE MOUTH AND NOSE

These cavities form the entrances to the digestive and respiratory tracts respectively. The nasal cavities connect with the throat. They are lined with blood vessels and membranes that secrete mucus to trap debris that enters the nose. Food enters the digestive tract via the mouth, which leads into the gullet (oesophagus). The epiglottis, a flap at the back of the throat, prevents food from entering the windpipe (trachea).

Structure of the mouth and nose

The nostrils lead into the two nasal cavities, which are lined with mucous membranes and blood vessels. The nasal cavities connect directly with the top of the throat, which is at the back of the mouth.

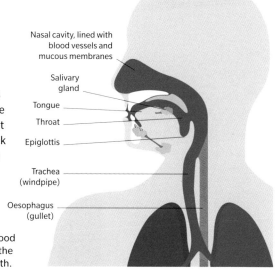

Nasal cavity, lined with blood vessels and mucous membranes

Salivary gland

Tongue

Throat

Epiglottis

Trachea (windpipe)

Oesophagus (gullet)

SPLINTER

YOUR AIMS

- To remove the splinter
- To minimise the risk of infection

Small splinters of wood, metal or glass may enter the skin. They carry a risk of infection because they are rarely clean. Often a splinter can be successfully withdrawn from the skin using tweezers. However, if the splinter is deeply embedded, lies over a joint, or is difficult to remove, you should leave it in place and advise the casualty to seek medical help.

WHAT TO DO

1 Gently clean the area around the splinter with soap and warm water.

2 Holding the tweezers near the end for a better grip, grasp the splinter as close to the skin as possible.

3 Draw the splinter out in a straight line at the same angle that it went into the skin; make sure it does not break.

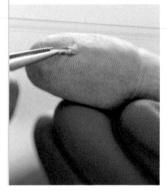
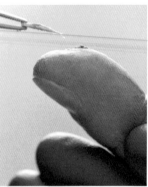

4 Carefully squeeze the wound to encourage a little bleeding. This will help to flush out any remaining dirt. Clean and dry the wound and cover it with a dressing.

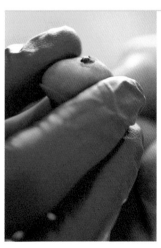

SPECIAL CASE
EMBEDDED SPLINTER

If a splinter is embedded or difficult to dislodge, do not probe the area with a sharp object, such as a needle, or you may introduce infection. Pad around the splinter until you can bandage over the top without pressing on it, and seek medical help.

EMBEDDED FISH-HOOK

A fish-hook that is embedded in the skin is difficult to remove because of the barb at the end of the hook. If possible, you should ensure that the hook is removed by a healthcare professional. Only attempt to remove a hook yourself if medical help is not readily available. Embedded fish-hooks carry a risk of infection, including tetanus.

WHAT TO DO

1 Support the injured area. If possible, cut off the fishing line as close to the hook as possible.

2 If medical help is readily available, build up pads of gauze around the hook until you can bandage over the top without pushing it in further. Bandage over the padding and the hook and arrange to take or send the casualty to hospital.

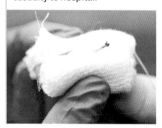

3 If medical help is not available, you can try to remove the hook if you can see the barb. Cut off the barb with wirecutters, then carefully withdraw the hook back through the skin by its eye.

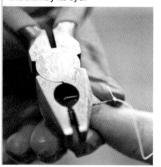

4 Clean and dry the wound and cover with a dressing.

CAUTION
- Do not try to pull out a fish-hook unless you can cut off the barb. If you cannot, seek medical help.

Ask the casualty about tetanus immunisation. Seek medical advice if they:
- Have a dirty wound.
- Have never been immunised.
- Are uncertain about the number or timings of immunisations.

YOUR AIMS
- To obtain medical help
- To minimise the risk of infection
- If help is delayed, to remove the fish-hook without causing a casualty any further injury and pain

SWALLOWED FOREIGN OBJECT

An adult may swallow a bone by mistake or ingest objects on purpose and children put small items in their mouths when playing. Most objects will pass through the digestive system, but some can cause a blockage or perforation. Ingestion of a button battery can cause serious injury as they are highly corrosive.

WHAT TO DO

1 Reassure the casualty and find out what they swallowed.

2 Seek medical advice. Call 999/112 for emergency help if necessary.

CAUTION
- Do not let the casualty make themselves vomit.

YOUR AIM
- To obtain medical advice as soon as possible

FOREIGN OBJECT IN THE EYE

Foreign objects such as grit, a loose eyelash or a contact lens that are floating on the surface of the eye can easily be rinsed out. However, you must not attempt to remove anything that sticks to the eye or penetrates the eyeball because this may damage the eye. Instead, make sure that the casualty receives urgent medical attention.

RECOGNITION

There may be:

- Blurred vision
- Pain or discomfort
- Redness and watering of the eye
- Eyelids screwed up in spasm

YOUR AIM

- To prevent injury to the eye

SPECIAL CASE IF OBJECT IS UNDER UPPER EYELID

Ask the casualty to grasp the lashes on the upper eyelid and pull the upper lid over the lower one; the lower lashes may brush the particle clear. If this is unsuccessful, ask them to try blinking under water since this may also make the object float off. Do not attempt to do this if the object is large or abrasive.

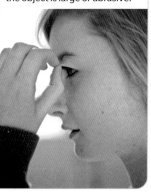

WHAT TO DO

1 **Advise the casualty not to rub their eye.** Ask them to sit down facing a light.

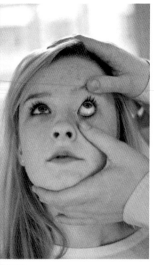
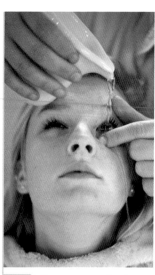

2 **Stand beside,** or just behind, the casualty. Gently separate the casualty's eyelids with your thumbs or finger and thumb. Ask them to look right, left, up and down. Examine every part of their eye as they do this.

3 **If you can see a foreign object** on the white of the eye, wash it out by pouring clean water from a glass or jug, or by using a sterile eyewash if you have one. Put a towel around the casualty's shoulders. Hold their eye open and pour the water from the inner corner so that it drains on to the towel.

4 **If this is unsuccessful,** try lifting the object off with a moist swab or the damp corner of a clean handkerchief or tissue. If you still cannot remove the object, seek medical help.

FOREIGN OBJECT IN THE EAR

If a foreign object becomes lodged in the ear, it may cause temporary deafness by blocking the ear canal. In some cases, a foreign object may damage the eardrum. Young children frequently push objects into their ears. The tips of cotton wool buds are often left in the ear. Insects can fly or crawl into the ear and may cause distress.

WHAT TO DO

1 **Arrange to take or send** the casualty to hospital as soon as possible. Do not try to remove a lodged object yourself.

2 **Reassure the casualty** during the journey or until medical help arrives.

YOUR AIMS

- To prevent injury to the ear
- To remove a trapped insect
- To arrange transport to hospital if a foreign object is lodged in the casualty's ear

SPECIAL CASE INSECT INSIDE THE EAR

Reassure the casualty and ask them to sit down. Support their head with the affected ear uppermost. Gently flood the ear with tepid water; the insect should float out. If this flooding does not remove the insect, seek medical help.

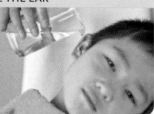

FOREIGN OBJECT IN THE NOSE

Young children may push small objects up their noses. Objects can block the nose and cause infection. If the object is sharp it can damage the tissues, and "button" batteries can cause burns and bleeding. Do not try to remove a foreign object; you may cause injury or push it further into the airway.

WHAT TO DO

1 **Try to keep the casualty** quiet and calm. Tell them to breathe through their mouth at a normal rate. Advise them not to poke inside their nose in an attempt to remove the object themselves.

2 **Arrange to take** or send the casualty to hospital, so that the object can be safely removed by medical staff.

RECOGNITION

There may be:

- Difficult or noisy breathing through the nose
- Swelling of the nose
- Smelly or blood-stained discharge, indicating that an object may have been lodged for a while

YOUR AIM

- To arrange transport to hospital

HOW POISONS AFFECT THE BODY

A poison (toxin) is a substance that, if taken into or absorbed into the body in sufficient quantity, can cause either temporary or permanent damage.

Poisons can be swallowed, absorbed through the skin, inhaled, splashed into the eyes or injected. Once in the body, they may enter the bloodstream and be carried swiftly to all organs and tissues. Signs and symptoms of poisoning vary with the poison. They may develop quickly or over a number of days. Vomiting is common, especially when the poison has been ingested. Inhaled poisons often cause breathing difficulties.

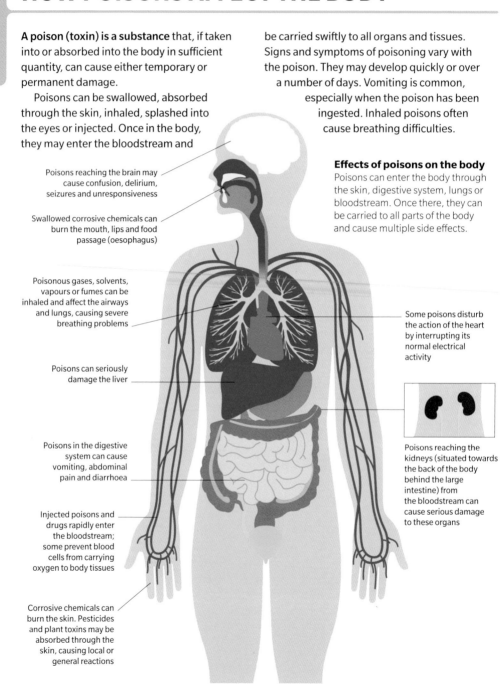

Poisons reaching the brain may cause confusion, delirium, seizures and unresponsiveness

Swallowed corrosive chemicals can burn the mouth, lips and food passage (oesophagus)

Poisonous gases, solvents, vapours or fumes can be inhaled and affect the airways and lungs, causing severe breathing problems

Poisons can seriously damage the liver

Poisons in the digestive system can cause vomiting, abdominal pain and diarrhoea

Injected poisons and drugs rapidly enter the bloodstream; some prevent blood cells from carrying oxygen to body tissues

Corrosive chemicals can burn the skin. Pesticides and plant toxins may be absorbed through the skin, causing local or general reactions

Effects of poisons on the body
Poisons can enter the body through the skin, digestive system, lungs or bloodstream. Once there, they can be carried to all parts of the body and cause multiple side effects.

Some poisons disturb the action of the heart by interrupting its normal electrical activity

Poisons reaching the kidneys (situated towards the back of the body behind the large intestine) from the bloodstream can cause serious damage to these organs

TYPES OF POISON

Some poisons are synthetic – for example, chemicals and drugs – and these are found in the home as well as in industry. Almost every household contains substances that are potentially poisonous, such as bleach and paint stripper, as well as prescribed or over-the-counter medicines, which may be dangerous if taken in excessive amounts.

Other poisons occur in nature: for example, plants produce poisons that may irritate the skin or cause more serious symptoms if ingested, and various insects and creatures produce venom in their bites and stings. Contamination of food by bacteria may result in food poisoning – one of the most common forms of poisoning.

RECOGNISING THE EFFECTS OF POISONING

ROUTE OF ENTRY INTO BODY	POISON	POSSIBLE EFFECTS	ACTION
Swallowed (ingested)	● Drugs and alcohol ● Cleaning products ● DIY and gardening products ● Plant poisons ● Bacterial food poisons ● Viral food poisons	● Nausea and vomiting ● Abdominal pain ● Seizures ● Irregular, or fast or slow heartbeat ● Impaired level of response	● Monitor casualty ● Call emergency help ● Commence CPR if necessary (pp.56–89) ● Use a face mask to protect yourself if you need to give rescue breaths
Absorbed through the skin	● Cleaning products ● DIY and gardening products ● Industrial poisons ● Plant poisons	● Pain ● Swelling ● Rash ● Redness ● Itching	● Remove contaminated clothing ● Wash with cold water for 20 minutes ● Seek medical help ● Commence CPR if necessary (pp.56–89)
Inhaled	● Fumes from cleaning and DIY products ● Industrial poisons ■ Fumes from fires	● Difficulty breathing ● Hypoxia ● Grey-blue skin (cyanosis)	● Help casualty into the fresh air ● Call emergency help ● Commence CPR if necessary (pp.56–89)
Splashed in the eye	● Cleaning products ● DIY and gardening products ● Industrial poisons ● Plant poisons	● Pain and watering of the eye ● Blurred vision	● Irrigate the eye for 20 minutes (p.182) ● Call emergency help ● Commence CPR if necessary (pp.56–89)
Injected through the skin	● Venom from stings and bites ● Drugs	● Pain, redness and swelling at injection site ● Blurred vision ● Nausea and vomiting ● Difficulty breathing ● Seizures ● Impaired level of response ● Anaphylactic shock	For sting/venom: ● Remove sting, if possible ● Call emergency help ● Commence CPR if necessary (pp.56–89) For injected drugs: ● Call emergency help ● Commence CPR if necessary (pp.56–89)

SWALLOWED POISONS

Chemicals that are swallowed may harm the digestive tract, or cause more widespread damage if they enter the bloodstream and are transported to other parts of the body. Hazardous chemicals include some household substances such as bleach and paint stripper, which are poisonous or corrosive if swallowed.

Drugs, both prescribed or those bought over the counter, can also be harmful if an overdose is taken. Some plants and their berries, and fungi can also be poisonous.

WHAT TO DO

1 **If the casualty is responding,** ask what they have swallowed, and if possible how much and when. Look for clues – for example, poisonous plants, berries or empty containers. Try to reassure them.

2 Call 999/112 for emergency help. Give the call handler as much information as possible about the poison. This information will assist the medical team to treat the casualty.

RECOGNITION

- History of ingestion/exposure

Depending on what has been swallowed, there may be:

- Vomiting, sometimes bloodstained, later diarrhoea
- Cramping abdominal pains
- Pain or a burning sensation
- Empty containers in the vicinity
- Impaired level of response
- Seizures

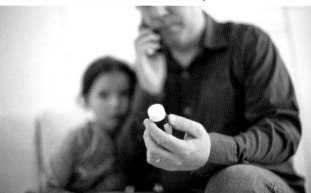

YOUR AIMS

- To maintain an open airway, breathing and circulation
- To remove any contaminated clothing
- To identify the poison
- To arrange urgent removal to hospital

3 **Monitor and record** the casualty's vital signs (pp.54–55) while waiting for help. Keep samples of any vomited material. Give these samples, containers and any other clues to the ambulance crew.

SPECIAL CASE IF LIPS ARE BURNT

If the casualty's lips are burnt by corrosive substances, give them frequent sips of cold milk or water while waiting for help to arrive.

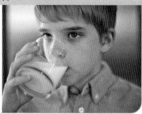

SEE ALSO Alcohol poisoning **p.204** | Chemical burn **p.181** | Drug poisoning **opposite** | Inhalation of fumes **pp.100–10** | Swallowed foreign object **p.197** | The unresponsive casualty **pp.56–89**

DRUG POISONING

Poisoning can result from an **overdose** of prescribed drugs, or drugs that are bought over the counter. It can also be caused by drug abuse or drug interactions. The effects vary depending on the drugs and how they are taken (below). When you call the emergency services, give as much information as possible. While waiting for help to arrive, look for containers that might help you to identify the drugs.

CAUTION

- Do not induce vomiting.
- Take care not to prick yourself on any needles found on or near the casualty (p.16).
- If the casualty becomes unresponsive, open the airway and check breathing (The unresponsive casualty, pp.56–89).

WHAT TO DO

1 If the casualty **is responding,** help them into a comfortable position and ask them what they have taken. Reassure them while you talk to them.

2 Call 999/112 for emergency help. Tell the call handler you suspect drug poisoning. Monitor and record the casualty's vital signs (pp.54–55) while waiting for medical help to arrive.

3 Keep samples **of any vomited** material. Look for evidence that helps identify the drug, such as empty containers. Give evidence or samples to the ambulance personnel.

YOUR AIMS

- To maintain breathing and circulation
- To arrange removal to hospital

RECOGNISING THE EFFECTS OF DRUG POISONING

CATEGORY	DRUG	EFFECTS OF POISONING
Painkillers	● Aspirin (swallowed)	● Upper abdominal pain, nausea and vomiting ● Ringing in the ears ● "Sighing" when breathing ● Confusion and delirium ● Dizziness
	● Paracetamol (swallowed)	● Little effect at first, but abdominal pain, nausea and vomiting may develop ● Irreversible liver damage may occur within three days (alcohol and malnourishment increase the risk)
Nervous system depressants and tranquillisers	● Benzodiazepines (swallowed) ● Antidepressants (swallowed) ● Antipsychotics (swallowed)	● Lethargy and sleepiness, leading to unresponsiveness ● Shallow breathing ● Weak, irregular or abnormally slow or fast pulse
Stimulants and hallucinogens	● Amphetamines (including ecstasy) and LSD (swallowed) ● Cocaine (inhaled or injected) ● "Legal highs"	● Excitable, hyperactive behaviour, agitation ● Sweating ● Tremor of the hands ● Chest pain ● Hallucinations in which the casualty may claim to "hear voices" or "see things" ● Dilated pupils
Narcotics	● Morphine, heroin (commonly injected) ● Opioids (swallowed and patches)	● Small pupils ● Sluggishness and confusion, and casualty may become unresponsive ● Slow, shallow breathing, which may stop altogether ● Needle marks which may be infected ● Nausea and vomiting ● Headaches
Solvents	● Glue, lighter fuel (inhaled)	● Hallucinations ● Casualty may be unresponsive ● Rarely, cardiac arrest
Anaesthetic	● Ketamine	● Drowsiness ● Shallow breathing ● Hallucinations

SEE ALSO The unresponsive casualty **pp.56–89** |

ALCOHOL POISONING

RECOGNITION

There may be:

- A strong smell of alcoholic drink
- Empty bottles or cans
- Impaired level of response: the casualty may respond if roused, but will quickly relapse
- Flushed and moist face
- Deep, noisy breathing
- Full, bounding pulse

In the later stages:

- Shallow breathing
- Weak, rapid pulse
- Dilated pupils that react poorly to light
- No response to stimuli

YOUR AIMS

- To maintain an open airway
- To assess for other conditions
- To seek medical help if necessary

Alcohol is a drug that depresses the activity of the central nervous system – in particular, the brain (pp.144–45). Prolonged or excessive intake of alcohol can severely impair all physical and mental functions, and the casualty may become unresponsive.

There are other risks to a casualty from alcohol poisoning, for example: an unresponsive casualty may inhale and choke on vomit; alcohol widens (dilates) the blood vessels so the body loses heat, and hypothermia may develop.

An unresponsive casualty who smells of alcoholic drink may be misdiagnosed and not receive appropriate treatment for the underlying cause of their condition, such as a head injury, stroke, heart attack or hypoglycaemia.

WHAT TO DO

1 **Cover the casualty with a coat** or blanket to protect them from the cold and reassure them.

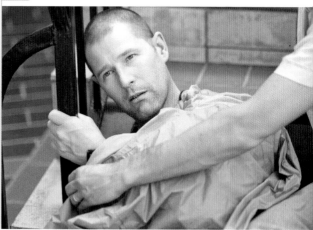

2 **Assess the casualty** for any injuries, especially head injuries, or other medical conditions.

3 **Monitor and record vital signs** (pp.54–55) until the casualty recovers or is placed in the care of a responsible person. If you are in any doubt about the casualty's condition, call 999 / 112 for emergency help.

SEE ALSO Head injury **pp.146–147** | Heart attack **p.213** | Hypoglycaemia **p.217** | Hypothermia **pp.188–190** Stroke **pp.214–215** | The unresponsive casualty **pp.56–89**

ANIMAL AND HUMAN BITES

Bites from sharp, pointed teeth cause deep puncture wounds that can damage tissues and introduce germs. Bites also crush the tissue. Any bite that breaks the skin needs prompt first aid because there is a high risk of infection.

A serious infection risk is rabies, a potentially fatal viral infection of the nervous system. The virus is carried in the saliva of infected animals. If bitten in an area where there is a risk of rabies, seek medical advice since the casualty must be given anti-rabies injections. Try to identify the animal.

Tetanus is also a potential risk following any animal bite. There is probably only a small risk of hepatitis viruses being transmitted through a human bite – and an even smaller risk of transmission of other blood borne viruses (p.16). However, medical advice should be sought straight away.

CAUTION

- If you suspect rabies, arrange to take or send the casualty to hospital immediately.

Ask the casualty about tetanus immunisation. Seek medical advice if they:

- Have a dirty wound.
- Have never been immunised.
- Are uncertain about the number and timing of immunisations.

WHAT TO DO

1 **Wash the bite wound** thoroughly with soap and warm water in order to minimise the risk of infection.

2 **Support the injured area** and pat wound dry with clean gauze swabs. Then cover with a sterile wound dressing secured with a bandage or tape. Check circulation after bandaging (p.247).

YOUR AIMS

- To control bleeding
- To minimise the risk of infection
- To seek medical help if necessary

SPECIAL CASE
FOR A DEEP WOUND

If the wound is deep, control bleeding by applying direct pressure over a sterile dressing. Once bleeding is under control, secure it with a bandage, tying the knot over the wound to help maintain pressure. Treat casualty for shock and call 999/112 for emergency help.

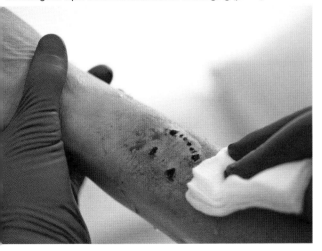

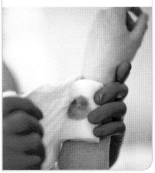

3 **Arrange to take or send** the casualty to hospital if the wound is over a joint and/or it is large or deep or if bleeding persists.

SEE ALSO Cuts and grazes **p.121** | Infected wound **p.122** | Severe external bleeding **pp.116–117** | Shock **pp.114–115**

INSECT STING

Usually, a sting from a bee, wasp or hornet is painful rather than dangerous. An initial sharp pain is followed by mild swelling, redness and soreness.

However, multiple insect stings can produce a serious reaction. A sting in the mouth or throat is potentially dangerous because swelling can obstruct the airway. With any bite or sting, it is also important to watch for signs of an allergic reaction, which can lead to anaphylactic shock (p.227).

RECOGNITION

- Pain at the site of the sting
- Redness and swelling around the site of the sting

YOUR AIMS

- To relieve swelling and pain
- To arrange removal to hospital if necessary

SPECIAL CASE
STINGS IN THE MOUTH AND THROAT

If a casualty has been stung in the mouth, there is a risk that swelling of tissues in the mouth and/or throat may occur, causing the airway to become blocked. To help prevent this, give the casualty an ice cube to suck or a glass of cold water to sip. Call 999/112 for emergency help if swelling starts to develop.

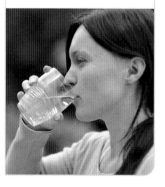

WHAT TO DO

1 Reassure the casualty. If the sting is visible, brush or scrape it off sideways with the edge of a credit card or your fingernail as quickly as you can.

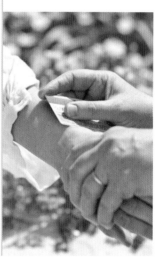

2 Raise the affected part and apply a cold compress such as an ice pack (p.245) to minimise swelling. Advise the casualty to keep the compress in place for up to 20 minutes. Tell them to seek medical advice if the pain and swelling persist.

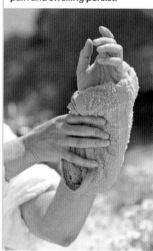

3 Monitor and record the casualty's vital signs (pp.54–55). Watch for signs of an allergic reaction, such as wheezing and/or reddened, swollen, itchy skin.

TICK BITE

Ticks are tiny, spider-like creatures found in grass or woodlands. They attach themselves to passing animals (including humans) and bite into the skin to suck blood. When sucking blood, a tick can swell to about the size of a pea, and it can then be seen easily. Ticks can carry infections such as Lyme disease, so they should be removed as soon as possible.

CAUTION

- Do not try to remove the tick with butter or petroleum jelly or burn or freeze it, since it may regurgitate infective fluids into the casualty.

WHAT TO DO

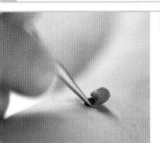

1 Using tweezers or tick remover, grasp the tick's head as close to the casualty's skin as you can. Gently pull the head upwards using steady even pressure. Do not jerk the tick as this may leave the mouth parts embedded in the casualty's skin, or cause it to regurgitate infective fluids into the skin.

YOUR AIM

- To remove the tick

2 Save the tick for identification; place it in a sealed plastic bag and give it to the casualty. The casualty should seek medical advice; tell them to take the tick with them since it may be required for analysis.

OTHER BITES AND STINGS

Scorpion stings as well as bites from some spiders and mosquitoes can cause serious illness, and may be fatal.
   Bites or stings in the mouth or throat are potentially dangerous because the resulting swelling can obstruct the airway. Be alert to an allergic reaction, which may lead the casualty to suffer anaphylactic shock (p.227).

CAUTION

- Call 999/112 for emergency help if a scorpion or a redback or funnel web spider has stung the casualty, or if the casualty is showing signs of anaphylactic shock (p.227).

WHAT TO DO

1 Reassure the casualty and help them to sit or lie down.

2 Raise the affected part if possible. Place a cold compress such as an ice pack (p.245) on the affected area for no more than 20 minutes to minimise the risk of swelling.

3 Monitor and record the casualty's vital signs (pp.54–55). Watch for signs of an allergic reaction, such as wheezing and/or reddened, swollen, itchy skin.

RECOGNITION

Depends on the species, but generally:

- Pain, redness and swelling at site of sting
- Nausea and vomiting
- Headache

YOUR AIMS

- To relieve pain and swelling
- To arrange removal to hospital if necessary

SNAKE BITE

RECOGNITION

There may be:

- A pair of puncture marks – the bite may be painless
- Severe pain, redness and swelling at the bite; the whole limb may become swollen and bruised within 24 hours
- Nausea and vomiting
- Disturbed vision
- Increased salivation and sweating
- Laboured breathing; it may stop altogether

YOUR AIMS

- To prevent venom spreading
- To arrange urgent removal to hospital

Snake bites are uncommon in the UK. The only poisonous snake native to mainland Britain is the adder, and its bite is rarely fatal. However, poisonous snakes are sometimes kept as pets and people can be exposed to venomous snakes through travel.

While a snake bite is not usually serious, it is safer to assume that a snake is venomous. Serious reactions similar to anaphylaxis (p.227) are rare but can occur within minutes or several hours later. Immediate sharp pain is usually followed by a sensation of tingling and local swelling that spreads up the limb.

Note the time of the bite, as well as the snake's appearance to help the medical team to identify the correct antivenom. If possible (and it is safe), photograph it and email or message the image to the medical team. Take precautions to prevent others being bitten. Notify the authorities who will deal with the snake.

WHAT TO DO

1 **Help the casualty to sit down** and make them comfortable. Reassure them and advise them not to move their limbs to prevent venom spreading. Immobilise an upper limb in a sling and apply a broad-fold bandage around limb and body; secure a lower limb to the other leg with broad- and narrow-fold bandages (p.253). **Call 999/112 for emergency help.** Keep the casualty immobilised throughout.

2 **If the casualty sustains a painless bite** from an exotic snake, place a pad on the site and apply a pressure bandage on top; extend the bandage as far up the limb as possible. Do not interfere with clothing at the site as movement increases the absorption of the venom into the bloodstream.

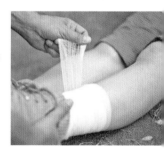

3 **Apply another pressure bandage** to extend from the bite as far up the limb as possible. Check circulation after bandaging (p.247). If possible, mark the site of the bite. Immobilise the limb by securing it to the other leg with broad- and narrow-fold bandages (p.253). If the bite is on the trunk a pressure bandage should still be applied.

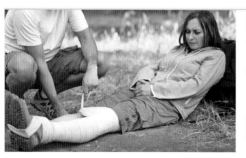

4 **Monitor and record** the casualty's vital signs (pp.54–55) while waiting for help to arrive.

STINGS FROM SEA CREATURES

Jellyfish, Portuguese men-of-war, sea anemones and corals can all cause stings. Their venom is contained in stinging cells that stick to the skin. Most marine species found in temperate regions of the world are not dangerous. However, some tropical marine creatures can cause severe poisoning. Occasionally, death results from paralysis of the chest muscles and, very rarely, from anaphylactic shock (p.227).

WHAT TO DO

1 **Encourage the casualty** to sit or lie down. Immerse the affected area in water as hot as can be tolerated for up to 30 minutes to inactivate venom; repeat every 30 minutes for pain relief. If there is no hot water, wash with plenty of sea water instead.

2 **Monitor and record** the casualty's vital signs (pp.54–55). Watch for signs of an allergic reaction, such as wheezing and itchy skin (p.226).

SPECIAL CASE
JELLYFISH STING

Pour copious amounts of vinegar or sea water over the area of the injury to incapacitate the stinging cells. Help the casualty to sit down and treat as for a snake bite (opposite). **Call 999/112 for emergency help.**

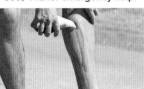

CAUTION

- If the injury is extensive or there is a severe reaction, **call 999/112 for emergency help.** Monitor and record vital signs (pp.54–55) while awaiting help.
- Do not scald the casualty; water temperature should be no more than 40°C (104°F).

RECOGNITION

Depends on the species, but generally:

- Pain, redness and swelling at site of sting
- Nausea and vomiting
- Headache

YOUR AIMS

- To relieve pain and discomfort
- To seek medical help if necessary

MARINE PUNCTURE WOUND

Many marine creatures have spines that provide a mechanism against attack from predators but that can also cause painful wounds if trodden on. Sea urchins and weever fish have sharp spines that can become embedded in the sole of the foot. Wounds may become infected if the spines are not removed. Immersing the affected area in hot water helps break down fish venom.

WHAT TO DO

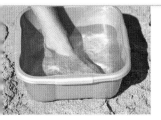

1 **Help the casualty to sit down.** Immerse the injured part in water as hot as they can tolerate (no higher than 40°C/104°F) for up to 30 minutes or as tolerated. This can be repeated at 30-minute intervals for pain relief.

CAUTION

- Do not bandage the wound.
- Do not scald the casualty; water temperature should be no more than 40°C (104°F).

YOUR AIM

- To relieve pain and discomfort

2 **Take or send** the casualty to hospital so that the spines can be safely removed.

10 MEDICAL CONDITIONS

Many everyday conditions, such as fever and headache, need prompt treatment and respond well to first aid. However, minor complaints can be the start of a serious illness, so you should seek medical advice if you are in doubt about the casualty's condition. There is also advice here on helping a casualty with a mental health crisis, where early signposting can reduce the risk of longer-term difficulties.

Other conditions such as heart attack, stroke, diabetes-related hypoglycaemia (lower than normal blood sugar levels), severe allergic reaction (anaphylaxis) and sepsis are potentially life-threatening and require urgent medical attention.

Childbirth is a natural process that often takes several hours. When a person goes into labour unexpectedly, while it is important to call for emergency help, there is usually plenty of time to get them to hospital. In the rare event of a baby arriving quickly, do not try to deliver them – the birth will happen naturally.

Miscarriage, however, is potentially serious due to the risk of severe bleeding. A person who is miscarrying needs urgent medical help.

AIMS AND OBJECTIVES

- To assess the casualty's condition quietly and calmly
- To comfort and reassure the casualty
- To call 999/112 for emergency help if you suspect a serious illness

ANGINA

RECOGNITION

- Dull, heavy or vice-like central chest pain, which may spread to the jaw and down one or both arms
- Pain that eases with rest
- Shortness of breath
- Tiredness, which is often sudden and extreme
- Feeling of anxiety

YOUR AIMS

- To ease strain on the heart by ensuring that the casualty rests
- To help the casualty with any medication
- To obtain medical help if necessary

The term angina literally means a constriction of the chest. Angina occurs when coronary arteries that supply the heart muscle with blood become narrowed and cannot carry sufficient blood to meet increased demands during exertion or excitement. An attack forces the casualty to rest; the pain should ease soon afterwards.

WHAT TO DO

1 Help the casualty to stop what they are doing and sit down. Make sure that they are comfortable and reassure them; this should help the pain to ease.

2 If the casualty has angina medication, such as tablets or a pump-action or aerosol spray, let them administer it themselves. If necessary, help the casualty to take it.

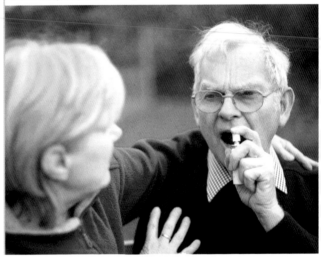

3 If the pain is not relieved 5 minutes after taking the angina medication, advise the casualty to take a second dose.

4 Encourage the casualty to rest, and keep any bystanders away from them.

5 If the casualty is still in pain 5 minutes after the second dose, or the pain returns, suspect a heart attack (opposite). Call 999/112 for emergency help.

6 If the pain subsides within 15 minutes after rest and/or medication, the casualty will usually be able to resume what they were doing. If they are concerned, tell them to seek medical advice.

HEART ATTACK

A **heart attack** is most commonly caused by a sudden obstruction of the blood supply to part of the heart muscle – for example, because of a clot in a coronary artery (coronary thrombosis). It can also be called a myocardial infarction. The main risk is that the heart will stop beating.

The effects of a heart attack depend on how much of the heart muscle is affected; many casualties recover completely. Aspirin can be used to try to restrict the size of the clot.

Coronary thrombosis

Coronary arteries supply blood to the heart muscle. When an artery is blocked, for example by a blood clot, the muscle beyond the blockage is deprived of oxygen and other nutrients carried by the blood and begins to die.

Coronary arteries

Site of blockage in coronary artery

Area deprived of oxygen and nutrients

WHAT TO DO

1 Call 999/112 for emergency help. Tell the call handler that you suspect a heart attack.

2 Make the casualty as comfortable as possible to ease the strain on the heart. A half-sitting position, with head and shoulders supported and knees bent, is often best. Place cushions both behind the casualty and under their knees.

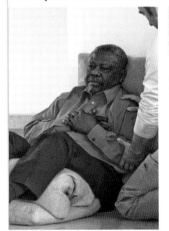

3 Assist the casualty to take one full-dose aspirin tablet (300 mg in total). Advise them to chew it slowly.

4 If the casualty has angina medication, for example, tablets or a pump-action or aerosol spray, let them administer it; help them if necessary. Encourage the casualty to rest.

5 Monitor and record vital signs (pp.54–55) while waiting for help to arrive. Stay calm to avoid undue stress.

RECOGNITION

- Persistent, dull, heavy vice-like central chest pain, which may spread to the jaw and down one or both arms. Unlike angina (opposite), the pain does not ease when the casualty rests
- Breathlessness
- Discomfort occurring high in the abdomen, which may feel similar to severe indigestion
- Collapse, often without any warning
- Sudden faintness or dizziness
- Casualty feels a sense of impending doom
- "Ashen" skin and blueness at the lips
- A rapid, weak or irregular pulse
- Profuse sweating
- Extreme gasping for air ("air hunger")

YOUR AIMS

- To ease the strain on the heart by ensuring that the casualty rests
- To call for urgent medical help without delay

SEE ALSO The unresponsive casualty **pp.56–89**

STROKE

RECOGNITION

- Facial weakness – the casualty is unable to smile evenly and the mouth or eye may be droopy
- Arm weakness – the casualty is only able to raise one arm
- Speech problems – the casualty is unable to speak clearly

There may also be:

- Sudden weakness or numbness of the face, arm or leg on one or both sides of the body
- Sudden loss or blurring of vision in one or both eyes
- Sudden difficulty with speech or understanding the spoken word
- Sudden confusion
- Sudden severe headache with no apparent cause
- Dizziness, unsteadiness or sudden fall

YOUR AIMS

- To arrange urgent admission to hospital
- To reassure and comfort the casualty

Causes of a stroke

Any disruption to the flow of blood to the brain starves the affected part of the brain of oxygen and nutrients. This can cause temporary or permanent loss of function in that area of the brain. A stroke can result from a blood clot that blocks an artery supplying blood to the brain (right), or from a burst blood vessel that causes bleeding which presses on the brain (far right).

A stroke is a medical emergency that occurs when the blood supply to the brain is disrupted. Strokes are the third most common cause of death in the UK and many people live with long-term disability as a result of a stroke. This condition is more common later in life and is associated with disorders of the circulatory system, such as high blood pressure.

The majority of strokes are caused by a clot in a blood vessel that blocks the flow of blood to part of the brain. However, some strokes are the result of a ruptured blood vessel that causes bleeding into the brain. If a stroke is due to a blood clot, it may be possible to give drugs to limit the extent of damage to the brain and improve recovery. **Call 999/112 for emergency help** immediately if you think a casualty has had a stroke.

Use the FAST (Face–Arm–Speech–Time) guide if you suspect a casualty has had a stroke:

F – Facial weakness – the casualty is unable to smile evenly and the mouth or eye may be droopy.

A – Arm weakness – the casualty is only able to raise one of their arms.

S – Speech problems – the casualty is unable to speak clearly or may not understand the spoken word.

T – Time to **call 999/112 for emergency help** if you suspect that the casualty has had a stroke.

TRANSIENT ISCHAEMIC ATTACK (TIA)

A transient ischaemic attack, or TIA, is sometimes called a mini-stroke. It is the same as a stroke, except that the symptoms and signs usually last for a shorter time, often just a few minutes, and disappear completely. A casualty with a TIA should be seen as an emergency as they are at risk of developing a full stroke in the near future and need specialist assessment and treatment, ideally within 24 hours. Do not wait to see if the symptoms go away. If there is any doubt, assume that it is a stroke.

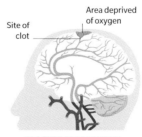

Site of clot

Area deprived of oxygen

BLOCKED BLOOD VESSEL

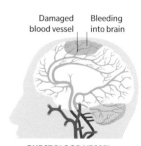

Damaged blood vessel

Bleeding into brain

BURST BLOOD VESSEL

WHAT TO DO

1 **Look at the casualty's face.** Ask them to smile: if they have had a stroke they may only be able to smile on one side – the other side of the mouth may droop.

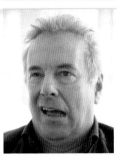

2 **Ask the casualty to raise both arms:** if they have had a stroke, they may only be able to lift one arm fully.

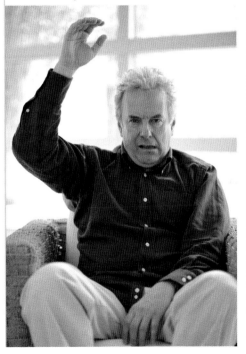

3 **Find out whether the person can speak** clearly and understand what you say. When you ask a question do they respond appropriately?

4 **Call 999/112 for emergency help** and tell the call handler that you have used the FAST guide and you suspect a stroke.

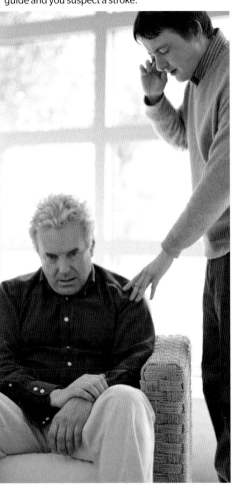

5 **Keep the casualty comfortable** and supported. If the casualty is responding, you may help them to lie down. Reassure them that help is on its way.

6 **Regularly monitor and record** the casualty's vital signs (see pp. 54–55) while you are waiting for help to arrive. Do not give the casualty anything to eat or drink because it may be difficult for them to swallow and there is a risk of choking.

DIABETES MELLITUS

This is a long-term (chronic) condition in which the body fails to produce sufficient insulin. Insulin is a chemical produced by the pancreas (a gland that lies behind the stomach), which regulates the blood sugar (glucose) level in the body. This condition can result in higher than normal blood sugar (hyperglycaemia) or lower than normal blood sugar (hypoglycaemia). If a person with diabetes is unwell, giving them sugar will rapidly correct hypoglycaemia and is unlikely to do harm in cases of hyperglycaemia.

TYPES OF DIABETES
The two most common types of diabetes are known as Type 1 and Type 2. Gestational diabetes may occur in pregnancy; the cause is unknown, but there are recognised risk factors.

Type 1 diabetes often develops in childhood or in the teenage years. In Type 1, also called insulin-dependent diabetes, the body's immune system destroys the cells in the pancreas that produce insulin, leaving the body without sufficient insulin to function normally. Insulin can be administered via daily injections (with an insulin pen) or a pump. This is a small portable device that is attached to the person's body, which delivers insulin continuously via a piece of tubing that leads from the device to a needle that sits just under the person's skin.

Type 2 diabetes occurs when the body does not produce enough insulin or it develops resistance to insulin produced by the pancreas. This type is usually linked with obesity and lifestyle factors and the risk of developing it is increased if it runs in your family. It used to be called maturity onset diabetes because it was more common in people over the age of 40, but it has now become much more common in younger age groups. It can normally be controlled with diet, weight loss and regular exercise. However, oral medication and, in some cases, insulin injections may be needed.

HYPERGLYCAEMIA

CAUTION
- If the casualty becomes unresponsive, open the airway and check breathing (The unresponsive casualty, pp.56–89).

High blood sugar (hyperglycaemia) may develop slowly over a period of hours or days. If it is not treated, hyperglycaemia will result in the person becoming unresponsive (diabetic coma). The person will require urgent treatment in hospital. People with diabetes may wear medical warning bracelets, cards or medallions alerting a first aider to the condition.

RECOGNITION
- Warm, dry skin
- Rapid pulse and breathing
- Fruity sweet breath and excessive thirst
- Medical warning bracelet
- Drowsiness, leading to unresponsiveness if untreated

YOUR AIM
- To arrange urgent removal to hospital

WHAT TO DO

1 Call 999/112 for emergency help; tell the call handler that you suspect hyperglycaemia.

2 Monitor and record the casualty's vital signs (pp.54–55) while waiting for help to arrive.

HYPOGLYCAEMIA

This condition occurs when the blood sugar level falls below normal. It is characterised by a rapidly deteriorating level of response. Hypoglycaemia (hypo) develops if the insulin–sugar balance is incorrect; for example, when a person with diabetes misses a meal or takes too much exercise. It is common in a person with newly diagnosed diabetes while they are learning to balance sugar levels. More rarely, it may develop following an epileptic seizure (pp.218–219) or after an episode of binge drinking.

People with diabetes normally carry their own blood-testing kits to check their blood sugar levels, as well as their insulin medication and sugary food for use in an emergency. For example, a person may have sugar lumps or a tube of glucose gel.

If the hypoglycaemic episode is at an advanced stage, a casualty's level of response may be affected (p.54) and you must call 999/112 for emergency help.

CAUTION

- If the person is not fully alert (p.52), do not give them anything to eat or drink.
- If the casualty becomes unresponsive, open the airway and check breathing (The unresponsive casualty, pp.56–89).

RECOGNITION

There may be:

- A history of diabetes – the casualty may recognise the onset of a hypoglycaemic episode, or "hypo", themselves
- Weakness, faintness or hunger
- Confusion and irrational behaviour
- Sweating with cold, clammy skin
- Rapid pulse
- Palpitations and muscle tremors
- Deteriorating level of response
- Medical warning bracelet and/or necklace and glucose gel or sweets for emergency use
- Medication such as an insulin pen or tablets and a glucose testing kit

YOUR AIMS

- To raise the sugar content of the blood as quickly as possible
- To obtain appropriate medical help

WHAT TO DO

1 **Help the casualty to sit down.** If they have an emergency sugar supply such as glucose gel, help them to take it. If not give them the equivalent of 15–20 g of glucose – for example, a 150 ml glass of non-diet fizzy drink or fruit juice, 3 teaspoons of sugar (or sugar lumps) or 3 sweets such as jelly babies.

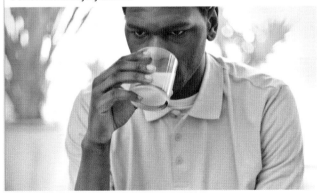

2 **If the casualty responds quickly,** give them more sugary food or drink and let them rest until they feel better. Help them find their glucose testing kit so that they can check their glucose level. Monitor them until they have completely recovered.

3 **If the casualty's condition does not improve,** look for other possible causes. **Call 999/112 for emergency help** and monitor and record their vital signs (pp.54–55) while waiting for help to arrive.

SEIZURES IN ADULTS

A seizure – also called a convulsion or fit – consists of involuntary contractions of many of the muscles in the body. The condition is due to a disturbance in the electrical activity of the brain. Seizures usually result in the person becoming unresponsive or their response is impaired. The most common cause is epilepsy. Other causes include head injury, some brain-damaging diseases, shortage of oxygen or glucose in the brain and the intake of certain poisons, including alcohol or drugs.

Epileptic seizures result from recurrent, major disturbances of brain activity and they can be sudden and dramatic. Just before a seizure, a casualty may experience a brief warning (aura) with, for example, a strange feeling or a special smell or taste.

No matter what the cause of the seizure, care must always include maintaining an open, clear airway and monitoring of the casualty's vital signs (pp.54–55) until they recover or help arrives. You will also need to protect the casualty from further harm during a seizure and arrange appropriate aftercare once they have recovered.

RECOGNITION

In epilepsy, the following sequence is common:

- Sudden loss of responsiveness
- Casualty becomes rigid, arching their back
- Breathing may be noisy and become difficult – the lips may show a grey-blue tinge (cyanosis)
- Convulsive movements begin
- Saliva may appear at the mouth and may be bloodstained if the lips or tongue have been bitten
- Possible loss of bladder or bowel control
- Muscles relax and breathing becomes normal; the casualty recovers and is responsive again, usually within a few minutes. They may feel dazed or act strangely. They may be unaware of their actions
- After a seizure, the casualty may feel tired and fall into a deep sleep

SPECIAL CASE ABSENCE SEIZURES

Some people experience a mild form of epilepsy known as absence seizures, during which they appear distant and unaware of their surroundings. This tends to affect children more than adults and a full seizure may follow. A casualty may suddenly "switch off" and stare blankly ahead. You may notice slight or localised twitching or jerking of the lips, eyelids, head or limbs and/or odd "automatic" movements, such as lip-smacking or making noises.

- Help the casualty to sit down in a quiet place.
- Remove any potentially dangerous items such as hot drinks or sharp objects.
- Talk to them in a calm and reassuring way and stay with them until they have fully recovered.
- Advise them to seek medical advice if they are unaware of the condition or do not recover fully.

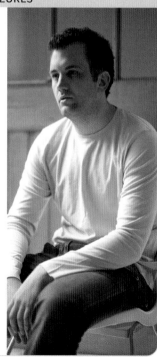

WHAT TO DO

1 Make space around the casualty; ask bystanders to move away. Remove potentially dangerous items, such as hot drinks and sharp objects. Note the time that the seizure started.

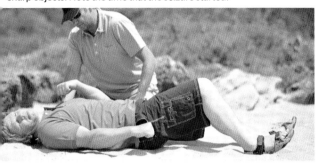

2 Protect the casualty's head from objects nearby; place soft padding such as rolled towels underneath or around their head and neck if possible. Loosen tight clothing around their neck if necessary.

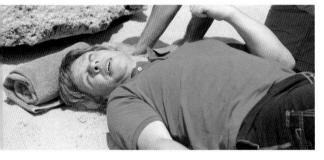

3 When the convulsive movements have ceased, open the casualty's airway and check breathing. If they are breathing, place them in the recovery position.

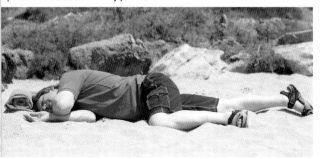

4 Monitor and record vital signs (pp.54–55) until they recover completely. Make a note of how long the seizure lasted.

YOUR AIMS

- To protect the casualty from injury during the seizure
- To care for the casualty when they are responsive and arrange removal to hospital if necessary

IMPORTANT

If a wheelchair user is having a seizure

- Apply the brakes to prevent the chair moving
- Leave the person in the chair unless they have a care plan stating otherwise
- If the casualty is wearing a seatbelt or harness, leave it secured. If there is no seatbelt or harness, gently support the casualty to prevent them falling
- Gently support and cushion the casualty's head to minimise the risk of injury
- When convulsive movements have ceased, check the casualty's airway and breathing and place in the recovery position if necessary. Monitor and record the casualty's vital signs (pp.54–55) until they recover completely.
- Make a note of how long the seizure lasts

SEIZURES IN CHILDREN

RECOGNITION

- Loss of or impaired response
- Vigorous shaking, with clenched fists and an arched back

There may also be:

- Obvious signs of fever: hot, flushed skin and sweating
- Twitching of the face and fixed, squinting or upturned eyes
- Breath-holding, with red, "puffy" face and neck and drooling at the mouth
- Vomiting and/or loss of bowel or bladder control

YOUR AIMS

- To protect the child from injury
- To cool the child
- To reassure the parents
- To arrange removal to hospital

In young children, seizures – sometimes called convulsions or fits – are most often the result of a raised body temperature associated with a throat or ear infection or other infections. This type of seizure, also known as a febrile seizure, occurs because the electrical systems in the brain are not mature enough to deal with the body's high temperature.

Although seizures can be alarming, they are rarely dangerous if properly dealt with. However, you should always seek medical advice for the child to rule out any serious underlying condition.

WHAT TO DO

1 **Place pillows or soft padding** around the child so that even violent movement will not result in injury. Do not restrain the child in any way.

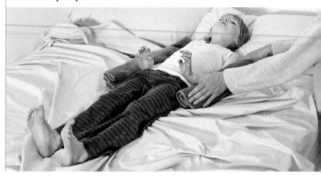

2 **Cool the child.** Remove any bedding and clothes, for example T-shirt or pyjama top; you may have to wait until the seizure stops. Ensure a good supply of fresh air, but be careful not to overcool the child.

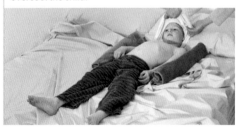

3 **Once the seizure has stopped,** place the child in the recovery position to maintain an open airway. Call 999/112 for emergency help.

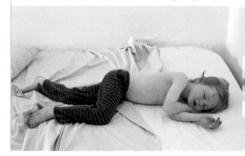

4 **Reassure the child** as well as the parents or carer. Monitor and record the child's vital signs (pp.54–55) until emergency help arrives.

FEVER

A sustained body temperature above the normal level of 37°C (98.6°F) is known as fever. It is usually caused by a bacterial or viral infection, and may be associated with earache, sore throat, measles, chickenpox, meningitis (p.223) or a local infection, such as an abscess. The infection may have been acquired during overseas travel.

In young children, a temperature above 39°C (102.2°F) can be dangerous and may trigger seizures (opposite). If you are in any doubt about a casualty's condition, seek medical advice.

CAUTION

- If you are concerned about the casualty's condition, seek medical advice.
- Do not over- or underdress a child with fever; do not sponge a child to cool them as there is a risk of overcooling.
- Do not give aspirin to any person under 16 years of age.

WHAT TO DO

1 **Keep the casualty cool and comfortable** – preferably in bed with a light covering.

2 **Give them plenty of cool drinks** to replace any body fluids lost through sweating.

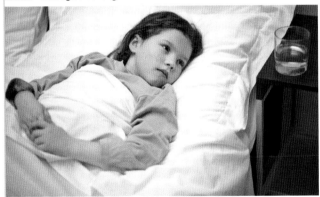

RECOGNITION

- Raised body temperature above 37°C (98.6°F)
- Pallor – casualty may feel cold with goose pimples, shivering and chattering teeth

Later:
- Hot, flushed skin and sweating
- Headache
- Generalised aches and pains

YOUR AIMS

- To bring down the fever
- To obtain medical aid if necessary

3 **If a child appears distressed or unwell,** they may have the recommended dose of paracetamol suspension (not aspirin). An adult may take the recommended dose of paracetamol.

4 **Monitor and record** the casualty's vital signs (pp.54–55) until they recover.

SEPSIS

RECOGNITION

Suspect sepsis if a person with a known or suspected infection develops any of the symptoms and signs below – note they are usually not all present at the same time, but include:

- Severe breathlessness and/or rapid shallow breathing (more than 22 breaths per minute)
- Extreme pain or discomfort
- Casualty has not passed urine all day
- Skin is pale, mottled and discoloured
- Hands and feet are cold
- Person says they feel like they are going to die
- Speech becomes slurred and person is confused and drowsy

In children you may also notice:

- Rapid breathing
- Mottled, blue or pale skin
- Cold hands and feet
- No recent wet nappies
- Seizure
- Child is very lethargic or difficult to rouse

YOUR AIM

- To obtain urgent medical help

This is a life-threatening complication that can develop when the body's response to an acute infection causes it to injure its own tissues and organs. It is important to recognise the difference between infection, which is common, and sepsis, which is an uncommon complication that can occur when an infection does not respond to treatment. Sepsis is responsible for one in five of all deaths globally, including most of the deaths associated with HIV/Aids, pneumonia, urinary and other infections acquired in the community and in hospitals. It can also be caused by diarrhoeal illnesses, abdominal conditions such as peritonitis, and infections such as meningitis (opposite) that affect the central nervous system.

Sepsis can affect anyone, but it is most common in the very young and very old and those with conditions that impair their immune system. It is often difficult to recognise because the early signs and symptoms are non-specific. Survival depends on prompt recognition of the condition and early treatment with antibiotics. Mortality rates from sepsis are high, the greater the delay in recognition and treatment, the higher the rate.

WHAT TO DO

1 **If you suspect sepsis** seek urgent medical advice without delay. Call 999/112 for emergency help. Do not wait for all of the signs or symptoms to develop as by that stage, the casualty will be critically ill.

2 **Reassure the casualty** and keep them cool by treating the fever. Monitor and record their vital signs (see pp.54–55) while waiting for help to arrive.

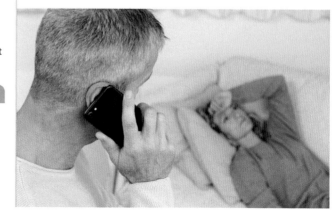

MENINGITIS

An infection of the membranes (called meninges) that surround the brain and spinal cord, meningitis can be caused by bacteria or viruses. Bacterial meningitis is an important but uncommon cause of sepsis that can rapidly become fatal and/or lead to severe disability in those who survive. Rapid deterioration is common, especially in children. Treat as for sepsis opposite.

WHAT TO DO

1 Seek urgent medical advice if you notice any of the signs of meningitis; for example, shielding eyes from the light. Do not wait for all the symptoms and signs to appear because they may not all develop. Treat the fever (p.221).

2 Check the child for signs of a rash. On dark skin, check on lighter parts of the body, such as the inner eyelids, palms of the hands or fingertips. If you see any signs, call 999/112 for emergency help even if the child has already seen a doctor.

3 While waiting for help to arrive, reassure the casualty and keep them cool. Monitor and record vital signs (pp.54–55).

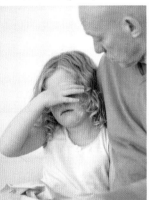

RECOGNITION

Suspect meningitis if you observe any of the following – note they are usually not all present at the same time:

- Any of the signs and symptoms of sepsis, opposite
- Flu-like illness with a high temperature
- Severe headache
- Neck stiffness (the casualty will not be able to touch their chest with their chin)
- Vomiting
- Casualty's eyes have become sensitive to any light
- In infants, there may also be high-pitched moaning or a whimpering cry, floppiness and a tense or bulging fontanelle (soft part of the skull)
- In later stages, a distinctive rash of red or purple spots that does not fade when pressed – the casualty is critically ill at this stage

IMPORTANT: CHECKING FOR MENINGITIS RASH

Most rashes will fade if you press the side of a glass firmly against them. Accompanying the later stage of meningitis is a distinctive red or purple rash that does not fade if you press it. If a rash does not fade, call 999/112 for emergency help.

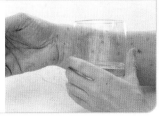

YOUR AIM

- To obtain urgent medical help

MENTAL HEALTH CRISIS

RECOGNITION

The person may:

- Describe feelings of worthlessness, entrapment, hopelessness and/or lack of social support
- Complain of disturbed sleep and/or changes in appetite
- Experience feelings of depression or anxiety

There may also be:

- Physical symptoms such as a pounding heart, sweating, trembling and shaking, chest pain or discomfort, feeling faint, hyperventilation, numbness or tingling in fingers or legs
- Casualty describing feelings of being detached from themselves, fears of losing control, being hated and loathsome, of dying and/or of a wish to not live anymore
- Attempts at self-harming, substance abuse or suicide

YOUR AIM

- To preserve life if a person may be at risk of significant harm to themselves or others
- To provide help to prevent the crisis worsening and to promote recovery
- To identify a problem early to reduce the time of an untreated crisis

Mental health is a state of well-being through which every individual copes with the normal stresses of life – but on average, one person in four experiences some form of mental health issue. Stress is a normal part of living, but it can become harmful when excessive. Chronic (long term) stress can be triggered in many ways. It can lead to a range of mental health problems from depression, anxiety or eating disorders, to psychosis and substance misuse.

Physical stress can arise from illness or injury and acute or chronic pain. Environmental stress can be caused by poor housing, social isolation, employment issues or financial problems. Emotional stress can result from relationship problems, peer pressure, marriage difficulties, life events, bereavement, physical or sexual abuse. By identifying the signs of chronic stress or a potential mental health crisis early, and encouraging a person to seek help, the severity and duration of a mental illness can be reduced, which can prevent the situation worsening.

WHAT TO DO

1 **Listen with empathy** and encourage the person to talk freely. Reassure them that they are not being judged. Always respect their privacy and confidentiality. Offer calm, emotional support and understanding and let them know that effective help is available.

2 **Encourage them to seek appropriate professional support.** Advise them to talk to their doctor, seek counselling or referral to mental health services, and, where appropriate, medication.

3 **Encourage the person to try self-help and coping methods,** for example talking to supportive family and friends, contacting support groups, and/or to seek assistance with employment, schooling, income and accommodation. Encourage strategies such as reducing caffeine and/or alcohol intake, taking regular exercise, engaging in leisure activities, maintaining adequate sleep and good nutrition and practising relaxation techniques.

4 **If the person has self-harmed,** or is attempting to self-harm, do not criticise them for their actions. Offer to treat any wound if they want you to do so. Recommend that they seek help for their self-harming.

5 **If the person is feeling suicidal** help them to call a close friend, family member and/or health professional. If they have attempted to act upon their feelings, call 999/112 for emergency help.

SEE ALSO Drug poisoning **p.203** | Hyperventilation **p.103** | Severe external bleeding p**p.116–117**
Swallowed poisons **p.202** | The unresponsive casualty **pp.56–89**

FAINTING

A faint is a brief loss of responsiveness caused by a temporary reduction of the blood flow to the brain. It may be a reaction to pain, exhaustion, lack of food or emotional stress. Fainting is also common after long periods of physical inactivity, such as standing or sitting still, especially in a warm atmosphere. This inactivity causes blood to pool in the legs, reducing the amount of blood reaching the brain.

When a person faints, the pulse rate becomes very slow. However, the rate soon picks up and returns to normal. A casualty who has fainted usually makes a rapid and complete recovery. Do not advise a person who is feeling faint to sit on a chair with their head between their knees because if they faint they may fall off the chair and injure themselves. If the casualty is in the late stage of pregnancy, help them to lie down so that they are leaning towards their left side to prevent the pregnant uterus restricting blood flow back to the casualty's heart.

CAUTION

- If the casualty does not regain responsiveness quickly, open the airway and check breathing (The unresponsive casualty, pp.56–89).

RECOGNITION

- Brief period of unresponsiveness that causes the casualty to fall to the ground
- A slow pulse
- Pale, cold skin and sweating

YOUR AIMS

- To improve blood flow to the brain
- To reassure the casualty and make them comfortable

WHAT TO DO

1 **When a casualty feels faint,** advise them to lie down. Kneel down, raise their legs, supporting the ankles on your shoulders, to improve blood flow to the brain. Watch the face for signs of recovery.

2 **Make sure that the casualty** has plenty of fresh air; ask someone to open a window if you are indoors. In addition, ask any bystanders to stand clear.

3 **As the casualty recovers,** reassure them and help them to sit up gradually. If the casualty starts to feel faint again, advise them to lie down again, and raise and support the legs until they are fully recovered.

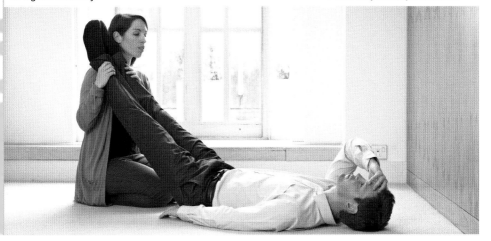

ALLERGY

An allergy is an abnormal reaction of the body's defence system (immune response) to a normally harmless "trigger" substance (or allergen). An allergy can present itself as a mild itching, swelling, wheezing or digestive condition, or can progress to full-blown anaphylaxis, or anaphylactic shock (opposite), which can occur within seconds or minutes of exposure to an offending allergen.

Common allergy triggers include pollen, dust, nuts, shellfish, eggs, wasp and bee stings, latex and certain medications. Skin changes can be subtle, absent or variable in some instances.

RECOGNITION

Features of mild allergy vary depending on the trigger. There may be:

- Red, itchy rash or raised areas of skin (weals)
- Red, itchy eyes
- Wheezing and/or difficulty breathing
- Swelling of hands, feet and/or face
- Abdominal pain, vomiting and diarrhoea

YOUR AIMS

- To assess the severity of the allergic reaction
- To seek medical advice if necessary

WHAT TO DO

1 **Assess the casualty's signs and symptoms.** Ask if they have any known allergies.

2 **Remove the trigger** if possible, or move the casualty away from the trigger.

3 **Treat any symptoms.** Allow the casualty to take their own medication for a known allergy.

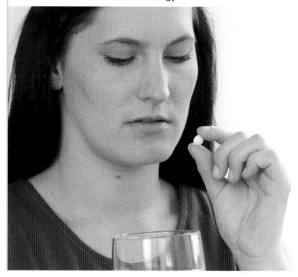

4 **If you are at all concerned** about the casualty's condition, seek medical advice.

ANAPHYLACTIC SHOCK

This is a severe allergic reaction affecting the whole body. It may develop within seconds or minutes of contact with a trigger and is potentially fatal. In an anaphylactic reaction, chemicals are released into the blood that widen (dilate) blood vessels. This causes blood pressure to fall and air passages to narrow (constrict), resulting in breathing difficulties. In addition, the tongue and throat can swell, obstructing the airway. The amount of oxygen reaching the vital organs can be severely reduced, causing hypoxia (p.94). Common triggers include: nuts, shellfish, eggs, wasp and bee stings, latex and certain medications.

A casualty with anaphylactic shock needs emergency treatment with adrenaline by injection.

CAUTION

- If a pregnant casualty needs to lie down, lean them towards their left side to prevent the pregnant uterus restricting blood flow back to the heart.
- If the casualty becomes unresponsive, open the airway and check breathing (The unresponsive casualty, pp.56–89).

WHAT TO DO

1 Call 999/112 for emergency help; tell them you suspect anaphylaxis.

2 If the casualty has an adrenaline auto-injector, help them to use it. If they are unable to administer it, and you have been trained, do it for them. Pull off the safety cap and, holding the auto-injector with your fist, push the tip firmly against the casualty's thigh until it clicks, releasing the medication (it can be delivered through clothing). Hold it in place for 3 seconds (or as instructed on the auto-injector), then remove it.

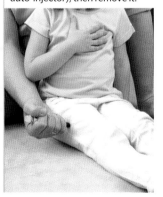

3 Help the casualty to sit up in the position that best relieves any breathing difficulty. If they become pale with a weak pulse, help them to lie down with legs raised and treat for shock (pp.114–115).

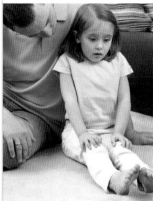

4 Monitor and record the casualty's vital signs (pp.54–55) while waiting for help to arrive. Repeated doses of adrenaline can be given at 5-minute intervals if there is no improvement or the symptoms return.

RECOGNITION

Features of allergy (opposite) may be present:

- Red, itchy rash or raised areas of skin (weals)
- Red itchy, watery eyes
- Swelling of hands, feet and/or face
- Abdominal pain, vomiting and diarrhoea

There may also be:

- Difficulty breathing, ranging from a tight chest to severe difficulty, causing the casualty to wheeze and gasp for air
- Pale or flushed skin
- Visible swelling of tongue and throat with puffiness around the eyes
- Feeling of terror
- Confusion and agitation
- Signs of shock, leading to collapse and unresponsiveness

YOUR AIMS

- To ease breathing
- Treat shock
- To arrange urgent removal to hospital

SEE ALSO Hypoxia p.94 | Shock pp.114–115 | The unresponsive casualty pp.56–89

HEADACHE

A headache may accompany any illness, particularly a feverish ailment such as flu. It may develop for no reason, but can often be traced to tiredness, tension, stress or undue heat or cold. Mild "poisoning" caused by a stuffy or fume-filled atmosphere, or by excess alcohol or any other drug, can also induce a headache. However, a headache may also be the most prominent symptom of meningitis or a stroke.

YOUR AIMS

- To relieve the pain
- To seek medical advice if needed

WHAT TO DO

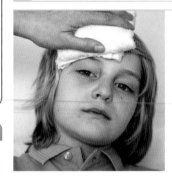

1 Help the casualty to sit or lie down in a quiet place. Give them a cold compress to hold against their head (p.245).

2 An adult may take the recommended dose of paracetamol or their own painkillers. A child may have the recommended dose of paracetamol suspension (not aspirin).

MIGRAINE

Migraine attacks are severe, "sickening" headaches and can be triggered by a variety of causes, such as allergy, stress or tiredness. Other triggers include lack of sleep, missed meals, alcohol and some foods – for example, cheese or chocolate. Individuals who suffer from migraines usually know how to recognise and deal with attacks and may carry medication.

RECOGNITION

- Possible disturbance of vision such as flickering lights and/or a "blind patch" just before onset
- Intense throbbing headache, which may be on just one side of the head
- Abdominal pain, nausea and vomiting
- Inability to tolerate bright light or loud noise

YOUR AIMS

- To relieve the pain
- To seek medical advice if needed

WHAT TO DO

1 Help the casualty to take any medication that they may have for migraine attacks. Advise them to lie down or sleep for a few hours in a quiet, dark room. Provide them with towels and a container in case they vomit.

2 If this is the first attack, advise the casualty to seek medical advice.

SORE THROAT

The most common sore throat is a "raw" feeling caused by inflammation, which is often the first sign of a cough or cold. Tonsillitis occurs when the tonsils at the back of the throat are infected. The tonsils become red and swollen and white spots of pus may be seen. Swallowing may be difficult and the glands at the angle of the jaw may be enlarged and sore.

WHAT TO DO

1 Give the casualty plenty of fluids to help ease the pain and stop the throat from becoming dry.

2 An adult may take the recommended dose of paracetamol or their own painkillers. A child may have the recommended dose of paracetamol suspension (not aspirin).

YOUR AIMS

- To relieve the pain
- To obtain medical advice if necessary

EARACHE AND TOOTHACHE

Earache can result from inflammation of the outer, middle or inner ear, and is often caused by an infection associated with a cold, tonsillitis or flu. It can also be caused by a boil, an object stuck in the ear canal or transmitted pain from a tooth abscess. There may also be temporary hearing loss. Earache often occurs when flying as a result of the changes in air pressure during ascent and descent. Infection can cause pus to collect in the middle ear and the eardrum may rupture, allowing the pus to drain, which temporarily eases the pain.

Toothache can develop when pulp inside a tooth becomes inflamed due to dental decay. If untreated, the pulp becomes infected, leading to an abscess, which causes a throbbing pain. Infection may cause swelling around the tooth or jaw.

YOUR AIMS

- To relieve the pain
- To obtain medical or dental advice if necessary

WHAT TO DO

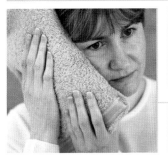

1 An adult may take the recommended dose of paracetamol or their painkillers. A child may have the recommended dose of paracetamol suspension (not aspirin).

2 Give them a source of heat, such as a hot-water bottle wrapped in a towel, to hold against the affected side.

3 In addition for toothache, you can soak a plug of cotton wool in oil of cloves to hold against the affected tooth.

4 Advise the casualty to seek medical advice if you are concerned, particularly if the casualty is a child. If a casualty has toothache, advise them to see their dentist.

SEE ALSO Foreign object in the ear **p.199**

ABDOMINAL PAIN

YOUR AIMS

- To relieve pain and discomfort
- To obtain medical help if necessary

Pain in the abdomen often has a relatively minor cause, such as food poisoning. The pain of a stitch usually occurs during exercise and is sharp. Distension (widening) or obstruction of the intestine causes colic – pain that comes and goes in waves – which often makes the casualty double up in agony and may be accompanied by vomiting.

Occasionally abdominal pain is a sign of a serious disorder affecting the organs and other structures in the abdomen. If the appendix bursts, or the intestine is damaged, the contents of the intestine can leak into the abdominal cavity, causing inflammation of the cavity lining. This life-threatening condition, called peritonitis, causes intense pain, which is made worse by movement or pressure on the abdomen, and will lead to shock developing (pp.114–115).

An inflamed appendix (appendicitis) is especially common in children. Symptoms include pain (often starting in the centre of the abdomen and moving towards their lower right side), loss of appetite, nausea, vomiting, bad breath and fever. If the appendix bursts, peritonitis will develop. The treatment is urgent surgical removal of the appendix.

SPECIAL CASE STITCH

This common condition is a form of cramp, usually associated with exercise, which occurs in the trunk or the sides of the chest. The most likely cause is a build-up of chemical waste products, such as lactic acid, in the muscles during physical exertion. Help the casualty to sit down and reassure them. The pain usually eases quickly. If it does not disappear within a few minutes, or if you are concerned about the casualty's condition, seek medical advice.

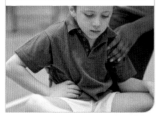

WHAT TO DO

1 **Reassure the casualty** and make them comfortable. Prop them up if they find breathing difficult. Give them a container to use if they are feeling sick or vomiting.

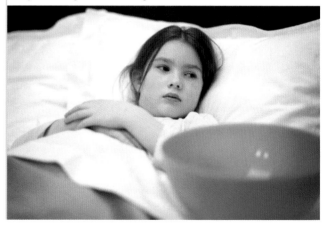

2 **Give the casualty a hot-water bottle** wrapped in a towel to hold against their abdomen. If in doubt about the casualty's condition, seek medical advice.

VOMITING AND DIARRHOEA

These problems are usually due to irritation of the digestive system. Diarrhoea and vomiting can be caused by a number of different organisms, including viruses, bacteria and parasites. They usually result from eating contaminated food or drinking contaminated water, but infection can be passed directly from person to person. Cleanliness and good hand hygiene (p.17) help prevent the spread of infectious diarrhoea.

Vomiting and diarrhoea may occur either separately or together. Both conditions can cause the body to lose vital fluids and salts, resulting in dehydration. When they occur together, the risk of dehydration is increased and can be serious, especially in infants, young children and elderly people.

The aim of treatment is to prevent dehydration by advising the casualty to have frequent sips of water, oral rehydration solution, or water containing rehydration powders even if they are still vomiting – when added to water, the powders provide the correct balance of water and salt to replace those lost through the vomiting and diarrhoea. If none of these is available, offer a non-fizzy drink. Food should be avoided while symptoms are active. When symptoms settle, introduce light, easily digestible foods.

CAUTION

- Do not give anti-diarrhoea medicines.
- If you are concerned about a casualty's condition, particularly if the vomiting or diarrhoea is persistent, or the casualty is a young child or an older person, seek medical advice.

RECOGNITION

There may be:
- Nausea
- Vomiting and later diarrhoea
- Stomach pains
- Fever

YOUR AIMS

- To reassure the casualty
- To restore lost fluids and salts

WHAT TO DO

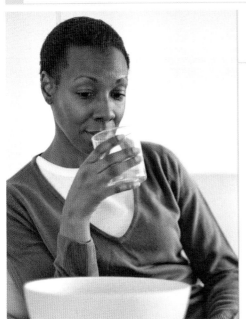

1 **Reassure the casualty** if they are vomiting. Give them a warm damp cloth so they can wipe their face.

2 **Help the casualty to sit down** and give them water, rehydration powders in water or a non-fizzy drink and advise them to sip the fluid slowly and often.

3 **When the symptoms have settled** and the casualty is hungry again, advise them to eat easily digested foods such as pasta, bread or potatoes for the first 24 hours.

4 **Advise the casualty** to stay away from work (or school) until they have been clear of all symptoms (vomiting and diarrhoea) for two days.

CHILDBIRTH

YOUR AIMS

- To obtain medical help or arrange for the woman to be taken to hospital
- To ensure privacy, reassure the woman and make them comfortable
- To prevent infection in the mother, baby and yourself
- To care for the baby during and after delivery

Childbirth is a natural and often lengthy process that normally occurs at about the 40th week of pregnancy. There is usually plenty of time to get a person to hospital, or get help to them, before the baby arrives. Most mothers-to-be are aware of what happens during childbirth, but if they go into labour early or unexpectedly they may be very anxious. You will need to reassure them and make them comfortable. Miscarriage, however, is potentially serious because there is a risk of severe bleeding. A person who is miscarrying needs urgent medical help (p.130).

There are three distinct stages to childbirth. In the first stage, the baby gets into position for the birth. The baby is born in the second stage, and in the third stage, the afterbirth (placenta and umbilical cord) is delivered.

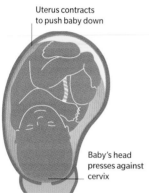

Uterus contracts to push baby down

Baby's head presses against cervix

Uterus continues to contract

Birth canal fully dilated

Baby emerges

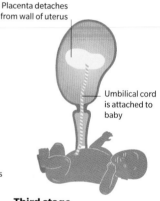

Placenta detaches from wall of uterus

Umbilical cord is attached to baby

First stage
In this stage, the body begins to experience contractions, which, together with the pressure of the baby's head, cause the cervix (neck of the uterus/womb) to open. The contractions become stronger and more frequent until the cervix is fully dilated (open) – about 10 cm (4 in) – and ready for the baby to be born. During this first stage, the mucus plug that protects the uterus from infection is expelled and the amniotic fluid surrounding the baby leaks out from the vagina. This stage can take several hours for a first baby, but is normally shorter in any subsequent pregnancies.

Second stage
Once the cervix is fully dilated, the baby's head will press down on the pelvic floor, triggering a strong urge to push. The birth canal (vagina) stretches as the baby travels through it. The baby's head normally emerges first, and the body is delivered soon afterwards. This stage of labour normally lasts about an hour.

Third stage
About 10–30 minutes after the baby is born, the placenta (the organ that nourishes the unborn baby) and the umbilical cord will be expelled from the uterus. The uterus begins to contract again, pushing the placenta out, then it closes down the area where it was attached; this reduces the bleeding.

EMERGENCY CHILDBIRTH

In the rare event of a baby arriving quickly, you should not try to "deliver" the baby; the birth will happen naturally without intervention. Your role is to comfort and listen to the wishes of the mother and care for them and their baby.

CAUTION

- Do not give the mother anything to eat because there is a risk that they may vomit. If they are thirsty give them sips of water.
- Do not pull on the baby's head or shoulders during delivery.
- If the umbilical cord is wrapped around the baby's neck as they are born, check that it is loose, and then very carefully ease it over the head to protect the baby from strangulation.
- If the baby does not cry, open the airway and check breathing (Unresponsive infant, pp.82–85) – do not smack the baby.
- Do not pull or cut the umbilical cord, even when the placenta has been delivered.

WHAT TO DO

1 Call 999/112 for emergency help. Give the call handler details of the stage that the mother has reached, the length of each contraction and the intervals between them. Call the mother's midwife too if they request it.

2 During the first stage, help the mother sit or kneel on the floor in a comfortable position. Support them with cushions or let them move around. Stay calm, and encourage them to breathe deeply during their contractions.

3 Massage the lower back gently using the heel of your hand. They may find having their face and hands wiped soothing, or spray their face with cool water and offer them ice cubes to suck.

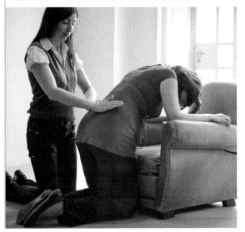

4 When the second stage starts, the mother will want to push. Make sure that the surroundings are as clean as possible to reduce the risk of infection. The mother should remove any items of clothing that could interfere with the birth. Put clean sheets or towels under them – they may also want to be covered. Encourage them to stay as upright as possible.

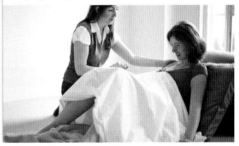

5 As the baby is born, handle them carefully; newborn babies are slippery. Give the baby to the mother; lay them on the mother's stomach or wrap them in a clean cloth, towel or blanket.

6 As the third stage begins, reassure the mother. Support them as they deliver the afterbirth; do not cut the cord. Keep the placenta and the umbilical cord intact as the midwife, doctor or ambulance crew need to check that it is complete. If the bleeding or pain is severe, treat for shock (pp.114–115). Help the mother to lie down with their legs raised.

SEE ALSO Shock **pp.114–115** | Vaginal bleeding **p.130**

11 TECHNIQUES AND EQUIPMENT

This chapter outlines the techniques and procedures that underpin first aid, including moving a casualty and applying dressings and bandages. Usually, a first aider is not expected to move an injured person, but in some circumstances – such as when a casualty is in immediate danger – it may be necessary. The key principles for moving casualties are described here. Information is also given on making an assessment of the risks involved in moving a casualty or assisting a casualty to safety.

A guide to the equipment and materials commonly found in a first aid kit is given, with information on how and when to use them. Applying dressings and bandages effectively is an essential part of first aid: wounds usually require a dressing, and many injuries benefit from the support that a bandage can give.

AIMS AND OBJECTIVES

- To assess the casualty's condition
- To comfort and reassure the casualty
- To maintain a casualty's privacy and dignity
- To use a first aid technique relevant to the injury
- To use dressings and bandages as needed
- To apply good handling techniques if moving a casualty
- To obtain appropriate help: call 999/112 for emergency help if you suspect serious injury or illness

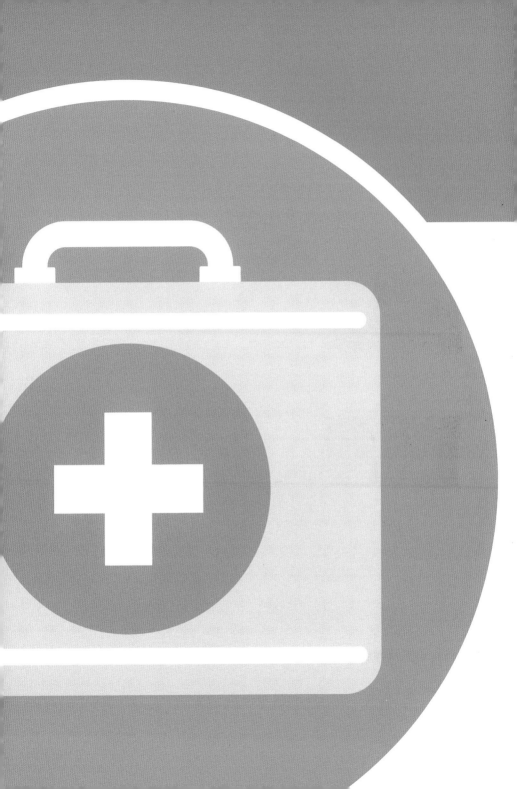

REMOVING CLOTHING

To make a thorough examination of a casualty, obtain an accurate diagnosis or give treatment, you may have to remove some of their clothing. This should be done with the minimum of disturbance to the casualty and with their agreement if possible. Remove as little clothing as possible and do not damage clothing unless it is necessary. If you need to cut a garment, try to cut along the seams, keeping the clothing clear of the casualty's injury. Maintain the casualty's privacy and prevent exposure to cold. Stop if removing clothing increases the casualty's discomfort or pain.

REMOVING CLOTHING IN LOWER BODY INJURIES

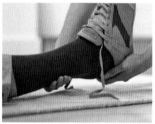 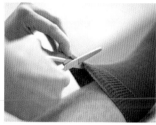 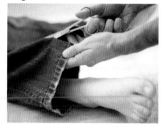

Shoes
Untie any laces, support the ankle and carefully pull the shoe off by the heel. To remove long boots, you may need to cut them down the back seam.

Socks
Remove socks by pulling them off gently. If this is not possible, lift each sock away from the leg and cut the fabric with a pair of scissors.

Trousers
Gently pull up the trouser leg to expose the calf and knee or pull down from the waist. If you need to cut clothing, lift it clear of the casualty's injury.

REMOVING CLOTHING IN UPPER BODY INJURIES

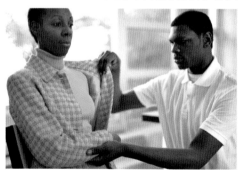 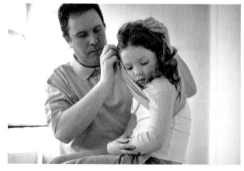

Jackets
Support the injured arm. Undo any fastenings on the jacket and gently pull the garment off the casualty's shoulders. Remove the arm on the uninjured side from its sleeve. Pull the garment round to the injured side of the body and ease it off the injured arm.

Sweaters and sweatshirts
With clothing that cannot be unfastened, begin by easing the arm on the uninjured side out of its sleeve. Next, roll up the garment and stretch it over the casualty's head. Finally, slip off the other sleeve of the garment, taking care not to disturb the arm on the injured side.

REMOVING HEADGEAR

Protective headgear, such as a riding hat or a motorcyclist's crash helmet, is best left on; it should be removed only if absolutely necessary, for example, if you cannot maintain an open airway. If the item does need to be removed, the casualty should do this themselves if possible; otherwise, you and a helper should remove it. Take care to support the head and neck at all times and keep the head aligned with the spine.

> **CAUTION**
> - Do not remove a helmet unless absolutely necessary.

REMOVING AN OPEN-FACE OR RIDING HELMET

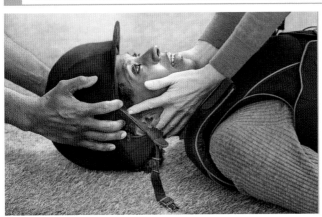

1 **Undo or cut through** the chinstrap. Support the casualty's head and neck. Place one hand on each side of the casualty's head and keep head and neck aligned with their spine; do not cover the ears.

2 **Ask a helper to grip** the sides of the helmet and pull them apart to take pressure off the head, then lift the helmet upwards and backwards.

REMOVING A FULL-FACE HELMET

1 **Undo or cut the straps.** Working from the base of the helmet, ease your fingers underneath the rim. Support the back of the neck with one hand and hold the lower jaw firmly. Ask a helper to hold the helmet with both hands.

2 **Continue to support the casualty's neck** and lower jaw. Ask your helper, working from above, to tilt the helmet backwards (without moving the head) and gently lift the front of the helmet clear of the casualty's chin.

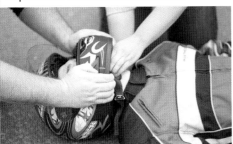

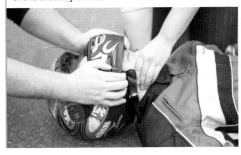

3 **Maintain support on the head and neck.** Ask your helper to tilt the helmet forwards slightly so that it will pass over the base of the skull, and then to lift it straight off the casualty's head.

CASUALTY HANDLING

CAUTION

- Do not approach a casualty if doing so puts your own life in danger.
- Do not move a casualty unless there is an emergency situation that demands you take immediate action.

When giving first aid you should leave a casualty in the position in which you find them until medical help arrives. Only move them if they are in imminent danger, and even then only if it is safe for you to approach and you have the training and equipment to carry out the move. A casualty should be moved quickly if they are in imminent danger from:

- Drowning (pp.36–37 and 102).
- Fire or an area that is filling with smoke (pp.32–33 and 100–101).
- Explosion or gunfire (pp.38–39).
- A collapsing building or other structure.

ASSESSING THE RISK OF MOVING A CASUALTY

If it is necessary to move a casualty, consider the following before you start.

- **Is the task necessary?** Usually, the casualty can be assessed and treated in the position in which you find them.
- **What are their injuries or conditions,** and will a move make them worse?
- **Can the casualty move themselves?** Ask the casualty if they feel able to move.
- **The weight and size** of the casualty.

- **Can anyone help?** If so, are you and any helpers trained and physically fit?
- **Will you need protective equipment** to enter the area, and do you have it?
- **Is there any equipment available** to assist with moving the casualty and are you trained to use it?
- **Is there enough space** around the casualty to move them safely?
- **What sort of ground** will you be crossing?

ASSISTING A CASUALTY SAFELY

If you need to move a casualty, take the following steps to ensure safety.

- **Select a method relevant** to the situation, the casualty's condition and the help and equipment that is available.
- **Use a team.** Appoint one person to coordinate the move and make sure that the team understands exactly what they are doing.
- **Plan your move** carefully and make sure that everyone is prepared.
- **Prepare any equipment** and make sure that the team and equipment are in position.
- **Use the correct technique** to avoid injuring the casualty, yourself or any helpers.
- **Ensure the safety** and comfort of the casualty, yourself and any helpers.

- **Always explain** to the casualty what is happening, and encourage them to cooperate as much as possible.
- **Position yourself** as close as possible to the casualty's body.
- **Adopt a stable base,** with your feet shoulder-width apart, so that you remain well balanced and maintain good posture at all times during the procedure.
- **Use the strongest muscles** in your legs and arms to power the move. Bend from your knees not your back.
- **If at any time you experience discomfort** or pain, stop and reassess what you are doing and request more support and assistance.

FIRST AID MATERIALS

All workplaces, leisure centres, homes and cars should have first aid kits (p.241). The kits for workplaces or public places must conform to legal requirements and be clearly marked in a green box with a white cross and easily accessible. For home or the car, you can either buy a kit or put together first aid items yourself and keep them in a clean, waterproof container. Any first aid kit must be kept in a dry place, and checked and replenished regularly.

The items on these pages form the basis of a first aid kit for the home. You may wish to add personal protective equipment (overleaf) and pain-relief tablets such as paracetamol.

STERILE DRESSINGS

Wound dressings

The most useful dressings consist of a dressing pad attached to a bandage, and are sealed in a protective wrapping. They are easy to apply, so are ideal in an emergency. Individual sealed sterile wound dressing pads may need to be secured with tape or bandages. For severe lacerations haemostatic dressings, impregnated with blood clotting agents are useful.

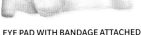

DRESSING WITH BANDAGE ATTACHED

WOUND PAD

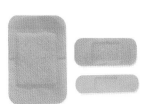

EYE PAD WITH BANDAGE ATTACHED

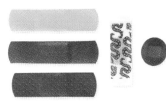

HAEMOSTATIC DRESSING

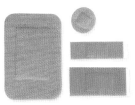

FABRIC PLASTERS

WATERPROOF PLASTERS

NOVELTY PLASTERS FOR CHILDREN

Adhesive dressings or plasters

These are applied to small cuts and grazes and are made of fabric or waterproof plastic. Use hypoallergenic plasters for anyone who is allergic to the adhesive in regular ones. People who work with food are required to use blue plasters. Special gel plasters can protect blisters.

CLEAR PLASTERS

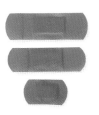

BLUE CATERING PLASTERS

GEL BLISTER PLASTER

continued ⟫

⟪ FIRST AID MATERIALS

BANDAGES

Roller bandages

This type of bandage can be used to secure dressings in position and maintain pressure on wounds to help control bleeding. Avoid using crepe bandages.

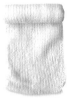

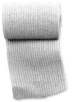

| CONFORMING ROLLER BANDAGE | OPEN-WEAVE ROLLER BANDAGE | SUPPPORT ROLLER BANDAGE | SELF-ADHESIVE BANDAGE |

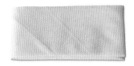
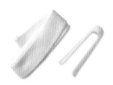

FOLDED TRIANGULAR BANDAGE

TUBE GAUZE BANDAGE WITH APPLICATOR

FINGER BANDAGE ROLL

Triangular bandages

Made of cloth, these items can be used folded as bandages or slings. If they are sterile and individually wrapped, they may also be used as dressings for large wounds and burns.

Tubular bandages

Gauze tubular bandages can be used to secure dressings on fingers and toes. Some have an applicator and need to be cut to size, others are simply rolled over the digit.

PROTECTIVE ITEMS

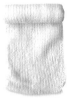

Face covering

Wear a surgical face mask to protect both the casualty and yourself from cross-infection.

Face mask and shield

Use a plastic face shield or a pocket mask to protect you and the casualty from cross infection when giving rescue breaths.

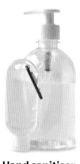
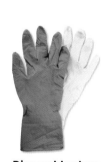
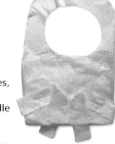

POCKET MASK

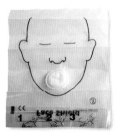

Hand sanitiser

Carry a bottle of alcohol-based hand sanitiser to clean your hands when there is no water available. Do not leave bottles of santiser in a car.

Disposable gloves

Wear disposable gloves, if available, when you dress a wound or handle body fluids or other waste materials. Use latex-free (nitrile) gloves because some people are allergic to latex.

Disposable apron

A plastic apron can help protect you from contact with body fluids.

FACE SHIELD

ADDITIONAL ITEMS

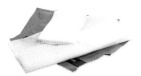

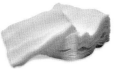

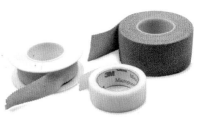

Cleansing wipes
Alcohol-free wipes can be used to clean skin around wounds.

Gauze pads
Use these pads as dressings, as padding, or as swabs to clean around wounds.

Adhesive tape
Use tape to secure dressings or the loose ends of bandages. If the casualty is allergic to the adhesive on the tape, use a hypoallergenic tape.

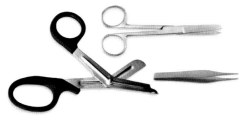

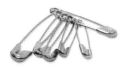

Scissors, shears and tweezers
Choose items that ideally are blunt-ended so that they will not cause injuries. Use shears to cut clothes.

Safety pins
Use these to secure the ends of bandages.

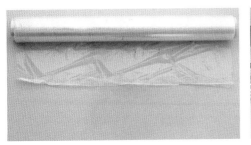

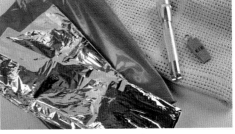

Kitchen film
Kitchen film (or clean plastic food bags) can be used to dress burns and scalds.

For use outdoors
A blanket can protect a casualty from cold. Compact survival bags can keep a person warm and dry in an emergency. A torch helps visibility, and a whistle can be used to summon help.

MATERIALS FOR A FIRST AID KIT

- Easily identifiable watertight box
- Assorted adhesive dressings
- Medium and large sterile wound dressings
- Sterile eye pad
- Triangular bandages
- Roller bandages

- Safety pins
- Disposable gloves, surgical face mask, disposable plastic apron and hand sanitiser
- Scissors, tweezers and tough-cut shears
- Alcohol-free cleansing wipes
- Adhesive tape

- Plastic face shield or pocket mask
- Roll of plastic kitchen film
- Notepad and pencil

Other useful items:

- Blanket, survival bag, torch, whistle
- Warning triangle and high visibility jacket for the car

DRESSINGS

You should always **cover a wound** with a dressing because this helps to prevent infection. With severe bleeding, dressings are used to help the blood-clotting process by exerting pressure on the wound. Use a pre-packed sterile wound dressing with a bandage attached (opposite), or use a sealed sterile pad, secured in place with a bandage (p.240) or adhesive tape (p.244). Alternatively, any clean pad of material can be used to improvise a dressing (p.244). Protect small cuts and grazes with an adhesive dressing (p.245).

GUIDELINES FOR APPLYING DRESSINGS

When handling or applying a dressing, there are a number of guidelines to follow. These enable you to apply dressings correctly. Dressings can also protect the casualty and yourself from cross-infection (p.16).

- **Wash your hands** or, if this is not possible, use hand sanitiser, then put on a pair of disposable gloves.
- **Cover the wound** with a dressing that extends beyond the wound's edges.
- **Hold the edge of the dressing,** keeping your fingers well away from the area that will be in contact with the wound.
- **Place the dressing** directly on top of the wound; do not slide it on from the side.
- **Remove and replace** any dressing that slips out of position.

- **If you only have one sterile dressing,** use it to cover the wound, and put other clean materials on top of it.
- **If blood seeps through** the initial dressing, remove it and reapply direct pressure over a fresh dressing or pad, making sure that you put pressure over the bleeding point. Secure the new dressing with a bandage only once the bleeding is controlled (pp.116–117).
- **After treating a wound,** dispose of gloves, used dressings and other soiled items (including your apron, mask and googles if you have used them) in a suitable plastic bag, ideally a clinical waste bag (below and p.18). Keep your gloves on until you have finished handling materials that may be contaminated then wash or sanitise your hands.

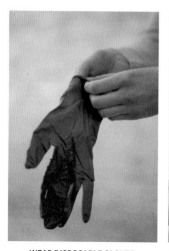

WEAR DISPOSABLE GLOVES

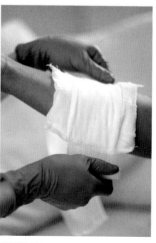

USE DRESSING LARGER THAN WOUND

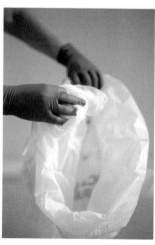

DISPOSE OF WASTE

| **SEE ALSO** Cuts and grazes **p.121** | First aid materials **pp.239–241** | Severe external bleeding **pp.116–117**

HOW TO APPLY A STERILE DRESSING WITH BANDAGE

This type of dressing consists of a dressing pad attached to a roller bandage. The pad may be a standard wound dressing or a piece of gauze backed with a layer of cotton wool or padding.

Sterile dressings are available individually wrapped in various sizes. They are sealed in protective wrappings to keep them sterile. Once the seal on this type of dressing has been broken, the dressing is no longer sterile.

CAUTION

- If the dressing slips out of place, remove it and apply a new dressing.
- Take care not to impair the circulation beyond the bandage (p.247).

WHAT TO DO

1 Break the seal and remove the wrapping. Unwind some of the bandage, taking care not to drop the roll or touch the dressing pad.

2 Unfold the dressing pad, and lay it directly on the wound. Hold the bandage on each side of the pad as you place it over the wound.

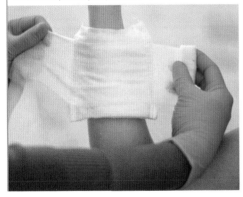

3 Wind the short end of the bandage once around the limb and the pad to secure the dressing.

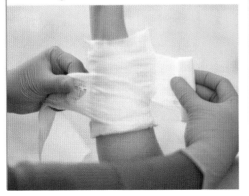

4 Wind the other end (head) of the bandage around the limb to cover the whole pad. Leave the short end of the bandage hanging free.

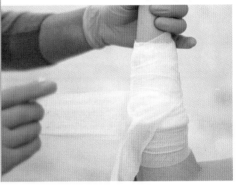

5 To secure the bandage, tie the ends in a reef knot (p.254). Tie the knot directly over the pad to maintain firm pressure on the wound.

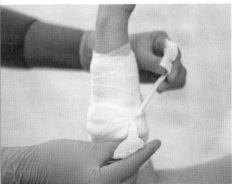

6 Once you have secured the bandage, check the circulation in the limb beyond it (p.247). Loosen the bandage if it is too tight, then reapply. Re-check the circulation every 10 minutes.

continued »

DRESSINGS

WOUND DRESSINGS AND GAUZE PADS

CAUTION

- Never apply adhesive tape all the way around a limb or digit as this can impair circulation.
- Check that the casualty is not allergic to the adhesive before using tape; if they have an allergy, use hypoallergenic tape or a bandage to secure the pad.

Wound dressings in the form of individually wrapped sterile pads, which often have a non-adherent surface on one side, are placed over the wound; if the seal is broken they are no longer sterile. Make sure the pad is large enough to extend well beyond the edges of the wound. Hold the dressing face down; never touch the part of the dressing that will be in contact with a wound. Secure the dressing with tape or a bandage if you need to maintain pressure to control bleeding. If there is no sterile wound dressing available, you can use pads of gauze or improvise.

WHAT TO DO

1 **Hold the dressing by its edges** and place it directly on to the wound.

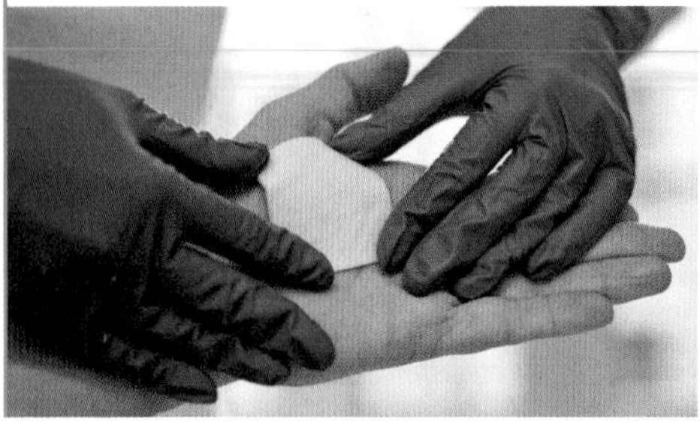

2 **Secure the dressing** with adhesive tape or a roller bandage.

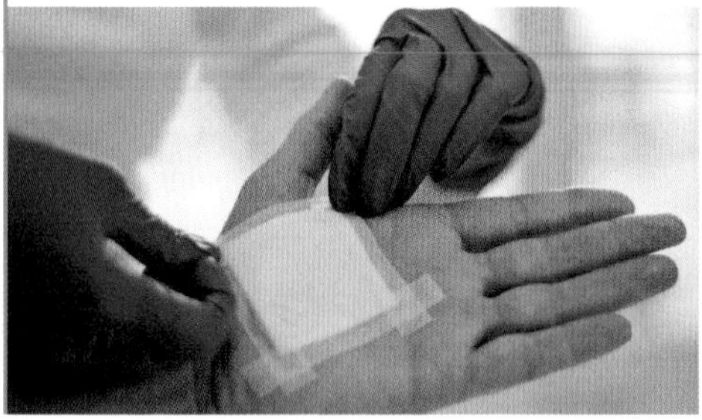

IMPROVISED DRESSINGS

If you have no dressings, use a pad of material such as a tea towel, scarf, handkerchief or a small towel. If using a piece of folded cloth always place the clean, inner, side against the wound.

WHAT TO DO

1 **Hold the material** by the edges. Open it out and refold it so that the inner surface faces outwards.

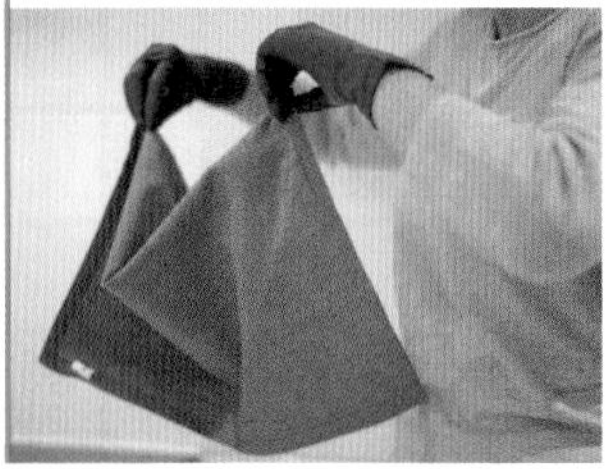

2 **Place the cloth pad** directly on to the wound. If necessary, cover the pad with more material.

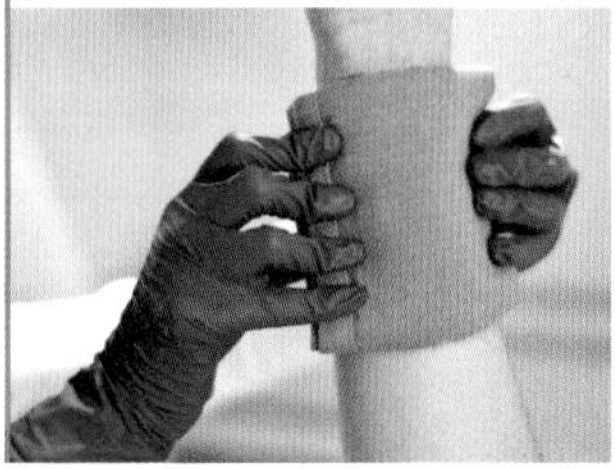

3 **Secure the pad** with a bandage or a clean strip of cloth, such as a scarf. Tie the ends in a reef knot (p.254).

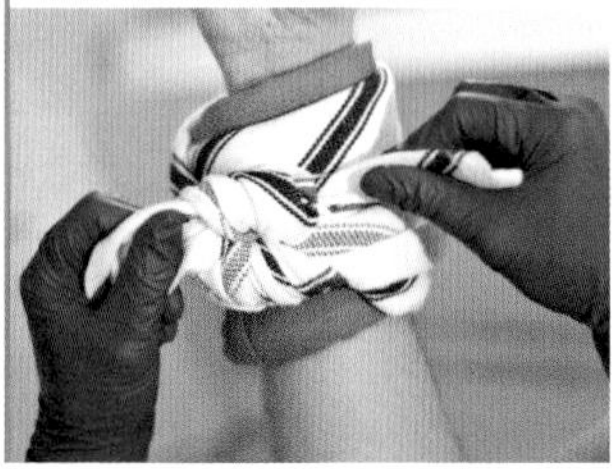

ADHESIVE DRESSINGS

Plasters, or adhesive dressings, are useful for covering small cuts and grazes. They consist of a gauze or cellulose pad with an adhesive backing, and are wrapped singly in sterile packs. There are several sizes available, as well as special shapes for use on fingertips, heels and elbows; some types are waterproof. Blister plasters have an oval cushioned pad. People who work with food must cover any wounds with visible, blue, waterproof plasters.

CAUTION

- Check that the casualty is not allergic to the adhesive dressings. If they are, use a pad and hypoallergenic tape or a bandage (opposite).

WHAT TO DO

1 **Clean and dry the skin around the wound.** Unwrap the plaster and hold it by the protective strips over the backing, with the pad side facing downwards.

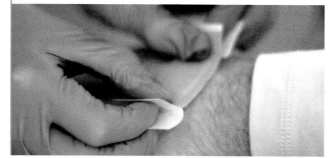

2 **Peel back the strips** to expose the pad, but do not remove them. Without touching the surface of the pad, place it on the wound.

3 **Carefully pull away** the protective strips, then press the edges of the plaster down.

COLD COMPRESSES

Cooling an injury such as a bruise or sprain can reduce swelling and pain. There are two types of compress: cold pads, which are made from material dampened with cold water, and ice packs. An ice pack can be made using bags of ice cubes or packs of frozen peas or other small vegetables wrapped in a dry cloth. Gently place a compress on the injury; a casualty may be able to do this.

CAUTION

- To prevent cold injuries, always wrap an ice pack in a cloth.
- Do not leave a compress on the skin for more than 20 minutes.

COLD PAD

1 **Soak a clean flannel** or towel in cold water. Wring it out lightly and fold it into a pad. Hold it firmly against the injured area (right).

2 **Re-soak the pad** in cold water every few minutes to keep it cold. Cool the injury for no more than 20 minutes.

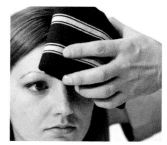

USING A COLD COMPRESS

ICE PACK

1 **Partly fill a plastic bag** with small ice cubes or crushed ice, or use a pack of frozen vegetables. Wrap the bag in a dry cloth.

2 **Hold the pack firmly** on the injury (left) and cool it for no more than 20 minutes; top up the ice as needed.

PRINCIPLES OF BANDAGING

There are a number of different first aid uses for bandages: they can be used to secure dressings, control bleeding, support and immobilise limbs and reduce swelling in an injured limb. There are three main types of bandage. Roller bandages secure dressings and support injured limbs. Tubular bandages hold dressings on fingers or toes, or support injured joints. Triangular bandages can be used as large dressings, as slings to secure dressings or folded to immobilise limbs. If you have no bandages available, you can improvise from everyday items; for example, you can fold a square of fabric, such as a headscarf, diagonally to make a triangular bandage (p.253).

GUIDELINES FOR APPLYING BANDAGES

- **Reassure the casualty** before applying a bandage and explain clearly what you are going to do.
- **Help the casualty** to sit or lie down in a comfortable position.

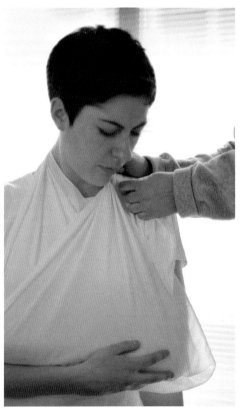

- **Support the injured part** of the body while you are working on it. Ask the casualty or a helper to assist.
- **Work from the front of the casualty,** and from the injured side where possible.
- **Pass the bandages** through the body's natural hollows at the ankles, knees, waist and neck, then slide them into position by easing them back and forth under the body.
- **Apply bandages firmly,** but not so tightly that they interfere with circulation to the area beyond the bandage (opposite).
- **Fingers or toes** should be left exposed, if possible, so that you can check the circulation in the affected area afterwards.
- **Use reef knots** to tie bandages (p.254). Ensure that the knots do not cause the casualty any discomfort, and do not tie the knot over a bony area. Tuck loose ends under a knot if possible, to provide additional padding.
- **Check the circulation** in the area beyond the bandage (opposite) every 10 minutes once the bandage is secure. If necessary, unroll the bandage until the blood supply returns, and reapply it more loosely.

IMMOBILISING A LIMB

When applying bandages to immobilise a limb you also need to use soft, bulky material, such as towels or clothing, as padding. Place the padding between the legs, or between an arm and the body, so that the bandaging does not displace broken bones or press bony areas against each other. Use folded triangular bandages and tie them at intervals along the casualty's limb, avoiding the injury site. Secure with reef knots (p.254) tied on the uninjured side. If both sides of the casualty's body are injured, tie knots in the middle or where there is least chance of causing further damage.

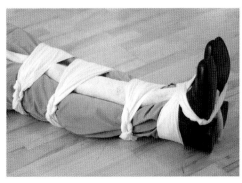

TIE KNOTS ON THE UNINJURED SIDE

CHECKING CIRCULATION AFTER BANDAGING

When bandaging a limb or applying a sling, you must check the circulation in the hand or foot beyond the bandage or sling immediately after you have finished applying it, and again every 10 minutes thereafter. These checks are essential because limbs can swell after an injury, and a bandage can rapidly become too tight and restrict blood circulation to the area beyond it. If this occurs, you need to undo the bandage and reapply it more loosely.

If circulation is impaired there may be:

- A swollen and congested limb
- Blue skin with prominent veins
- A feeling that the skin is painfully distended

Later there may be:

- Pale skin
- Skin is cold to touch
- Casualty complains of numbness and tingling followed by severe pain
- Casualty is unable to move affected fingers or toes

WHAT TO DO

1 Press one of the nails, or the skin beyond the bandage, for 5 seconds until it turns pale, then release the pressure. If the colour does not return within 2 seconds, the bandage is too tight.

2 Loosen a tight bandage by unrolling enough turns for warmth and colour to return to the skin; the casualty may feel a tingling sensation. Reapply the bandage more loosely. Check again every 10 minutes.

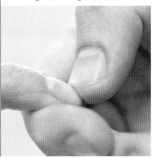

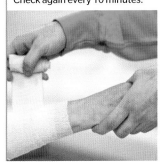

ROLLER BANDAGES

This type of bandage can be made of cotton, gauze, elasticated fabric or linen and is wrapped around the injured part of the body in spiral turns, working from below the injury up a limb. There are three main types :

- **Open-weave bandages** are used to hold dressings in place. Because of their loose weave they allow good ventilation, but they cannot be used to exert direct pressure on the wound to control bleeding or to provide support to joints.
- **Self-adhesive support bandages** are used to support muscle (and joint) injuries and do not need pins or clips.
- **Conforming bandages** are used to give firm, even support to injured joints.

SECURING ROLLER BANDAGES

There are several ways to fasten the end of a roller bandage. Safety pins or adhesive tape are usually included in commercially available first aid kits. If you do not have any pins or tape, a simple tuck (right) should keep the bandage end in place.

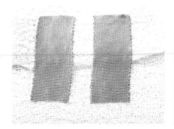

Adhesive tape
The ends of bandages can be folded under and then stuck down with small strips of adhesive tape.

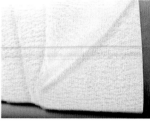

Tucking in the end
If you have no fastening, secure the bandage by passing the end around the limb once and tucking it in under the previous layer.

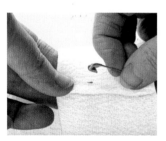

Safety pin
These pins can secure all types of roller bandage. Fold the end of the bandage under, then put your finger under the previous layer of bandage to prevent injury as you insert the pin (left). Make sure that, once fastened, the pin lies flat (right).

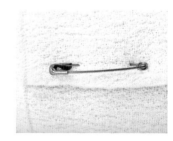

CHOOSING THE CORRECT SIZE OF BANDAGE

Before applying a roller bandage, check that it is tightly rolled and of a suitable width for the injured area. Small areas such as fingers require narrow bandages of approximately 2.5 cm (1 in) wide, while wider bandages of 10–15 cm (4–6 in) are more suitable for large areas such as legs. It is better for a roller bandage to be too wide than too narrow. Smaller sizes may also be needed for a child.

APPLYING A ROLLER BANDAGE

Follow the general rules below when applying a roller bandage to an injury.

- **Keep the rolled** part of the bandage (the "head") uppermost as you work. (The unrolled short end is called the "tail".)
- **Position yourself** in front of the casualty, on the injured side.
- **Support the injured** part while you apply the bandage.

CAUTION

- Once you have applied the bandage, check the circulation in the limb beyond it (p.247). This is especially important if you are applying an elasticated or conforming bandage since these mould to the shape of the limb and may become tighter if the limb swells.

WHAT TO DO

1 **Place the tail of the bandage** below the injury. Working from the inside of the limb outwards, make two straight turns with the bandage to anchor the tail in place.

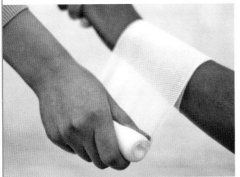

2 **Wind the bandage in spiralling turns** working from the inner to the outer side of the limb, and work up the limb. Cover one half to two-thirds of the previous layer of bandage with each new turn.

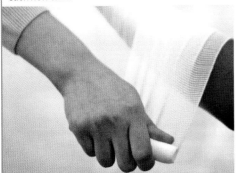

3 **Finish with one straight turn.** If the bandage is too short, apply another one in the same way so that the injured area is covered.

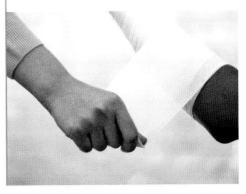

4 **Secure the end of the bandage,** then check the circulation beyond the bandage (p.247). If necessary, unroll the bandage until the blood supply returns, and reapply it more loosely. Re-check every 10 minutes.

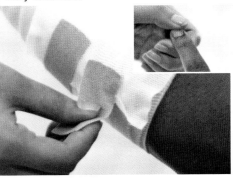

ROLLER BANDAGES

ELBOW AND KNEE BANDAGES

Roller bandages can be used on elbows and knees to support soft tissue injuries such as strains or sprains. To ensure that there is effective support, flex the joint slightly, then apply the bandage in figure-of-eight turns rather than the standard spiralling turns (p.249). Work from the inside to the outside of the upper surface of the joint. Extend the bandaging far enough on either side of the joint to exert an even pressure.

WHAT TO DO

1 **Support the injured limb** in a comfortable position for the casualty, with the joint partially flexed. Place the tail of the bandage on the inner side of the joint. Pass the bandage over and around to the outside of the joint. Make one-and-a-half turns, so that the tail end of the bandage is fixed and the joint is covered.

2 **Pass the bandage** to the inner side of the limb, just above the joint. Make a turn around the limb, covering the upper half of the bandage from the first turn.

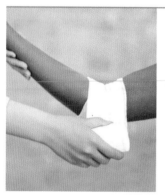

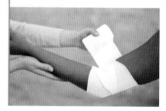

3 **Pass the bandage from** the inner side of the upper limb to just below the joint. Make one diagonal turn below the elbow joint to cover the lower half of the bandaging from the first straight turn.

4 **Continue to bandage** diagonally above and below the joint in a figure-of-eight. Increase the bandaged area by covering about two-thirds of the previous turn with each new layer of bandage.

5 **To finish bandaging the joint,** make two straight turns around the limb, then secure the end of the bandage (p.248). Check the circulation beyond the bandage as soon as you have finished, then re-check every 10 minutes (p.247). If necessary unroll the bandage and reapply more loosely.

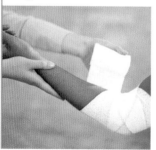

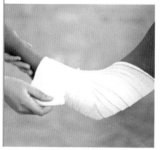

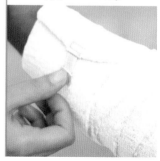

HAND BANDAGES

A roller bandage may be applied to hold dressings in place on a hand, or to support a wrist in soft tissue injuries. A support bandage should extend well beyond the injury site to provide pressure over the whole of the injured area.

WHAT TO DO

1 **Place the tail** of the bandage on the inner side of the wrist, below the base of the thumb. Make two straight turns around the wrist.

2 **Working from the inner side** of the wrist, pass the bandage diagonally across the back of the hand to the nail of the little finger, and across the front of the casualty's fingers.

3 **Pass the bandage diagonally** across the back of the hand to the outer side of the wrist. Take the bandage under the wrist. Then repeat the diagonal over the back of the hand.

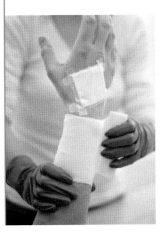

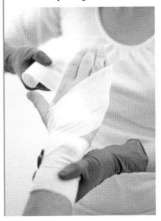

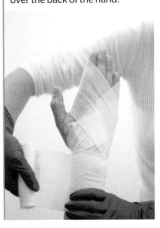

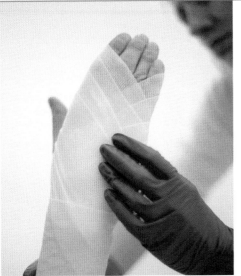

4 **Repeat the sequence** of figure-of-eight turns. Extend the bandaging by covering about two-thirds of the bandage from the previous turn with each new layer. When the main part of the hand is completely covered, finish with two straight turns around the casualty's wrist.

5 **Secure the end** (p.248). As soon as you have finished, check the circulation beyond the bandage (p.247), then re-check every 10 minutes. If necessary, unroll the bandage until the blood supply returns and reapply it more loosely.

TUBULAR GAUZE BANDAGES

CAUTION

- Do not encircle the finger completely with tape because this may impair circulation.

These are rolls of seamless tubular fabric. They may be supplied in the form of a small roll (p.240) or as lengths of tube gauze to be applied using with a special applicator (below). Tube gauze is used for securing dressings but not for controlling bleeding. Secure it with hypoallergenic tape if a casualty is allergic to adhesive tape.

WHAT TO DO

1 Cut a piece of tubular gauze about two-and-a-half times the length of the casualty's injured finger (or toe). Push the whole length of the tubular gauze on to the applicator, then gently slide the applicator over the finger and dressing.

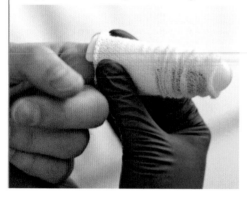

2 Holding the end of the gauze on the finger, pull the applicator slightly beyond the fingertip, leaving a layer of gauze bandage on the finger. Twist the applicator twice to seal the bandage over the end of the finger.

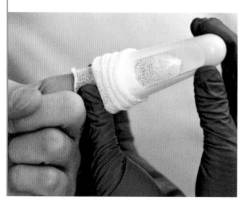

3 While still holding the gauze at the base of the finger, gently push the applicator back over the finger to apply a second layer of gauze. Once the gauze has been applied, remove the applicator from the finger.

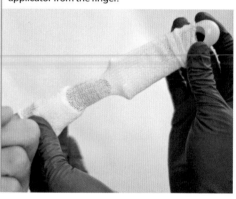

4 Secure the gauze at the base of the finger with adhesive tape that does not encircle the finger. Check the circulation to the finger (p.247), then again every 10 minutes. Ask the casualty if the finger feels cold or tingly. If necessary, remove the gauze and apply it more loosely.

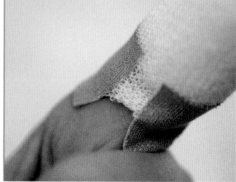

TRIANGULAR BANDAGES

This type of bandage may be supplied in a sterile pack as part of a first aid kit. You can also make one by cutting or folding a square metre of sturdy fabric (such as linen or calico) diagonally in half. The bandage can be used in the following three ways.

- **Folded as a broad-fold bandage or narrow-fold bandage** (below) to immobilise and support a limb or to secure a splint or bulky dressing.
- **Opened to form a sling,** or to hold a hand, foot or scalp dressing in place.
- **If from a sterile pack,** folded into a pad and used as a sterile dressing.

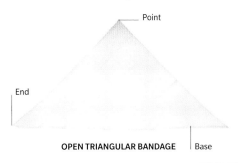

Point

End

Base

OPEN TRIANGULAR BANDAGE

MAKING A BROAD-FOLD BANDAGE

1 Open out a triangular bandage and lay it flat on a clean surface. Fold the bandage in half horizontally, so that the point of the triangle touches the centre of the base.

2 Fold the bandage in half again in the same direction, so that the first folded edge touches the base. The bandage should now form a broad strip of fabric.

MAKING A NARROW-FOLD BANDAGE

1 Fold a triangular bandage to make a broad-fold bandage (above).

2 Fold the bandage horizontally in half again. It should form a long, narrow, thick strip of material.

STORING A TRIANGULAR BANDAGE

Keep triangular bandages in their packs so that they remain sterile until you need them. Alternatively, fold them as shown (right) so that they are ready-folded for use as a pad or bandage, or can be shaken open for use as a sling.

1 Start by folding the triangle into a narrow-fold bandage (above right). Bring the two ends of the bandage into the centre.

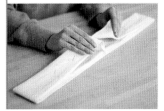

2 Continue folding the ends into the centre until the bandage is a convenient size for storing. Keep the bandage in a dry place.

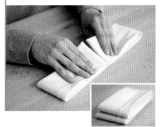

REEF KNOTS

When securing a triangular bandage, always use a reef knot. It is secure and will not slip, it is easy to untie and it lies flat, so it is more comfortable for the casualty. Avoid tying the knot around or directly over the injury, since this may cause discomfort to the casualty.

TYING AND UNTYING A REEF KNOT

1 **Pass the left end** (blue) over and under the right end of the bandage (light blue).

2 **Lift both ends** of the bandage above the rest of the material.

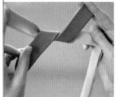

3 **Pass the end** in your right hand (blue) over and under the other end (light blue).

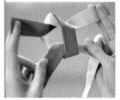

4 **Pull the ends** to tighten the knot, then tuck them under the bandage.

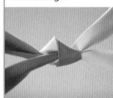

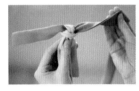

Untying a reef knot
Pull one end and one piece of bandage from the same side of the knot firmly so that the piece of bandage straightens. Hold the knot and pull the straightened end through it.

HAND AND FOOT COVER BANDAGE

An open triangular bandage can be used to hold a dressing in place on a hand or foot, but it will not provide enough pressure to control bleeding. The method for covering a hand (right) can also be used for a foot, with the bandage ends tied in a reef knot at the ankle.

1 **Lay the bandage flat.** Place the casualty's hand on the bandage, fingers towards the point. Fold the point down over the hand.

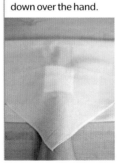

2 **Cross the ends** over the hand, then pass the ends around the wrist in opposite directions. Tie the ends in a reef knot (above) at the wrist.

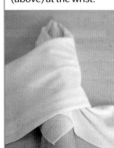

3 **Pull the point** gently to tighten the bandage. Fold the point up over the knot and tuck it in.

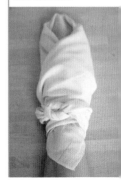

ARM SLING

An arm sling holds the forearm in a slightly raised or horizontal position. It provides support for an injured upper arm, wrist or forearm, on a casualty whose elbow can be bent, or to immobilise the arm for a rib fracture (p.156). An elevation sling (p.256) is used to keep the forearm and hand raised in a higher position, for example to control bleeding.

WHAT TO DO

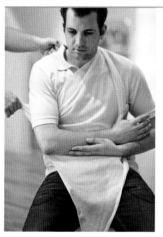

1 **Ensure that the injured arm** is supported with the hand slightly higher than the elbow. Fold the base of the bandage under to form a hem. Place the bandage with the base parallel to the casualty's body and level with their little finger nail. Slide the upper end under the injured arm and pull it around the neck to the opposite shoulder.

2 **Fold the lower end** of the bandage up over the forearm and bring it to meet the upper end at the shoulder.

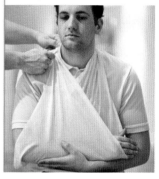

3 **Tie a reef knot** (opposite) on the injured side, at the hollow above the casualty's collar bone. Tuck both free ends of the bandage under the knot to pad it. Adjust the sling so that the front edge supports the hand – it should extend to the top of the casualty's little finger.

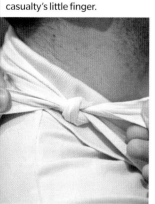

4 **Hold the point** of the bandage beyond the elbow and twist it until the fabric fits the elbow snugly, then tuck it in (inset). Alternatively, if you have a safety pin, fold the fabric and fasten it to the front.

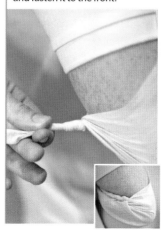

5 **As soon as** you have finished, check the circulation in the fingers (p.247). Check the fingers again every 10 minutes. If necessary, loosen and reapply the bandages and sling.

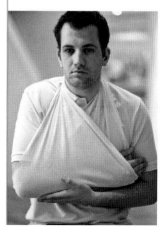

ELEVATION SLING

This form of sling supports the forearm and hand in a raised position, with the fingertips touching the casualty's shoulder. In this way, an elevation sling helps to control bleeding from wounds in the forearm or hand, and/or to minimise swelling. An elevation sling can also be used to support the arm in the case of an injured hand.

WHAT TO DO

1 **Ask the casualty** to support their injured arm across their chest, with the fingers resting on the opposite shoulder.

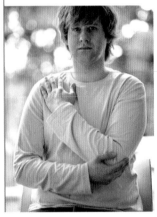

2 **Place the bandage** over the body, with one end over the shoulder on the uninjured side. Hold the point of the bandage just beyond their elbow.

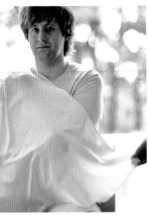

3 **Ask the casualty** to let go of their injured arm and tuck the base of the bandage under their hand, forearm and elbow; you may need to help.

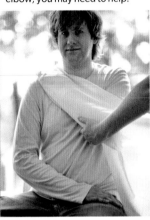

4 **Bring the lower end** of the bandage up diagonally across the back to meet the other end at the casualty's shoulder.

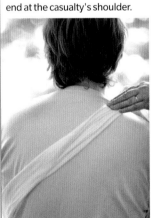

5 **Tie the ends** in a reef knot (p.254) at the hollow above the collarbone. Tuck the ends under the knot to pad it.

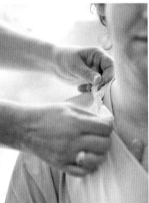

6 **Twist the point** until the bandage fits closely around the casualty's elbow (inset). Tuck the point in just above their elbow to secure it. If you have a safety pin, fold the fabric over the elbow and fasten the point at the corner. Check the circulation in the thumb every 10 minutes (p.247); loosen and reapply the sling if necessary.

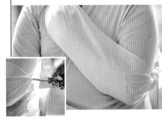

IMPROVISED SLINGS

If you need to support a casualty's injured arm but do not have a triangular bandage available, you can make a sling by using a square metre (just over one square yard) of any strong cloth (p.253). You can also improvise by using an item of the casualty's clothing (below). Check circulation after applying support (p.247) and check it again every 10 minutes.

CAUTION

If you suspect that the forearm is broken, use a cloth sling or a jacket corner to provide support. Do not use any other form of improvised sling as it will not provide enough support.

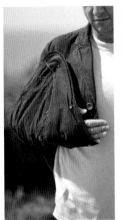

Jacket corner
Undo the casualty's jacket. Fold the lower edge on the injured side up over their arm. Secure the corner of the hem to the jacket breast with a large safety pin. Tuck and pin the excess material closely around the casualty's elbow.

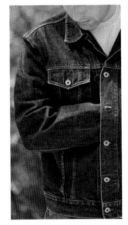

Button-up jacket
Undo one button of a jacket or coat (or waistcoat). Place the hand of the injured arm inside the garment at the gap formed by the unfastened button. Advise the casualty to rest their wrist on the button just beneath the gap.

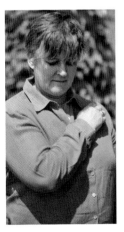

Long-sleeved shirt
Place the injured arm across the casualty's chest. Pin the cuff of the sleeve to the breast of the shirt. To improvise an elevation sling (opposite), pin the sleeve at the casualty's opposite shoulder, to keep their arm raised.

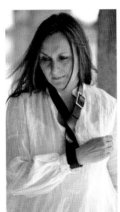

Belt or thin garment
Use a belt, a tie or a pair of braces or tights to make a "collar-and-cuff" support. Fasten the item to form a loop. Place it over the casualty's head, then twist it once to form a smaller loop at the front. Place the casualty's hand into the loop.

12 EMERGENCY FIRST AID

This chapter is designed as an easy-to-use, quick-reference guide to first aid treatment for casualties with serious illnesses or injuries. It begins with an action plan to help you assess a casualty and identify first aid priorities, using the primary survey (pp.46–47), followed by the secondary survey (pp.48–53) where appropriate.

The chapter goes on to show how to treat unresponsive casualties, whose care always takes priority over that of less seriously injured casualties. In addition, there is step-by-step essential first aid for potentially life-threatening illnesses and injuries that benefit from immediate first aid. These include asthma, sepsis, stroke, severe bleeding, shock, heart attack, burns, heatstroke, broken bones and spinal injuries. Each condition is described in more detail in the main part of the book and cross-referenced here so that the entry can easily be found if you need further advice and background information.

AIMS AND OBJECTIVES

- To protect yourself from danger and make the area safe
- To assess the situation quickly and calmly and summon appropriate help
- To assist casualties and provide necessary treatment with the help of bystanders
- To call 999/112 for emergency help if you suspect a serious illness or injury
- To be aware of your own needs

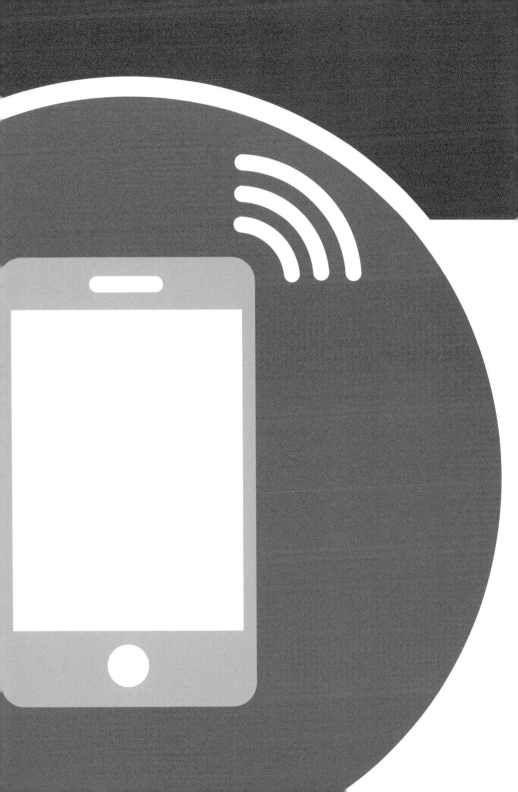

ACTION IN AN EMERGENCY

Use the **primary survey** (pp.46–47) to identify the most serious injury, and treat injuries in order of priority. Once these are managed carry out a secondary survey (pp.48–53).

START

DANGER
Make sure the area is safe before you approach. *Is anyone in danger?*

YES

NO

RESPONSE
Is the casualty responding? Try to initiate a response by asking questions and gently shaking their shoulders (p.46). *Is there a response?*

YES

NO

UNRESPONSIVE CASUALTY

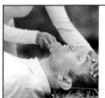

AIRWAY
Is the casualty's airway open and clear?

Open the airway
Tilt the head and lift the chin to open the airway.

CPR/CIRCULATION
Ask a helper to **call 999/112 for emergency help** and bring an AED if possible. Begin cardiopulmonary resuscitation/CPR (adult p.262, child p.264, infant p.264).

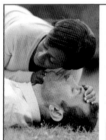

BREATHING
Is the casualty breathing normally?

NO

NO

Are you on your own?

YES

Check breathing
Look along the chest, and listen and feel for breaths.

YES

CPR/CIRCULATION
If the casualty is a child or infant, give FIVE initial rescue breaths and cardiopulmonary resuscitation/CPR for one minute (child p.264, infant p.264). **Call 999/112 for emergency help**, then continue CPR. Take a child or infant to the phone if necessary. If the casualty is an adult, **call 999/112 for emergency help** first, then begin CPR (p.262).
Do not leave any casualty (adult or child) alone to search for an AED.

CIRCULATION
Check for and treat life-threatening conditions, such as severe bleeding.

Call 999/112 for emergency help.
Maintain an open airway. If necessary, place the casualty on their side in the recovery position.

CHEST-COMPRESSION-ONLY CPR
If you have not had training in CPR, you are unwilling or unable to give rescue breaths, or guidelines advise against giving them, you can give chest compressions only. The emergency services will give instructions for chest-compression-only CPR (p.262).

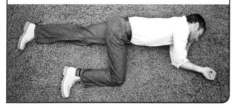

If it is not safe, do not approach.
Call 999/112 for emergency help.

RESPONSIVE CASUALTY

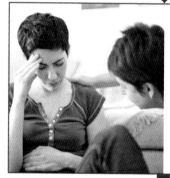

AIRWAY AND BREATHING

If a person is alert and talking to you, it follows that their airway is open and clear and they are breathing. A casualty's breathing may be fast, slow, easy or difficult. Assess and treat any problem found.

CIRCULATION

Are there life-threatening conditions, such as severe bleeding or heart attack?

YES

NO

TREAT LIFE-THREATENING INJURIES OR ILLNESSES

Call 999/112 for emergency help. Monitor and record a casualty's vital signs (pp.54–55) while waiting for help to arrive.

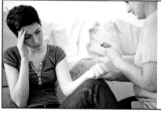

CARRY OUT A SECONDARY SURVEY

Assess the level of response using the scale described on p.54 and carry out a head-to-toe survey to check for signs of illness or injury (pp.52–53).

Call for appropriate help. **Call 999/112 for emergency help** if you suspect serious injury or illness. Monitor and record a casualty's vital signs (pp.54–55) while waiting for help to arrive.

CPR FOR AN ADULT

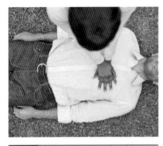 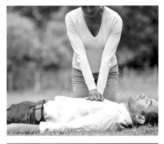 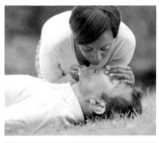

1 POSITION HANDS ON CHEST

Place the heel of one hand on the centre of the casualty's chest. Place the heel of your other hand on top of the first and interlock your fingers, but keep your fingers off the casualty's ribs.

2 GIVE 30 CHEST COMPRESSIONS

Lean directly over the casualty's chest and press down vertically about 5–6 cm (2–2½ in). Release the pressure, but do not remove your hands. Give 30 compressions at a rate of 100–120 per minute.

3 OPEN AIRWAY, BEGIN RESCUE BREATHS

Tilt the casualty's head with one hand and lift the chin with two fingers of your other hand. Pinch the nostrils closed, and allow their mouth to fall open. Take a breath, seal your lips over the casualty's mouth, and blow steadily until the chest rises.

CHEST-COMPRESSION-ONLY CPR

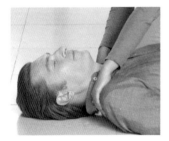 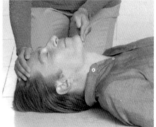 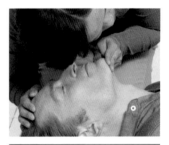

1 CHECK FOR RESPONSE

Check for a response. Gently shake the casualty's shoulders, and talk to them. If there is no response, go to the next step.

2 OPEN THE AIRWAY

Open the casualty's airway. Place one hand on the forehead and gently tilt the head – the mouth should fall open. Place the fingertips of your other hand on the chin and lift it.

3 CHECK BREATHING

Check breathing: put your ear as near to the casualty's mouth and nose as you can and look along the chest. Look, listen and feel for breathing for no more than 10 seconds. If they are not breathing call 999 / 112 for emergency help, then begin chest compressions.

FIND OUT MORE **pp.68–71**

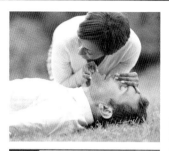

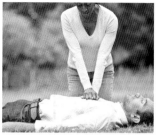

4 WATCH CHEST FALL

Maintaining the open airway, take your mouth away from the casualty's. Look along the chest and watch it fall. Repeat to give TWO rescue breaths; each full breath should take one second. Repeat 30 chest compressions followed by TWO rescue breaths.

5 CONTINUE CPR

Continue CPR (30:2) until: emergency help arrives; the casualty shows signs of becoming responsive – such as coughing, opening their eyes, speaking or moving purposefully – and starts breathing normally; or you are too exhausted to continue.

> **CAUTION**
> - If you have not had training in CPR, you are unwilling or unable to give rescue breaths or guidelines advise against giving them, give chest compressions only, see below. The emergency services give instructions for chest-compression-only CPR.
> - If the casualty vomits during CPR, roll them away from you onto their side, with the head turned towards the floor to allow vomit to drain. Clear the mouth, then immediately roll them onto their back again and restart CPR.
> - If there is more than one rescuer, change over every 1–2 minutes, with minimal interruption to CPR.
> - Ask a helper to fetch an AED.

FIND OUT MORE **pp.72–73**

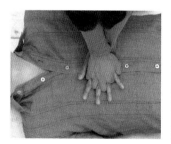

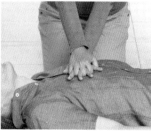

4 BEGIN CHEST COMPRESSIONS

Kneel level with the casualty's chest. Place the heel of one hand on the centre of the chest. Put the heel of your other hand on top of the first and interlock your fingers. Press down on the breastbone, to depress the chest 5–6 cm (2–2½ in), then release the pressure.

5 CONTINUE CHEST COMPRESSIONS

Give compressions at a rate of 100–120 per minute until: help arrives; the casualty shows signs of becoming responsive (coughing, opening their eyes, speaking or moving purposefully) and starts breathing normally; or you are too exhausted to continue.

> **CAUTION**
> - Follow these instructions if you have not had training in CPR, you are unwilling or unable to give rescue breaths, or guidelines advise against giving them. The emergency services give instructions for chest-compression-only CPR.
> - If the casualty vomits during CPR, roll them away from you onto their side, with the head turned towards the floor to allow vomit to drain. Clear the mouth, then roll them onto their back again and restart chest compressions.
> - If there is more than one rescuer, change over every 1–2 minutes, with minimal interruption to compressions.
> - Ask a helper to fetch an AED.

CPR FOR A CHILD ONE YEAR AND OVER

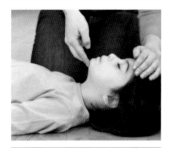

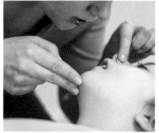

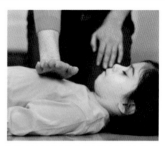

1 **CHECK THAT AIRWAY IS OPEN**

Tilt the child's head with one hand and lift the chin with two fingers of the other hand to ensure the airway is open.

2 **GIVE FIVE INITIAL RESCUE BREATHS**

Pinch the nose to close the nostrils. Allow the mouth to fall open. Take a breath and seal your lips over the child's mouth. Blow steadily until the chest rises, then watch it fall; a rescue breath should take one second. Give FIVE rescue breaths.

3 **GIVE 30 CHEST COMPRESSIONS**

Place the heel of one hand on the centre of the chest. Lean directly over the child's chest and press down to at least one third of its depth, then release the pressure, but do not remove your hand. Give 30 compressions at a rate of 100–120 per minute.

CPR FOR AN INFANT UNDER ONE YEAR

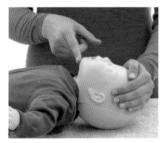

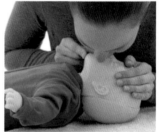

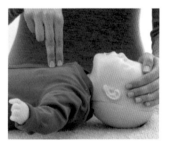

1 **CHECK THAT AIRWAY IS OPEN**

Place the infant on a firm surface or on the floor. Gently tilt the head with one hand and lift the chin with one finger of the other hand to ensure the airway is open.

2 **GIVE FIVE INITIAL RESCUE BREATHS**

Take a breath and place your lips over the infant's mouth and nose. Blow gently and steadily into the mouth and nose until the chest rises, then watch it fall. Each full breath should take about one second. Give FIVE rescue breaths.

3 **GIVE 30 CHEST COMPRESSIONS**

Place two finger tips of your lower hand on the centre of the infant's chest. Lean over their chest and press down vertically to at least one third of its depth. Release pressure but do not remove your fingers. Give 30 compressions at a rate of 100–120 per minute.

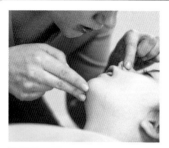

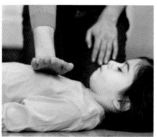

4 GIVE TWO RESCUE BREATHS

Return to the head and give TWO more rescue breaths. Repeat 30 chest compressions followed by TWO rescue breaths (30:2) for one minute. **Call 999/112 for emergency help** if this has not already been done. Take the child to the phone with you if necessary.

5 CONTINUE CPR

Continue CPR (30:2) until: emergency help arrives; the child shows signs of becoming responsive – such as coughing, opening their eyes, speaking or moving purposefully – and starts breathing normally; or you are too exhausted to continue.

CAUTION

- If you have not had training in CPR, you are unwilling or unable to give rescue breaths or guidelines advise against giving them, give chest compressions only. The emergency services will give instructions for chest-compression-only CPR.
- If the child vomits, roll them away from you onto their side, with the head turned towards the floor to allow vomit to drain. Clear the mouth, then roll them onto their back again immediately and restart CPR.
- If there is more than one rescuer, change over every 1–2 minutes, with minimal interruption to CPR.
- Ask a helper to fetch an AED, ideally with paediatric pads.

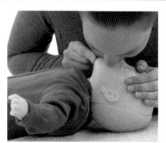

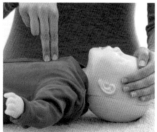

4 GIVE TWO RESCUE BREATHS

Return to the head and give TWO more rescue breaths. Repeat 30 chest compressions followed by TWO rescue breaths (30:2) for one minute. **Call 999/112 for emergency help** if this has not already been done. Take the infant to the phone if necessary.

5 CONTINUE CPR

Continue CPR (30:2) until: emergency help arrives; the infant shows signs of becoming responsive – such as coughing, opening their eyes, crying or moving purposefully – and starts breathing normally; or you are too exhausted to continue.

CAUTION

- If you have not had training in CPR , you are unwilling or unable to give rescue breaths or guidelines advise against giving them, give chest compressions only. The emergency services will give instructions for chest-compression-only CPR.
- If the infant vomits, roll them away from you onto their side, with the head turned towards the floor to allow vomit to drain. Clear the mouth, then roll them onto their back again immediately and restart CPR.
- If there is more than one rescuer, change over every 1–2 minutes, with minimal interruption to CPR.
- Do not use AED on an infant.

HEART ATTACK

RECOGNITION

There may be:

- Vice-like chest pain, spreading to one or both arms or jaw that does not ease with rest
- Breathlessness
- Discomfort, like indigestion, in upper abdomen
- Collapse, with no warning
- Sudden dizziness or faintness
- Casualty may have sense of impending doom
- "Ashen" skin and blueness of lips
- Rapid, weak or irregular pulse
- Profuse sweating
- Extreme gasping for air (air hunger)

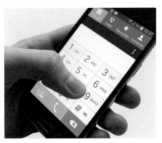

1 CALL FOR EMERGENCY HELP

Call 999 / 112 for emergency help. Tell the call handler that you suspect a heart attack.

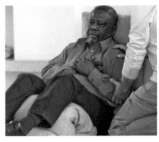

2 MAKE CASUALTY COMFORTABLE

Help the casualty into a comfortable position; a half-sitting position is often best. Support their head and shoulders and place cushions under their knees. Reassure the casualty.

STROKE

RECOGNITION

Use the FAST guide (p.214) to assess the casualty.

- Facial weakness – casualty is unable to smile evenly
- Arm weakness – casualty may only be able to move arm on one side of the body
- Speech problems

There may also be:

- Sudden weakness or numbness along one or both sides of body
- Sudden blurring or loss of vision
- Sudden difficulty understanding the spoken word
- Sudden confusion
- Sudden severe headache with no apparent cause
- Dizziness, unsteadiness or a sudden fall

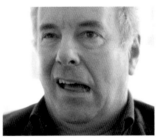

1 CHECK CASUALTY'S FACE

Keep the casualty comfortable. Ask them to smile. If they have had a stroke, they may only be able to smile on one side – the other side of the face may droop.

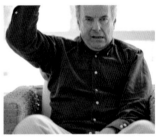

2 CHECK CASUALTY'S ARMS

Ask the casualty to raise their arms. If they have had a stroke, they may only be able to lift one arm fully.

FIND OUT MORE **p.213**

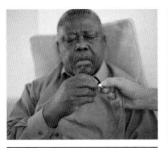

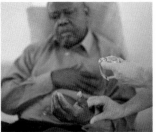

3 GIVE CASUALTY MEDICATION

Assist the casualty to take one full dose aspirin tablet (300mg in total); advise them to chew it slowly. If the casualty has tablets or a spray for angina, allow them to take it; help them if necessary.

4 MONITOR CASUALTY

Encourage the casualty to rest. Keep any bystanders away. Monitor and record the casualty's vital signs (pp.54–55) while waiting for help to arrive.

FIND OUT MORE **pp.214–215**

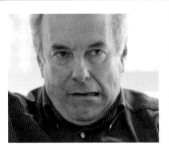

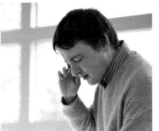

3 CHECK CASUALTY'S SPEECH

Ask the casualty some questions. Can they speak and/or understand what you are saying?

4 CALL FOR EMERGENCY HELP

Call 999/112 for emergency help. Tell the call handler that you suspect a stroke. Reassure the casualty and monitor and record their vital signs (pp.54–55) while waiting for help to arrive.

CHOKING ADULT

RECOGNITION

Ask the casualty: "Are you choking?"

For mild obstruction:

- Difficulty in speaking, coughing and breathing

For severe obstruction:

- Inability to speak, cough or breathe
- Eventually casualty will become unresponsive

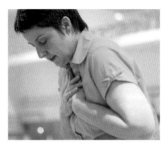

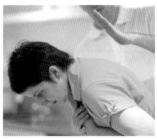

1 ENCOURAGE CASUALTY TO COUGH

If the casualty is breathing, encourage them to cough to try to remove the obstruction themselves. If this fails, go to step 2.

2 GIVE UP TO FIVE BACK BLOWS

If the casualty cannot speak, cough or breathe, bend them forward. Give up to five sharp blows between the shoulder blades with the heel of your hand. Check the mouth. If choking persists, proceed to step 3.

CHOKING CHILD ONE YEAR AND OVER

RECOGNITION

Ask the child: "Are you choking?"

For mild obstruction:

- Difficulty in speaking, coughing and breathing

For severe obstruction:

- Inability to speak, cough or breathe
- Eventually child will become unresponsive

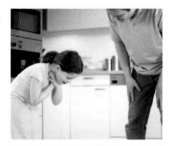

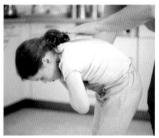

1 ENCOURAGE CHILD TO COUGH

If the child is breathing, encourage them to cough to try to remove the obstruction themselves. If this fails, go to step 2.

2 GIVE UP TO FIVE BACK BLOWS

If the child cannot speak, cough or breathe, bend them forward. Give up to five sharp blows between the shoulder blades with the heel of your hand. Check their mouth. If choking persists, proceed to step 3.

FIND OUT MORE **p.96**

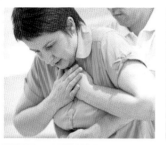

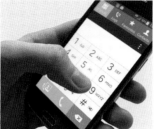

3 GIVE UP TO FIVE ABDOMINAL THRUSTS

Stand behind the casualty. Put both arms around them, and put one fist between the navel and the bottom of their breastbone. Grasp your fist with your other hand, and pull sharply inwards and upwards up to five times. Recheck the casualty's mouth.

4 CALL FOR EMERGENCY HELP THEN CONTINUE

If the obstruction has not cleared, call 999/112 for emergency help. Repeat steps 2 and 3 – rechecking the mouth after each step – until emergency help arrives, the obstruction is cleared or the casualty becomes unresponsive.

FIND OUT MORE **p.97**

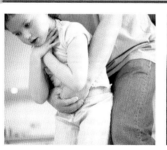

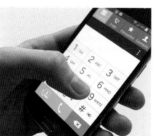

3 GIVE UP TO FIVE ABDOMINAL THRUSTS

Stand behind the child. Put both your arms around them, and put one fist between the navel and the bottom of their breastbone. Grasp your fist with your other hand, and pull sharply inwards and upwards up to five times. Recheck the child's mouth.

4 CALL FOR EMERGENCY HELP THEN CONTINUE

If the obstruction has not cleared, call 999/112 for emergency help. Repeat steps 2 and 3 – rechecking the mouth after each step – until emergency help arrives, the obstruction is cleared or the child becomes unresponsive.

269

CHOKING INFANT UNDER ONE YEAR

Mild obstruction:

- Able to cough but difficulty in breathing or making any noise

Severe obstruction:

- Inability to cough, make any noise or breathe
- Eventually infant will become unresponsive

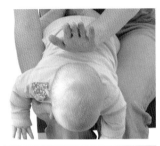

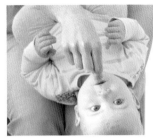

1 GIVE UP TO FIVE BACK BLOWS

If the infant is unable to cough, breathe or make any noise, lay them face down along your forearm and thigh, and support their head. Give up to five back blows between the shoulder blades with the heel of your hand.

2 CHECK INFANT'S MOUTH

Turn the infant over so that they are face up along your other leg, with your arm along the infant's back; support the head with your hand. Check their mouth – do not sweep the mouth with your finger – pick out any obvious obstructions. If choking persists, move to step 3.

ASTHMA

- Difficulty in breathing
- Wheezing
- Coughing
- Distress and anxiety
- Difficulty in speaking
- Grey-blue colouring in skin, lips, earlobes and nailbeds

In a severe attack:

- Exhaustion and casualty may become unresponsive

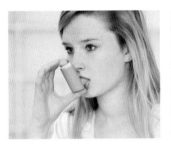

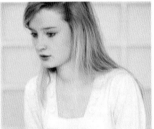

1 SEEK MEDICAL ADVICE

Keep calm and reassure the casualty. Sit the casualty down in the position they find most comfortable. Get them to take their usual dose of their reliever inhaler (it is usually blue); use a spacer device if they have one.

2 ENCOURAGE SLOW BREATHS

Tell them to breathe slowly and deeply. A mild attack should ease within a few minutes. If it does not ease, the casualty may take 1 to 2 puffs from their inhaler every 30–60 seconds until they have had 10 puffs. If they have a personal asthma plan they should follow it.

FIND OUT MORE **p.98**

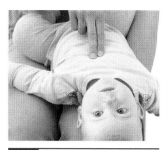

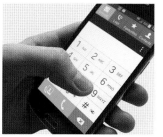

3 GIVE UP TO FIVE CHEST THRUSTS

With the infant lying on your leg, place two fingertips on the lower half of their breastbone, a finger's breadth below the nipples. Give up to five sharp downward thrusts, similar to chest compressions (p.264), but sharper and slower. Recheck the infant's mouth.

4 CALL FOR EMERGENCY HELP THEN CONTINUE

If the obstruction is still not clear, call 999/112 for emergency help. Take the infant with you to make the call if necessary. Repeat steps 1 to 3 until emergency help arrives, the obstruction is cleared or the infant becomes unresponsive (see caution, above right).

FIND OUT MORE **p.104**

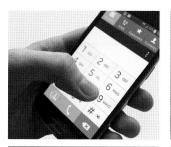

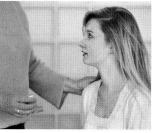

3 CALL FOR EMERGENCY HELP

Call 999/112 for emergency help if the attack is severe and one of the following occurs: the inhaler has no effect; breathlessness makes talking difficult; the casualty is becoming exhausted.

4 MONITOR CASUALTY

Monitor and record the casualty's vital signs (pp.54–55) until help arrives. If there is a delay of more than 15 minutes, repeat step 2. If they recover, advise the casualty to seek medical advice if they are concerned about the attack.

SEPSIS

RECOGNITION

Signs may not all be present

- Severe breathlessness and/or rapid shallow breathing (more than 22 breaths per minute)
- Extreme pain or discomfort
- Casualty has not passed urine
- Skin is pale, mottled and discoloured and hands and feet are cold
- Person says they feel like they are going to die
- Speech becomes slurred and person is confused and drowsy

In children you may also notice:

- Breathing is rapid and child is lethargic or difficult to rouse
- Mottled, blue or pale skin, and cold hands and feet
- No recent wet nappies and possible seizure

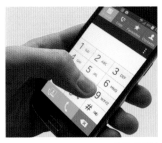

1 CALL FOR EMERGENCY HELP

If you suspect sepsis seek urgent medical advice without delay. **Call 999/112 for emergency help.** Do not wait for all of the signs or symptoms to develop as by that stage, the casualty will be critically ill.

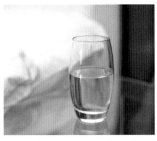

2 TREAT FEVER

Keep the casualty cool and give plenty of water to replace fluids lost through sweating. An adult may take the recommended dose of paracetamol tablets; a child may have the recommended dose of paracetamol suspension.

MENINGITIS

RECOGNITION

Some, but not all, of these signs and symptoms may be present:

- Signs and symptoms of sepsis
- Flu-like illness with a high temperature and severe headache
- Neck stiffness (casualty is unable to put their chin on their chest)
- Vomiting
- Casualty's eyes have become sensitive to any light
- In infants, there may also be a high-pitched moaning or a whimpering cry, floppiness and a tense or bulging fontanelle (soft part of the skull)
- In later stages, a distinctive rash of red or purple spots that does not fade when pressed

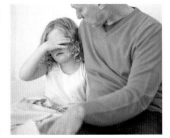

1 SEEK MEDICAL ADVICE

If you notice any signs of meningitis, left, such as the casualty shielding their eyes from light or if they have a stiff neck, seek urgent medical advice.

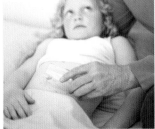

2 CHECK FOR SIGNS OF A RASH

Check the casualty for signs of the meningitis rash: press against the rash with the side of a glass. Most rashes will fade when pressed; if you can still see the rash through the glass, it is possibly meningitis.

FIND OUT MORE **p.222**

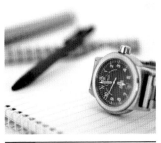

> **CAUTION**
> - If a casualty's condition is deteriorating, and you suspect sepsis, call 999/112 for emergency help even if they have already seen a doctor.

3 MONITOR CASUALTY

Monitor the casualty's vital signs (pp.54–55) while waiting for help to arrive.

FIND OUT MORE **p.223**

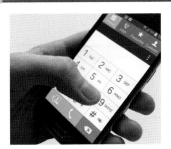

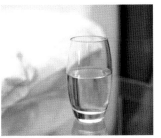

> **CAUTION**
> - If a casualty's condition is deteriorating, and you suspect meningitis, call 999/112 for emergency help even if they have already seen a doctor.

3 CALL FOR EMERGENCY HELP

Call 999/112 for emergency help if you see signs of the rash, or if medical help is delayed. Reassure the casualty. Keep them cool and monitor the casualty's vital signs (pp.54–55) while waiting for help to arrive.

4 TREAT FEVER

Keep the casualty cool and give plenty of water to replace fluids lost through sweating. An adult may take the recommended dose of paracetamol tablets; a child may have the recommended dose of paracetamol suspension.

SEVERE EXTERNAL BLEEDING

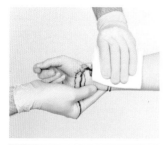

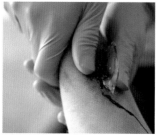

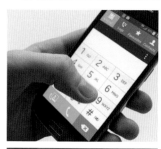

1 APPLY DIRECT PRESSURE TO WOUND

Apply direct pressure to the wound with your fingers or the palm of your hand over a sterile wound dressing or clean cloth pad. If you do not have a dressing or a pad, ask the casualty to apply direct pressure themselves. Remove or cut any clothing if necessary.

2 IF THERE IS AN OBJECT IN THE WOUND

Apply pressure either side of the embedded object to control bleeding. Do not press directly on the object and do not make any attempt to remove it.

3 CALL FOR EMERGENCY HELP

Call 999/112 for emergency help – ideally ask a helper to do this. Give the call handler details of the injury and extent of the bleeding.

SHOCK

RECOGNITION

- Rapid pulse
- Pale, cold, clammy skin
- Sweating

As shock develops:

- Rapid, shallow breathing
- Weak, "thready" pulse
- Grey-blue skin, especially inside lips
- Weakness and giddiness
- Nausea and vomiting
- Thirst

As the brain's oxygen supply weakens:

- Restlessness and aggressive behaviour
- Gasping for air
- Casualty will become unresponsive

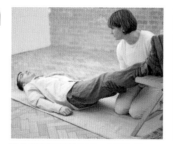

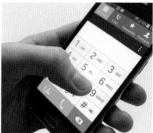

1 HELP CASUALTY TO LIE DOWN

Treat any cause of shock, such as bleeding (above) or burns (pp.280–281). Help the casualty to lie down, ideally on a blanket. Raise and support their legs above the level of their heart.

2 CALL FOR EMERGENCY HELP

Call 999/112 for emergency help – ideally ask a helper to do this for you. Tell the call handler that you suspect shock.

FIND OUT MORE **pp.116–117**

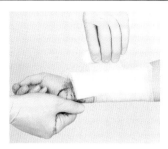

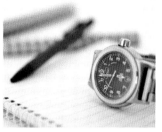

4 **APPLY BANDAGE AND TREAT FOR SHOCK**

Secure the pad over the wound with a bandage; tie the ends in a knot over the dressing pad. Check the circulation beyond the bandage (p.247) and re-check it every 10 minutes; loosen and reapply the bandage if necessary. Treat the casualty for shock, see below.

5 **MONITOR CASUALTY**

Monitor and record the casualty's vital signs (pp.54–55) while waiting for emergency help to arrive.

CAUTION

- If blood loss persists, remove the dressing and reapply direct pressure ensuring that you apply it directly over the injury.
- If bleeding is severe, use a haemostatic dressing (p.239) if there is one available.
- If bleeding on a limb cannot be controlled with direct pressure, consider using a tourniquet (p.117) if you have been trained in its use.
- Do not give the casualty anything to eat or drink as an anaesthetic may be needed.
- If the casualty becomes unresponsive, open the airway and check breathing (p.260). Be prepared to begin CPR (pp.262–265).

FIND OUT MORE **pp.114–115**

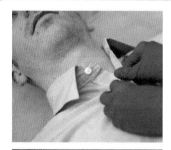

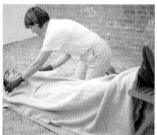

3 **LOOSEN TIGHT CLOTHING**

Loosen any tight clothing to reduce constriction at the neck, chest and waist.

4 **KEEP CASUALTY WARM**

Cover the casualty with a blanket to keep them warm. Advise the casualty not to move. Monitor and record the casualty's vital signs (pp.54–55) while waiting for help to arrive.

CAUTION

- Do not give the casualty anything to eat or drink because an anaesthetic may be needed.
- Do not leave the casualty unattended, unless you have to to call for emergency help.
- Do not let the casualty move.
- Do not try to warm the casualty with a hot-water bottle or any other form of direct heat.
- If the casualty is in the late stages of pregnancy, lean them towards their left side so the pregnant uterus does not restrict blood flow to the heart.
- If the casualty becomes unresponsive, open the airway and check breathing (p.260). Be prepared to begin CPR (pp.262–265).

ANAPHYLACTIC SHOCK

RECOGNITION

- Anxiety
- Red, itchy rash or raised areas of skin (weals) and/or red, itchy, watery eyes
- Swelling of hands, feet and/or face
- Puffiness around the eyes
- Abdominal pain, vomiting and diarrhoea
- Difficulty breathing, ranging from tight chest to severe difficulty, which causes wheezing and gasping for air
- Swelling of tongue and throat
- A feeling of terror
- Confusion and agitation
- Signs of shock (p.274) leading to collapse and the casualty becoming unresponsive

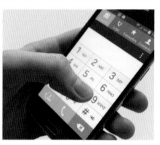

1 CALL FOR EMERGENCY HELP

Call 999/112 for emergency help. Ideally, ask someone to make the call while you treat the casualty. Tell the call handler that you suspect anaphylaxis.

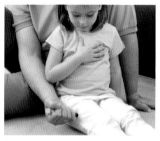

2 HELP CASUALTY WITH MEDICATION

If they have an adrenaline auto-injector, help them to use it. If you are trained you can give it to them. Hold the injector in your fist, pull off the safety cap and push the tip against the thigh until it clicks. Hold it for 3 seconds (or as instructed on the auto-injector) then remove it.

HYPOGLYCAEMIA

RECOGNITION

There may be:

- A history of diabetes – the casualty may recognise the onset of a hypoglycaemic (low blood sugar) episode
- Weakness, faintness or hunger
- Confusion and irrational behaviour
- Sweating with cold, clammy skin
- Rapid pulse
- Palpitations and muscle tremors
- Deteriorating level of response
- Medical warning bracelet or necklace and emergency sugar supply such as glucose gel or sweets
- Medication such as an insulin pen or tablets and a glucose testing kit

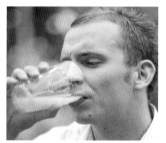

1 GIVE CASUALTY SUGAR

Help the casualty to sit down. If they have their emergency sugar, help them to take it. If not give them the equivalent of 15–20 g of glucose – a 150 ml glass of fruit juice or non-diet fizzy drink, 3 teaspoons of sugar or 3 sweets like jelly babies.

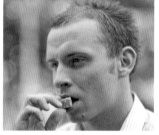

2 GIVE MORE SUGARY FOOD

If the casualty responds quickly, give them more food or drink and let them rest until they feel better. Help them find their glucose testing kit so that they can check their glucose levels.

FIND OUT MORE **pp.227**

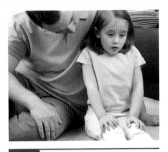

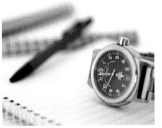

CAUTION

- An adrenaline autoinjector can be delivered through clothing.
- If the casualty becomes unresponsive, open the airway and check breathing (p.260). Be prepared to begin CPR (pp.262–265).
- If an obviously pregnant casualty needs to lie down, lean them towards their left side to prevent the pregnant uterus restricting blood flow back to the heart. Place a cushion or rolled clothing under the right hip to keep it slightly elevated.

3 MAKE CASUALTY COMFORTABLE

Reassure the casualty and help them to sit in a position that eases any breathing difficulties. If they become very pale with a weak pulse, lay them down with their legs raised and supported as for shock (pp.274–275).

4 MONITOR CASUALTY

Monitor and record the casualty's vital signs (pp.54–55) while waiting for help to arrive. Repeated doses of adrenaline can be given every 5 minutes if there is no improvement or the casualty's symptoms return.

FIND OUT MORE **p.216–217**

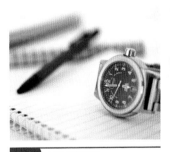

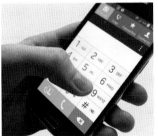

CAUTION

- If the casualty is not fully responsive do not give them anything to eat or drink.
- If the casualty becomes unresponsive, open the airway and check breathing (p.260). Be prepared to begin CPR (pp.262–265).

3 MONITOR CASUALTY

Monitor and record the casualty's vital signs (pp.54–55) until they have fully recovered.

4 CALL FOR EMERGENCY HELP

If the casualty's condition does not improve, look for other causes of their condition. **Call 999/112 for emergency help.** Continue to monitor the casualty's vital signs while waiting for help to arrive.

HEAD INJURY

RECOGNITION

There may be:

- Level of response may be impaired for a brief period
- Possible scalp wound
- Dizziness and/or nausea
- Loss of memory of events at the time of, or immediately before, the injury
- Headache
- Confusion

For severe injury:

- History of severe blow to the head
- Deteriorating level of response
- Casualty may become unresponsive
- Leakage of blood or bloodstained watery fluid from the ear or nose
- Unequal pupil size

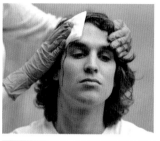

1 APPLY DIRECT PRESSURE TO ANY WOUND

Replace any displaced skin flaps over the wound. Put a sterile wound dressing or a clean, fabric pad over the wound. Apply firm, direct pressure with your hand to control the bleeding.

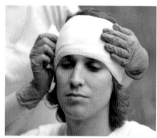

2 SECURE DRESSING WITH BANDAGE

Secure the dressing over the wound with a roller bandage to help maintain direct pressure on the injury.

SPINAL INJURY

RECOGNITION

- Can occur after a fall from a height onto the back, head or feet

There may be:

- Pain in neck or back
- Step, irregularity or twist in the normal curve of the spine
- Tenderness in the skin over the spine
- Weakness or loss of movement in the limbs
- Loss of sensation, or abnormal sensation
- Loss of bladder and/or bowel control
- Difficulty breathing

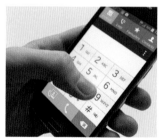

1 CALL FOR EMERGENCY HELP

Tell the casualty not to move and to maintain a stable head and neck position. **Call 999/112 for emergency help.** If possible, ask a helper to make the call. Tell the ambulance call handler that a spinal injury is suspected.

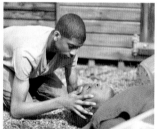

2 STEADY AND SUPPORT HEAD

If the casualty cannot maintain a stable head and neck position, sit or kneel behind their head and, resting your arms on the ground, grasp either side of the casualty's head and hold it still. Do not cover the casualty's ears.

FIND OUT MORE pp.146–147

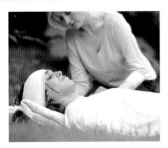

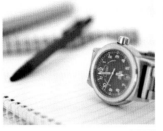

3 HELP CASUALTY TO LIE DOWN

Help the casualty to lie down, ideally on a blanket. Ensure that their head and shoulders are slightly raised. Make them as comfortable as possible.

4 MONITOR CASUALTY

Monitor and record the casualty's vital signs (pp.54–55). **Call 999/112 for emergency help** if there are any signs of severe head injury. Continue to monitor the casualty while waiting for help to arrive.

CAUTION

Seek medical advice if after the injury you notice signs of worsening head injury such as:

- Increasing drowsiness.
- Persistent headache.
- Confusion, dizziness, loss of balance and/or loss of memory.
- Difficulty speaking.
- Difficulty walking.
- Vomiting episodes.
- Double vision.
- Seizures.

FIND OUT MORE pp.159–161

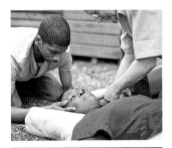

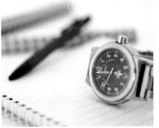

3 PLACE EXTRA SUPPORT AROUND HEAD

Continue to hold the casualty's head. Ask a helper to place rolled towels, or other padding, on either side of the casualty's head for extra support.

4 MONITOR CASUALTY

Monitor and record the casualty's vital signs (pp.54–55) while waiting for help to arrive.

CAUTION

- Do not move the casualty unless they are in danger.
- If the casualty is unresponsive, open the airway by gently lifting the jaw, but do not tilt the head, then check breathing (p.260). Be prepared to begin CPR (pp.262–265).
- If you need to place the casualty into the recovery position use the log-roll technique (p.161).

BROKEN BONES

- Deformity, swelling and bruising at the injury site
- Pain and difficulty in moving the injured part

There may be:

- Bending, twisting or shortening of a limb
- A wound, possibly with bone ends protruding

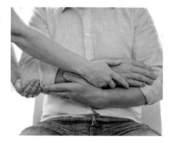

 SUPPORT INJURED PART

Help the casualty to support the affected part at the joints above and below the injury, in the most comfortable position for them.

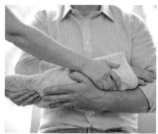

2 PROTECT INJURY WITH PADDING

Place padding, such as towels or cushions, around the affected part, and support it in a comfortable position.

BURNS AND SCALDS

RECOGNITION

There may be:

- Possible areas of superficial, partial-thickness and/or full-thickness burns
- Pain in the area of the burn
- Breathing difficulties if the airway is affected
- Swelling and blistering of the skin
- Signs of shock (p.274)

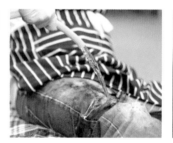

 START TO COOL BURN

Immediately flood the injury with cold water; cool for at least 20 minutes or until pain is relieved. Make the casualty comfortable by helping them to sit or lie down and protect the injured area from contact with the ground.

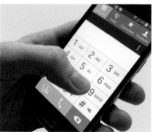

2 CALL FOR EMERGENCY HELP

Call 999/112 for emergency help if necessary. Tell the call handler that the injury is a burn. Explain what caused the burn and tell them the estimated size and depth.

FIND OUT MORE pp.138–140

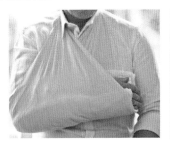

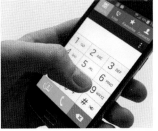

3 SUPPORT WITH SLINGS OR BANDAGES

For extra support or if help is delayed, secure the injured part to an uninjured part of the body. For upper body injuries, use a sling; for lower limb injuries, use broad- and narrow-fold bandages. Tie knots on the uninjured side. Check the circulation after bandaging (p.247).

4 TAKE OR SEND CASUALTY TO HOSPITAL

A casualty with an arm injury can be taken by car if not in shock. If they have a leg injury they should go by ambulance, so **call 999 / 112 for emergency help.** Treat for shock. Monitor and record the casualty's vital signs (pp.54–55) while waiting for help.

CAUTION

- Do not attempt to move an injured limb unnecessarily, or if it causes further pain.
- If there is an open wound, cover it with a sterile dressing or a clean cloth pad and bandage it in place.
- Do not give the casualty anything to eat or drink as an anaesthetic may be needed.
- If treating a casualty for shock, and they have a broken bone in their leg, do not raise the legs.

FIND OUT MORE pp.176–177

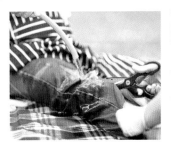

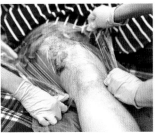

3 REMOVE ANY CONSTRICTIONS

While you are cooling the burn, carefully remove or cut away any clothing, watches, rings or other jewellery from the area before it starts to swell; a helper can do this for you. Do not remove anything that is sticking to the burn.

4 COVER BURN

When cooled, cover the burn with kitchen film placed lengthways over the injury, or use a clean plastic bag. Alternatively, cover it with a sterile wound dressing or clean pad of material. Monitor and record the casualty's vital signs (pp.54–55) while waiting for help to arrive.

CAUTION

- Do not apply lotions, ointment or fat to a burn; specialised burn dressings are also not recommended.
- Do not use adhesive dressings.
- Do not touch the burn or burst any blisters.
- If the burn is severe, treat the casualty for shock (pp.274–275).
- If the burn is on the face, do not cover it. Keep cooling with water until help arrives.
- If the burn is caused by contact with chemicals wear gloves and goggles to protect yourself from contact with the chemical.
- Watch the casualty for signs of smoke inhalation, such as difficulty breathing.

281

SEIZURES IN ADULTS

Seizures often follow a pattern:

- Sudden loss of responsiveness
- Rigidity and arching of the back
- Breathing may be noisy and become become difficult. The lips may show a grey-blue tinge (cyanosis)
- Convulsive movements begin
- Saliva (bloodstained if they have bitten their lip or tongue) may appear at the mouth
- Possible loss of bladder or bowel control
- Muscles relax and breathing becomes normal again
- After the seizure the casualty may be dazed and unaware of what has happened
- Casualty may fall into a deep sleep

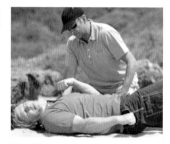

1 PROTECT CASUALTY

Try to ease the casualty's fall. Talk to them calmly and reassuringly. Clear away any potentially dangerous objects to prevent injury to the casualty. Ask bystanders to keep clear. Make a note of when the seizure began.

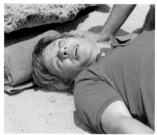

2 PROTECT HEAD AND LOOSEN TIGHT CLOTHING

If possible, cushion the casualty's head with soft material until the seizure ceases. Place padding around them to protect them from objects that cannot be moved. Loosen any tight clothing around the casualty's neck.

SEIZURES IN CHILDREN

- Loss of or impaired response
- Vigorous shaking with clenched fists and arched back

There may also be:

- Signs of fever, such as hot, flushed skin
- A twitching face and squinting, fixed or upturned eyes
- Breath-holding, with red, puffy face and neck
- Drooling at the mouth
- Possible vomiting
- Loss of bladder or bowel control

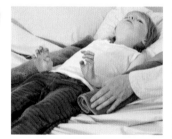

1 PROTECT CHILD FROM INJURY

Clear away any nearby objects and surround the child with soft padding, such as pillows or rolled towels, so that even violent movement will not result in injury.

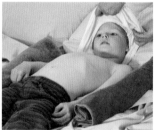

2 HELP THE CHILD COOL DOWN

Remove bedding and clothing, such as a vest or pyjama top; you may have to wait until the seizure stops to do this. Ensure a good supply of cool air, but do not let the child become too cold.

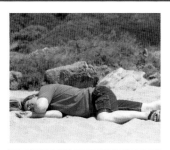

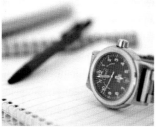

3 PLACE CASUALTY IN RECOVERY POSITION

Once the seizure has stopped the casualty may fall into a deep sleep. Open the casualty's airway and check breathing (p.260). If they are breathing normally, place them in the recovery position if necessary.

4 MONITOR CASUALTY'S RECOVERY

Monitor and record the casualty's vital signs (pp.54–55) until they recover. Make a note of the duration of the seizure.

CAUTION

- Do not attempt to restrain the casualty.
- Do not put anything in the casualty's mouth during a seizure.
- If the casualty is in a wheelchair, apply the brakes to prevent the chair moving, and leave them in the chair unless their care plan states otherwise.

Call 999 / 112 for emergency help **if the casualty:**

- Is having repeated seizures.
- Has a seizure that lasts more than 5 minutes.
- Is having their first seizure.
- Remains unresponsive for more than 10 minutes after the seizure has stopped.
- Has sustained an injury.

FIND OUT MORE **p.220**

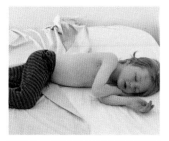

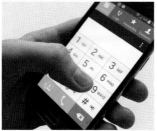

3 PLACE CHILD IN RECOVERY POSITION

Once the seizure has stopped, open the airway and check breathing (p.260). If the child is breathing normally, place them in the recovery position to maintain an open airway.

4 CALL FOR EMERGENCY HELP

Call 999 / 112 for emergency help. Reassure the parents or carer, if necessary. Monitor and record the child's vital signs (pp.54–55), including their temperature, while waiting for help to arrive.

CAUTION

- Do not let the child get too cold.
- Do not over or underdress a child with a fever.
- Do not sponge a child to cool them as there is a risk of overcooling them.
- If the child becomes unresponsive, open the airway and check breathing (p.260). Be prepared to begin CPR (pp.264–265).

SWALLOWED POISONS

RECOGNITION

- A history of ingestion/exposure to poison; evidence of poison nearby

Depending on what the casualty has taken, there may be:

- Vomit that may be bloodstained, and later diarrhoea
- Cramping abdominal pains
- Pain or burning sensation
- Empty containers near the casualty
- Impaired level of response
- Seizures

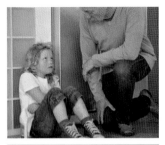

1 IDENTIFY THE POISON

Reassure the casualty. If they are responsive, ask them what they have swallowed and, if possible, how much and when. Look for clues such as poisonous leaves or berries, containers or pill bottles.

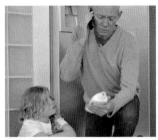

2 CALL FOR EMERGENCY HELP

Call 999/112 for emergency help. Give the call handler as much information as possible. This will help the medical team to give the casualty the correct treatment.

HEATSTROKE

RECOGNITION

There may be:

- Headache, dizziness and discomfort
- Restlessness and confusion
- Hot, flushed and dry skin
- Rapid deterioration in the level of response
- Full, bounding pulse
- Body temperature above 40°C (104°F)

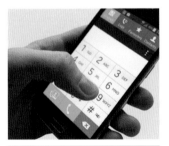

1 CALL FOR EMERGENCY HELP

Quickly move the casualty to a cool area. Remove as much of their outer clothing as possible. **Call 999/112 for emergency help;** ask a helper to do this if possible.

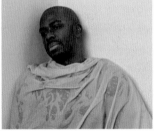

2 WRAP CASUALTY IN COLD, WET SHEET

Help the casualty to sit down, supported with cushions. Wrap them in a cold, wet sheet to start lowering their temperature. If there is no sheet available, fan the casualty, and/or sponge them with cold water.

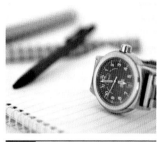

3 MONITOR CASUALTY

Monitor and record the casualty's vital signs (pp.54–55) while waiting for help to arrive. Keep samples of vomited material and any other clues and give them to the ambulance crew.

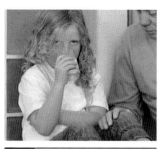

4 IF CASUALTY'S LIPS ARE BURNT

If the casualty has swallowed a substance that has burnt their lips, give them frequent sips of cool milk or water.

CAUTION

- Do not attempt to induce vomiting.
- If the casualty is contaminated with chemicals, wear protective equipment such as disposable gloves, a mask and goggles.
- If the casualty becomes unresponsive, make sure that there is no vomit or other matter in the mouth. Open the airway and check breathing (p.260). Be prepared to begin CPR (pp.262–265).
- If there are chemicals on the casualty's mouth, protect yourself by using a face shield or pocket mask when giving rescue breaths.

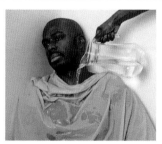

3 CONTINUE COOLING

Continue cooling the casualty until their temperature falls below 38°C (100.4°F). Keep the sheet wet by continually pouring cold water over it. Once the casualty's temperature appears to have returned to normal, replace the wet sheet with a dry one.

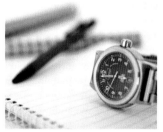

4 MONITOR CASUALTY

Monitor and record the casualty's vital signs (pp.54–55), including their temperature, while waiting for help to arrive. If the casualty's temperature begins to rise again, repeat the cooling process.

CAUTION

- If the casualty becomes unresponsive, open the airway and check breathing (p.260). Be prepared to begin CPR (pp.262–265).

FIRST AID REGULATIONS

First aid should be practised in any situation where injuries or illnesses occur. In many cases, the first person on the scene is a volunteer who wants to help, rather than someone who is medically trained. However, in certain circumstances the provision of first aid, and first aid responsibilities, is defined by statutes. In the UK, these regulations apply to incidents that occur in the workplace and at mass gatherings.

FIRST AID AT WORK

The Health and Safety (First-Aid) Regulations 1981 (as amended in 2018) place a duty on employers to make first aid provision for employees. The practical aspects of this statutory duty for employers and for the self-employed are set out in the Guidance on Regulations. In order to meet their regulatory requirements, employers have a responsibility to carry out an assessment of their first aid needs based on hazards and risks involved in their work, select a suitable training provider and undertake due diligence on that provider. Employers are also advised to consider the provision of mental health and well-being support when carrying out a needs assessment.

The Voluntary Aid Societies are cited in the Guidance on Regulations as the standard setters for currently accepted first aid at work. The training provided by the Voluntary Aid Societies meets the requirements of employers identified in the needs assessment. The Guidance on Regulations encourages all employers to assess their organisation's ability to meet certain first aid standards. The number of first aiders in a specific workplace is dependent on a needs assessment that should be carried out by your Health and Safety Representative. The checklist opposite will assist in determining the number and type of first aid personnel required.

Comprehensive advice can also be found at www.hse.gov.uk/firstaid/

ACCIDENT BOOK

An employer has the overall responsibility for an accident book, but it is the responsibility of the first aider or appointed person to look after and note details of incidents in the book.

If an employee is involved in an incident in the workplace, the following details should be recorded in the accident book:
- Date, time and place of incident.
- Name and job of the injured or ill person.
- Details of the injury/illness and what first aid was given.
- What happened to the person immediately afterwards (for example, went home or taken to hospital).
- Name and signature of the first aider or person dealing with the incident.

REPORTING OF INJURIES, DISEASES AND DANGEROUS OCCURRENCES

In the event of injury or ill health at work, an employer has a legal obligation to report the incident – Reporting of Injuries, Diseases and Dangerous Occurrences Regulations 2013 (RIDDOR) requires an employer to report the following:
- **Deaths.**
- **Major injuries.**
- **Injuries lasting more than seven days** where an employee or self-employed person is away from work or unable to perform their normal work duties for more than seven consecutive days.
- **Injuries to members of the public** or people not at work, where they are taken from the scene of an accident to hospital.
- **Some work-related diseases.**
- **Some dangerous occurrences** such as a near miss, where something happened that, although no injury occurred, could have resulted in an injury.

CHECKLIST FOR ASSESSMENT OF FIRST AID NEEDS

FACTORS TO CONSIDER	REQUIREMENTS AND CONSIDERATIONS
Is your workplace low risk (for example, shops, offices and libraries)?	**The minimum provision is:** An appointed person to take charge of first aid arrangements ● A suitably stocked first aid box. As there is a possibility of an accident or sudden illness, consider providing a qualified first aider. **First aider requirements:** For fewer than 25 employees, one appointed person ● For 25–50 employees, at least one first aider trained in Emergency First Aid at Work (EFAW) ● For more than 50 employees, one First Aid at Work (FAW) trained first aider for every 100 employees (or part thereof). **Where there are large numbers of employees consider:** Additional first aid equipment ● A first aid room.
Is your workplace higher risk (for example, light engineering and assembly work, food processing, warehousing, extensive work with dangerous machinery or sharp instruments, construction or chemical manufacture)? Do your work activities involve special hazards, such as hydrofluoric acid or confined spaces?	**The minimum provision is:** An appointed person to take charge of first aid arrangements ● A suitably stocked first aid box. **First aider requirements:** For fewer than five employees, one appointed person; for 5–50 employees, at least one first aider trained in Emergency First Aid at Work (EFAW) or First Aid at Work (FAW) depending on the type of injuries that could occur; for more than 50 employees, at least one First Aid at Work (FAW) trained first aider for every 50 employees (or part thereof). **Consider:** Additional training for first aiders to deal with injuries resulting from special hazards ● Additional first aid equipment ● Precise siting of first aid equipment ● Providing a first aid room ● Informing the emergency services if there are chemicals on site.
Are there inexperienced workers on site, or employees with disabilities or special health problems?	**Consider:** Additional training for first aiders ● Additional first aid equipment ● Local siting of first-aid equipment. Your first aid provision should cover any work-experience trainees.
What is your record of accidents and ill health? What injuries and illness have occurred and where?	Ensure your first aid provision caters for the type of injury and illness that might occur in your workplace. Monitor accidents and ill health and review your first aid provision as appropriate.
Do you have employees who travel a lot, work remotely or work alone?	**Consider:** Personal first aid kits ● Personal communicators or mobile phones for remote or lone workers.
Do any of your employees work shifts or work out of hours?	Ensure there is adequate first aid provision at all times while people are at work.
Are the premises spread out; for example, are there several buildings on the site or multi-floor buildings?	**Consider:** First aid provision in each building or on each floor.
Is your workplace remote from emergency medical services?	**Consider:** Special arrangements with the emergency services ● Informing the emergency services of your location.
Do any of your employees work at sites occupied by other employers?	Make arrangements with other site occupiers to ensure adequate provision of first aid. A written agreement between employers is strongly recommended.
Do you have sufficient provision to cover absences of first aiders or appointed persons?	**Consider what cover is needed for:** Annual leave and other planned absences ● Unplanned and exceptional absences.
Do members of the public visit your premises (for example, schools, places of entertainment, fairgrounds, shops)?	Under the regulations, there is no legal obligation to provide first aid for non-employees, but the Health and Safety Executive (HSE), strongly recommends that you consider the members of the public when planning your first aid provision.

INDEX

NOTES

ACKNOWLEDGMENTS

AUTHORS OF 11TH EDITION

St John Ambulance
Dr Margaret Austin DSTJ LRCPI LRSCI LM
Chief Medical Adviser

St Andrew's First Aid
Mr Rudy Crawford MBE BSC (HONS) MB CHB
FRCS (GLASG) FRCEM
Chairman of the Board

British Red Cross
Dr Barry Klaassen BSC (HONS) MB CHB FRCS (EDIN)
FRCEM
Chief Medical Adviser

CONTRIBUTORS TO 11TH EDITION

Alan Weir
Formerly Head of Clinical Operations,
St John Ambulance

Jim Dorman
Director of Campaigns & Public Engagement,
St Andrew's First Aid

Joe Mulligan
Head of First Aid Education, British Red Cross

TRIPARTITE COMMERCIAL COMMITTEE

St John Ambulance
Andrew New
Head of Education and Training Products
Deji Soetan
Marketing Manager

St Andrew's First Aid
Jim Dorman
Director of Campaigns & Public Engagement
Grant MacKintosh
National Sales Manager
Moyra Reid
Head of Marketing, Communications
and Fundraising

British Red Cross
Patrick Gollop
Director of Red Cross Training
Paul Stoddart
Marketing Manager, Red Cross Training

AUTHORS' ACKNOWLEDGMENTS

The authors would like to extend special thanks to – St John Ambulance: Mary Barrett. St Andrew's First Aid: Angela McCappin, Training Manager; and Stewart Simpson, Head of Volunteer Development. British Red Cross: Emily Oliver, First Aid Education Research Manager; Tracey Taylor, First Aid Education Development Manager; Pam Dwyer, First Aid Business Support Manager; and James Reed, Training Product Manager.

PUBLISHERS' ACKNOWLEDGMENTS

Dorling Kindersley would like to thank the following for their help with this 11th edition: Rohan Sinha and Sudakshina Basu for setting up the project; Francis Wong for work on the initial template; Rupanki Kaushik, George Thomas, Sonakshi Singh and Jessica Tapolcai for design assistance; Vikram Singh and Vishal Bhatia for DTP assistance; Mark Clifton for illustrations; XAB design for organising the photo shoot, Julie Stewart for assisting, and Source and Elliot Brown agencies for providing models; Ann Baggaley for proofreading.

Dorling Kindersley would also like to thank the following people who appear as models:

Lyndon Allen, Gillian Andrews, Kayko Andrieux, Mags Ashcroft, Nicholas Austin, Neil Bamford, Jay Benedict, Dunstan Bentley, Joseph Bevan, Bob Bridle, Gerard Brown, Helen Brown, Jennifer Brown, Val Brown, Michelle Burke, Tamlyn Calitz, Tyler Chambers, Evie Clark, Tim Clark, Junior Cole, Sue Cooper, Linda Dare, Julia Davies, Simon Davis, Tom Defrates, Louise Dick, Jemima Dunne, Maria Elia, Phil Fitzgerald, Alex Gayer, John Goldsmid, Nicholas Hayne, Stephen Hines, Nicola Hodgson, Spencer Holbrook, Jennifer Irving, Dan James, Megan Jones, Dallas Kidman, Carol King, Ashwin Khurana, Andrea Kofi-Opata, Andrews Kofi-Opata, Edna Kofi-Opata, Joslyn Kofi-Opata, Tim Lane, Libby Lawson, Wren Lawson-Fole Daniel Lee, Crispin Lord, Danny Lord, Harriet Lord, Phil Lord, Gareth Lowe, Mulkina Mackay, Ethan Mackay-Wardle, Ben Marcus, Catherine McCormick, Fiona McDonald, Alfie McMeeking, Cath McMeeking, Archie Midgley, David Midgley, Eve Mills, Erica Mills, Gary Moore, Sandra Newman, Matt Robbins, Dean Morris, Eva Mulligan, Priscilla Nelson-Cole, Rachel NG, Emma Noppers, Phil Ormerod, Julie Oughton, Rebekah Parsons-King, Stefan Podohorodecki, Tom Raettig, Andrew Roff, Ian Rowland, Phil Sergeant, Vicky Short, Lucy Sims, Gregory Small, Andrew Smith, Emily Smith, Sophie Smith, Bev Speight, Silke Spingies, Michael Stanfield, Alex Stewart, Adam Stoneham, David Swinson, Hannah Swinson, Laura Swinson, Becky Tennant, Laura Tester, Pip Tinsley, Daniel Toorie, Helen Thewlis, Fiona Vance, Adam Walker, Jonathan Ward, David Wardle, Dion Wardle, Francesca Wardell, Angela Wilkes, Liz Wheeler, Jenny Woodcock, Nigel Wright, Nan Zhang.

Picture credits Page 25 Alamy Stock Photo: Prostock-studio; page 31 Dorling Kindersley: Julesunlimited / Christophe Testi / Dreamstime.cc (t/Hazardous Signs)
All other images © Dorling Kindersley. For further information see www.dkimages.com